THE COMPLETE GUIDE TO

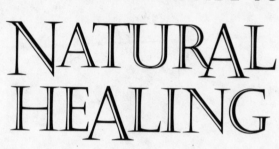

NATURAL HEALING

THE COMPLETE GUIDE TO
NATURAL HEALING

TOM MONTE

and the Editors of Natural Health *magazine*

A PERIGEE BOOK

This book is designed to provide accurate and authoritative information. The information provided in this book is not intended as a substitute for medical advice. The publisher and the author expressly disclaim responsibility for any unforeseen consequences arising from use of the information contained herein.

A Perigee Book
Published by The Berkley Publishing Group
200 Madison Avenue
New York, NY 10016

Copyright © 1997 by Boston Common Press
Book design by Irving Perkins Associates
Cover design by Elizabeth Sheehan
Interior illustrations by Hogie McMurtrie

First edition: August 1997

Perigee trade edition ISBN: 0-399-52312-X
Perigee hardcover edition ISBN: 0-399-52320-0

Published simultaneously in Canada.

The Putnam Berkley World Wide Web site address is
http://www.berkley.com

Library of Congress Cataloging-in-Publication Data

Monte, Tom.
    The complete guide to natural healing / Tom Monte and the editors of Natural health magazine. — 1st ed.
      p.   cm.
    Includes index.
    ISBN 0-399-52320-0. — ISBN 0-399-52312-X (pbk.)
    1. Alternative medicine.   2. Self-care, Health.   I. Natural health.   II. Title.
R733.M647   1997
615.5—dc21
                                                97-3527
                                                 CIP

Printed in the United States of America

10 9 8 7 6 5 4 3 2 1

CONTENTS

ACKNOWLEDGMENTS

No one produces such a compilation of diagnostic and healing tools as this book offers without considerable help from highly skilled and talented people. The first person I would like to thank with all my heart is my wife, Toby, who helped me research every entry in this book, and applied her more than 20 years of study and experience of natural healing to the book's overall content and quality. I also would like to thank Frank Head for his generous editorial support, research, and guidance; Mark Bittman for initiating this project and for his editorial support throughout the work; Chris Kimball for his ongoing support and his visionary approach to publishing; and John Duff for his princely patience, editorial guidance, and clarity of vision. I constantly marveled at John's ability to right the direction of this book whenever it drifted from its true spirit. Finally, I would like to thank all the professional healers who are restoring health to millions each day, while, at the same time, giving us a deeper understanding of the awesome mystery we call the human body. Their work is transforming the world.

PART I

A Guide to Natural Healing

When the first European settlers came to the New World, they marveled at the effectiveness of Native American healers and their medical armamentarium. Cotton Mather wrote that Native American "cures" were "truly stupendous." An early American historian of North Carolina reported in 1714 that the healing methods of Native Americans were "too many to repeat"; he went so far as to advocate intermarriage with native healers so that Europeans could gain "a true Knowledge of all the Indian's Skill in Medicine and Surgery." The British founder of Methodism, John Wesley, visited the United States in the early 1730s and noted that "diseases were extremely few" among the Native Americans and that their medicines were "quick, as well as generally infallible." Overall, European settlers marveled at the medical techniques of Native Americans. For every illness that they had previously encountered, Native American healers had found an answer in their own natural environment: in their foods, herbal plants, soil, water, and air. The effectiveness of Native healing baffled many Europeans, especially since they considered themselves far more civilized, intelligent, and scientific than the Indian population.

Today, we are witness to the rise of the medicinal and healing tools used by our ancestors, whether they be Asian, Native American, European, or African. And just as the European settlers marveled at the effectiveness of such simple methods, so do we. Every day, scientists are discovering that the old forms of treatment have great therapeutic value, whether they are healing foods, herbal plants, or simple poultices. To quote Ecclesiastes, "That which has been is that which will be, And that which has been done is that which will be done. So, there is nothing new under the sun."

This book is a guide to the use of natural healing methods in the treatment of more than 120 illnesses and disorders. The recommendations offered in this book are of two types. The first promotes health and prevents disease. Included in this group are general dietary recommendations, exercises, and meditation and relaxation techniques, all of which boost immune function and strengthen your ability to fight disease. The second type, made up primarily of herbs, homeopathic remedies, certain foods, and various kinds of physiotherapy, are powerful healing tools with therapeutic properties that address specific illnesses. As you will see after using the recommendations offered in this book, many natural healing methods can promote health, relieve symptoms of illness, and very often can heal the underlying causes of disease.

For the person who has had only a superficial encounter with traditional healing—or no exposure at all—the use of herbs, nutrition, acupuncture, and other natural healing methods may seem altogether foreign and even a bit frightening at first. After all, most of us are used to getting our medicines from drug stores, which, thanks to the pharmaceutical companies, present their pills and potions in appealing colors and tamper-proof containers. Our familiarity with these medicines give us the impression that they are safe and effective. Unfortunately, as we all know, the common pharmaceutical drugs are not always effective, nor are they always safe. Every drug has toxic effects on the body, which are commonly referred to as side effects. In addition, when used in conjunction with other medications, drugs can have extremely harmful results. Many are addictive, and some are even life-threatening.

This is not to say that natural medicines are entirely without side effects, however. As long as one follows the traditional recommendations, natural medicine has been free of toxic effects, in part because foods, herbs, and homeopathic remedies—just to name a few medicinal substances—are essentially plant-based foods with active, medicinal properties that are taken in small doses. Nevertheless, some herbs do cause negative side effects, particularly if they are taken in extremely high doses or for purposes other than those for which they are traditionally recommended. One such example is the herb known as *Ephedra sinica* (also known by its Chinese name, *ma huang*). When taken as recommended, ephedra can be effective in the treatment of a number of disorders, as this book points out. However, some people have taken ephedra for its effects on brain chemistry and as a natural stimulant, neither of which is recommended here. Its use in these areas has led to chronic overdosing by some people and to a variety of toxic side effects, including liver damage, high blood pressure, heart palpitations, and, in a very small number of people, even stroke. In other words, you can abuse a plant-based medicine, just as you can a drug. Still, research has consistently shown that in cases in which herbs have caused toxic side effects, the herb was taken in extremely high doses or for reasons that were outside its traditional use, such as for weight loss or for improvement in mood.

Part III, which describes each natural remedy and its common usage, provides information on the possible contraindications of a specific herb or natural remedy, especially when taken in high doses. *However, we strongly advise against taking any natural remedy for purposes other than those recommended in this book, or in doses that exceed those suggested here.*

If taken as advised, the healing methods offered in this book are both safe and effective.

ORTHODOX OR MODERN MEDICINE VERSUS TRADITIONAL; MODERN VERSUS ANCIENT

Throughout this book, we refer to the modern medical system as *orthodox* medicine, and natural healing techniques as *traditional* medicine. By *orthodox*, we mean the practices and techniques dispensed by medical doctors and the scientists who are part of our society's accepted medical establishment. *Traditional* refers to the medical systems of the ancient Chinese, Asian Indians, Greeks, and Native Americans; we also include relatively modern therapies, such as homeopathy and naturopathy, which originated largely in the last two hundred years but are based on ancient principles and practices. For the most part, traditional medicine has been handed down over thousands of years, both orally and as a written record. Modern medicine, of course, is about two hundred years old.

Orthodox and traditional medicine approach the human body from diametrically opposite points of view, and in that sense, they can be seen as complementary systems. Both systems have strengths and weaknesses. Wherever possible, we have tried to create a bridge between modern science and traditional medicine, especially in the places where the two overlap or where science validates traditional healing methods. Nevertheless, in their basic approach to the human body, the two medical systems represent opposite worldviews.

Medical doctors see the body as essentially a series of independent parts. They treat those parts only after they become diseased. Disease itself is regarded as an exceptional condition that must be dealt with directly, either by killing the disease-causing agent (usually with the use of antibiotics, chemotherapy, or radiation treatment) or by removing part of the body through surgery. For the most part, medicine has focused its efforts on the treatment of symptoms rather than on the causes of disease. Cold medications, for example, reduce fever, discomforts, and runny nose. They do not address the underlying causes of a cold, especially the weakened immune system that allowed the cold to manifest in the first place. In fact, a growing body of scientific evidence shows that antibiotics and other pharmaceutical drugs weaken the body's immune system and thus make us more susceptible to illness over the long run.

Only in the last twenty years has medicine's exclusive focus on symptoms begun to change. Ironically, as medicine's approach to health and illness changes, doctors invariably adopt the methods of more traditional healers, especially the use of diet, exercise, relaxation techniques, and many herbs.

A good example of this change in thinking is the treatment of coronary heart disease, caused when cholesterol plaques clog the coronary arteries and prevent optimal blood and oxygen from flowing to the heart. These cholesterol plaques, known as atherosclerosis, become unstable, erupt, and become even larger, eventually blocking blood flow to the heart or brain entirely, thus causing a heart attack or stroke. In the 1950s, '60s, and early '70s, doctors didn't believe the plaques themselves could be prevented, stabilized, or reversed. The medical establishment denied that diet could raise or lower blood cholesterol—doctors maintained that cholesterol was genetically controlled—and even if cholesterol could be lowered, it wouldn't have any effect on coronary heart disease. Since the cause of heart disease and stroke could not be prevented or treated, drugs were used instead to affect heart rate, or surgery was used to replace the coronary arteries entirely with unclogged vessels. No medical doctor attempted to restore the health of the arteries by changing a person's diet or lifestyle. That approach has dramatically changed in the past two decades as science has demonstrated that a diet low in fat and cholesterol lowers blood cholesterol, prevents heart attacks and strokes, and even reverses the underlying disease process, thus improving blood flow to the heart.

New research into cancer and the human immune system has brought about an even broader perspective in medicine. Scientists are discovering that certain foods promote the body's cancer-fighting abilities; others boost the immune system and the body's capacity to fight more than sixty common illnesses, such as colds and flu, cataracts and glaucoma, disorders of the nervous system, cancer, and heart disease. Increasingly, scientists are learning that the body's ability to conquer disease and restore health depends on how we live—meaning, the presence of certain immune-boosting and cancer-fighting foods and herbs in our diets, the absence of other foods that weaken the body's defenses and promote disease, and our ability to engage consistently in immune-boosting behaviors, thoughts, and emotions.

As science probes ever deeper into the mysteries of the human body, the links connecting the body, the mind, and the environment are being revealed. Indeed, one of the underappreciated ironies of today's medical research is that the more science understands the workings of the human body, the more evidence it provides to support the practices and approaches of traditional medicine.

WITHIN THE TISSUES, A LIVING ENERGY

Every form of traditional medicine, whether it be Chinese, Ayurvedic, Greek, or Japanese, shares the same philosophical foundation, which is that the human body is animated by an integrated and intelligent energy called the life force. The life force is understood as both a living energy that sustains the life of organs, tissues, and cells, but also as a spiritual entity that is linked inextricably to an infinite source, namely the creator. Each of us is a unique and singular manifestation of the creative force in the universe, a force that flows through each of us and sustains our lives. The Chinese refer to this life force within the body and outer environment as *qi,* or *chi,* the Hindus refer to it as *prana,* the Greeks call it *pneuma,* and the Japanese call it *ki.*

When this life energy flows freely throughout the body, there is optimal health, vitality, and the full expression of our inner selves. When the life force is blocked or weakened, organs, tissues, and cells are deprived of the energy they need to function at their full potential. The essence of the life force is energy, but it also manifests as blood, oxygen, nutrition, and the circulation of lymph. Many traditional healers practicing today would also include immune cells as a manifestation of the life force. In its essence, the life force is pure energy, but that energy animates every cell and organ in the body. In a sense, the entire body is a manifestation of the underlying life force.

This life energy flows through the body in an organized pattern, unifying all the body's parts in much the same way that integrated circuitry would unify all the parts of a computer. Block the electrical circuit in one part of the computer, and the whole machine fails to function properly. It's the same with the human body. Block the life force in one part, and the whole organism fails to function properly.

This is how the conditions for disease begin to manifest in the traditional view. With the blockage of the life force, the vitality of organs and tissues is reduced; oxygen supply is diminished; waste products accumulate; and organs and tissues degenerate and become deformed. The body awakens us to the diminution of the life force by manifesting symptoms of one kind or another. Symptoms are the body's way of communicating that the life force has been blocked or compromised. If the body's language is repressed by pharmaceutical drugs or if it is ignored, the degeneration of cells and organs continues, leading eventually to disease. A traditional healer views the disorder not so much as the disease itself, but as the conditions that are blocking the life force from flowing optimally through the body. Illness is the flower of the weakened soil, so to speak. It is the end result of a long line of events that began with a diminution of the life force. Healing begins when the blockages to the life force are removed and when the deficiency is restored. Once the life force flows optimally to the weakened organs or tissues, the body can heal itself.

BALANCE AS THE ESSENCE OF HEALTH

Blockages in the life force can be seen as a condition in which one part of the body is contracted, while another is expanded. Physical tension, for example, occurs when muscles contract, squeezing capillaries and preventing blood, lymph, and qi from flowing optimally to organs, tissues, and cells. Atherosclerosis, or the presence of cholesterol plaques in the coronary arteries, is a contraction within the blood vessels, preventing blood from flowing optimally to the heart.

A contraction in one part of the body causes an expansion in another. When muscles contract on blood vessels in one place, the vessels bulge in another. High blood pressure, for example, is often the result of the contraction of arteries in certain parts of the body. Such contractions cause vessels in other areas to bulge or form an aneurysm, which can sometimes burst. If an aneurysm bursts in the brain, the person suffers a stroke. Extreme contractions in one part of the body usually cause extreme expansions in others. Thus, the higher the blood pressure, the more likely a blood vessel will burst. This is but one example of how extremes in expansion and contraction lead to illness. One of the goals of traditional healing is to use natural medicine to restore balance to such conditions.

The life force flows maximally in such a state of balance, that is, in a condition in which there is an equilibrium of tensions between expansion and contraction, or what the Chinese refer to as a balance between yin and yang. The words *yin* and *yang* are used to characterize the polar opposites that exist in everything and make up the physical world. Yin is a general category for passivity, contraction, and the feminine nature. Things that are cool, moist, slow-moving or even stationary are said to be in a yin state. Nighttime, when life slows down and sleep occurs, is yin. Water and the moon are yin and thus are connected mythologically with the feminine in nature. The earth is yin, as is all space.

Yang is a general category for things that are in a state of activity, aggressiveness, and expansion. Fire is yang. So, too, are all things that are hot, dry, and fast-moving. The daylight hours, during which there is much activity, is yang. Time is yang. The sun is the great yang ball of fire in the sky. Yang is considered the masculine principle in nature. Thus, time and the sun are associated with the masculine, as in Father Time, or the sun as a masculine deity.

Those things that are close to the ground are yin, while those higher up are yang. The grass is more yin than the trees; people of low stature are more yin than those who are tall.

Because yin and yang can be used to understand many forms of opposites within a person's life, they can be used to understand the underlying sources of any illness. They can also be used to understand the influences in a person's life that may be the underlying causes of disease.

Once the healer understands that a person's condition stems from excesses of yin or yang influences, he or she can restore balance by applying the opposite conditions to the person's life. For example, if a person suffers from too much stress, usually understood as an overly yang condition, more yin conditions, such as relaxation, may be the appropriate antidote. As you will see when you read the section on Chinese medicine, there are many ways to use yin and yang to understand a person's physical condition, as well as to apply appropriate balance to restore health. Everything needed to restore health already exists in nature.

THE TOOLS OF BALANCE

The human body is made up of the elements of nature: the minerals, vitamins, and amino acids that make up our bones, teeth, muscles, and organic tissues were all in the natural environment before they were organized into a physical whole that is your body. Indeed, the same forces that created the natural environment and the universe itself have combined to create each of us. Traditional peoples believe the connection between the macrocosm and the individual human being never ceases. In a sense, an energetic umbilical cord exists between each of us and nature. Throughout time, healers have used the products of nature—plants, minerals, soil, water, and air—as the basis for medicine. Each form of medicine was assessed according to its energetic qualities, as well as its inherent medicinal properties. Foods and herbs are understood according to the environmental conditions in which they grow; the characteristics of their leaves, roots, and stems; growing cycles; moisture content; and their relative heartiness or fragility. On the basis of these and other characteristics, traditional healers would determine the energetic nature of plants and experiment with such substances as treatments for specific ailments. Over thousands of years, a medical pharmacopoeia developed in every culture, from the Asian to North and South American to European and African. Remarkably, when scientists examine the chemical properties of these so-called medicinal plants, they find that they contain powerful chemicals that do indeed treat the very illnesses that the traditional healer used them for.

For example, echinacea was traditionally used by Native American healers to treat infections. A scientific analysis of echinacea has found that it contains a powerful antibiotic. It has also been shown to boost immune response, as do many other healing herbs. Saw palmetto has been used traditionally to treat the liver, spleen, kidneys, and the prostate. When scientists test saw palmetto, they find that it does indeed shrink a swollen prostate, relieve the symptoms of prostatitis, and restore health.

In fact, scientists are discovering that the traditional uses of foods, herbs, and physical therapies, such as acupuncture, have profound healing effects, very often precisely those healing effects for which they have been used traditionally.

Just a cursory review of the most recent studies reveals how dramatic are the scientific revelations.

- Nearly a thousand studies have been published on the medicinal benefits of garlic and related plants, such as onions and scallions. Garlic has been consistently shown to lower total cholesterol; lower triglycerides; decrease platelet adhesiveness and thus reduce the risk of heart attack; increase detoxification of the blood by the liver; boost immune function, particularly against carcinogens and existing cancer cells; and lower blood pressure. Garlic is also a powerful antibiotic and antifungal agent.
- A family of compounds called phytoestrogens found in soybeans, soybean products (tofu, tempeh, soy milk), and many grains and fruits have the power to stop blood vessels from attaching to tumors, thus depriving cancer cells and tumors from receiving essential oxygen and nutrients needed to survive (*Proceedings of the National Academy of Sciences,* April 1993). Phytoestrogens are being touted as powerful tools in the prevention of premenstrual syndrome (PMS), osteoporosis, and breast cancer.
- *Ginkgo biloba,* an herb used for millennia by Chinese healers and today widely prescribed by physicians in Germany and France, is an effective remedy for peripheral vascular disease (claudication) and cerebral insufficiency (low blood supply to the brain), according to a study published in the British medical journal *The Lancet* (340:1136, 1992). Ginkgo results in an increase in blood flow, and a decrease in the stickiness of

the blood (viscosity). There have been no adverse effects and no known drug interactions.

- Harvard researchers have discovered that kuzu (also known as kudzu in the American southwest) is highly effective as a treatment for alcoholism in animal studies. Extracts from kuzu are now being trial-tested in human alcoholics (November 1993 issue of the *Proceedings of the National Academy of Sciences*).

- Hawthorn berries, leaves, and blossoms contain biologically active flavonoids that lower blood pressure and reduce chest pain (angina), according to research published in Japanese, American, and British medical journals (*Biochemical Pharmacology*, 33:3491, 1984; *The Lancet*, 342:1007, 1993).

- Gugulipid, a plant extract that is now widely available in health food stores, has been shown to lower cholesterol by 21 percent and triglycerides by 25 percent in three to eight weeks, Japanese scientists have discovered.

- Researchers at the M. D. Anderson Hospital in Houston, Texas, have found that turmeric inhibits cancer at several sites in the body by disrupting certain chemical processes that would otherwise lead to cancer and support its growth.

- Japanese green tea, rich in antioxidants, flavonoids, and substances called indoles, stimulates the body's production of enzymes that block tumor formation and boost immunity, according to researchers at the National Cancer Institute (NCI).

- NCI researchers have also found that the sweet-tasting plant licorice inhibits skin cancer in animal studies.

- Shiitake mushrooms, NCI scientists have discovered, is a powerful immune booster, cancer fighter, and cholesterol-lowering herb. Shiitake also has significant antiviral and antibacterial properties.

- Acupuncture is being used successfully at Lincoln Hospital in the Bronx in the treatment of cocaine addiction. Impressed by the hospital's remarkable results—acupuncture changes brain chemistry and reduces withdrawal pains—the National Institute on Drug Abuse has agreed to fund a study using acupuncture to treat drug addiction.

- NCI researchers have found that many common plant foods contain specific cancer-fighting compounds. Among the most effective are the cruciferous vegetables (broccoli, cabbage, kale, brussels sprouts, collard greens, and mustard greens), which contain phytoestrogens and indoles that may prevent tumor-causing estrogen from targeting the breast. Broccoli is a rich source of another cancer fighter, sulforanphane, called by scientists a "major and very potent" trigger for detoxifying tissues and blood and for promoting production of cancer-preventive enzymes.

- U.S. Department of Agriculture botanist and herb researcher Jim Duke, Ph.D., has discovered that more than a hundred common herbs possess powerful immune-boosting, anticancer, and healing properties. Among those Dr. Duke commonly recommends are: licorice, which not only is a powerful cancer fighter, but also prevents ulcers and liver disorders; milk thistle, which strengthens the liver and treats cirrhosis and hepatitis; peppermint plant, which prevents cancer, heart disease, stroke, and cataracts, and which improves memory; cinnamon, which boosts immunity and triples insulin's ability to metabolize blood sugar; astragalus, angelica, echinacea, goldenseal, ligustrum, and numerous other common herbs significantly boost immune response and promote healing.

MORE AND MORE PEOPLE ARE TURNING TO NATURAL MEDICINE

People of every walk of life are discovering the healing power of natural remedies. In ever-increasing numbers, people throughout the Western world, especially Americans, have been turning to traditional practices for answers to disease. A 1993 issue of the *New England Journal of Medicine* reported that one-third of Americans sought the advice of a holistic health practitioner during the previous year. CBS News estimated that 50 percent of Americans see holistic health practitioners each year, and that number is growing. Even among those who have never consulted a holistic health therapist, the vast majority of Americans surveyed (62 percent, according to the November 4, 1991, issue of *Time* magazine) say they would consider such an option if a medical doctor failed to help them. Once people apply such methods, however, the overwhelming majority are convinced of their efficacy. According to *Time,* 84 percent of those who have already consulted a holistic healer say they would return for more treatment, while only 10 percent say they would not return.

Medical science has not been blind to this remarkable shift in the public's embrace of traditional healing methods. The National Institutes of Health has launched a series of scientific studies designed to assess the efficacy of a wide array of ancient and traditional healing therapies, including herbology, homeopathy, various dietary therapies, and acupuncture. Meanwhile, Harvard Medical School is one of several prestigious institutions now offering courses in natural, holistic medicine.

The remarkable embrace of traditional medicine by people of all walks of life is occurring for many reasons, but perhaps the most important is that our understanding of health is expanding beyond the boundaries of the current orthodox medical model. Increasingly, people are asking themselves deeper and more meaningful questions, such as, *What is health and what does it mean to heal?*

If you asked a healer from the Chinese, Greek, Hindu, or Native American traditions about the meaning of health or how healing occurs, the healer would offer vastly different answers to these questions than a Western physician would.

Health, say traditional healers, is a condition of wholeness, a condition in which body, mind, and spirit direct one's life in equal proportion, so that there is a balance and a harmony among all aspects of our humanness. In such a state, health and healing flourish because the body is capable of healing itself when it is placed in a balanced condition. The healer merely manipulates the conditions to achieve such a balance.

The characteristics of health as defined in such a way are unmistakable. To be healthy means to have abundant energy, excellent appetite, restful sleep, to be keen of mind and balanced in temperament, to enjoy a healthy and satisfying sex life, to love and be loved, to grow in awareness and expression of one's own unique nature and talents, and to apply such abilities to the service of others. Health is that magical but altogether tenuous condition in which the physical, mental, emotional, and spiritual conditions all find expression and nourishment in our lives. This, said traditional peoples, is the basis for wholeness, integration, and spirituality. Health, therefore, was seen as far greater than merely the absence of a symptom or problem. Indeed, health has as much to do with your approach to a problem as it does with the problem's resolution.

BALANCE IN DAILY LIVING

One of the major characteristics of health and healing in traditional terms is the patient's responsibility in the healing process. No one can establish balance in another person's life. It is up to each of us to look at our lives honestly and dispassionately, to assess where our imbalances lie, and to make corrections where they are needed. A traditional healer can help us with the use of medicinal foods, herbs, and other techniques, as well as with counseling, but in the end, it is up to each of us to bring balance to our daily lives.

Achieving such a balance can begin by adopting a healthy way of eating; by getting sufficient physical activity; and by establishing equilibrium between work and play, stress and rest, self-reflection and recreation, anxiety and joy. Each of us needs time to be alone, to be with family, and for friends. Each of us needs a balance between introversion and extroversion. Balance affects every aspect of our lives. When we approach a problem with a balanced temperament, we are far more in control of ourselves and the events around us. Out of such a balance comes emotional equilibrium, good judgment, health, and joy.

HOW TO USE THIS BOOK

Part II of this book offers the traditional healing tools for more than 120 illnesses and disorders, each one listed in alphabetical order. Each illness is defined in both orthodox and traditional terms. After the definition, an array of natural remedies for that disorder are provided. Part III provides a fuller description of the herb or remedy suggested under Part II. Part III also contains instructions on how to use specific herbs and supplements (in the sections on herbology and supplementation, respectively); how to make herbal preparations, such as infusions and decoctions (see the section on herbology); and how to prepare poultices, compresses, and packs (in the section on hydrotherapy and physiotherapy). Part III also provides a deeper understanding of specific disciplines, such as nutrition and exercise, the use of supplements, and traditional healing systems, such as Chinese medicine, herbology, and homeopathy. The table of contents will direct you to each of these areas of the book.

If you want to know the traditional approach to bronchitis, for example, you would look up bronchitis in Part II. Among the suggested herbs to treat bronchitis, you will find yerba santa and lotus root tea, just two of the herbal recommendations. If you want to know more about these herbs or how to prepare them, you would look up yerba santa and lotus root tea in the section on herbology in Part III. There you will find directions for making teas from such herbs, as well. Also, Part III provides a more detailed explanation of the traditional systems, such as Chinese medicine or herbology. If you want to learn more about Chinese medicine or some other system, turn to Part III for an overview of that system.

Part IV provides a traditional approach to supporting and improving the health of specific organs, such as the liver, heart, spleen, small and large intestine, kidneys, and bladder.

As much as possible, we have tried to create a bridge between the East and West, the ancient and modern, the traditional and orthodox. We've tried to show where science has supported the traditional approaches and where it deviates considerably from traditional medicine. We expect every reader to do the same with his or her health. We encourage you to work with your medical doctor for the treatment of any and every illness but to use traditional medicine wherever it is prudent and possible. Share this information with your doctor. Create your own bridge between the modern and the traditional. Such understanding and cooperation will lead you inevitably to the best health care you will receive. More importantly, it will give you the best chance at the full restoration of your health.

PART II

SYMPTOMS, DISORDERS, AND ILLNESSES

ACNE

SYMPTOMS

Skin eruptions on the face, back, and elsewhere on the body. The eruptions, which can be blackheads, whiteheads, inflamed pustules, sacs, or cysts, occur when hair follicles from the sebaceous glands become blocked and infected. The infection can cause the pores to become permanently dilated or even lead to scarring.

WHAT IS ACNE?

From Modern Western Medicine

About 80 percent of teenagers suffer from some degree of acne. The ostensible cause appears to be an increase in androgens, or the male hormone, which in turn produces an increase in sebum, a fatty, waxy substance designed to keep the skin supple and healthy. The sebum can block pores and lead to acne.

Acne can be made worse by some drugs, including corticosteroids and androgens, which increase production of oil by the sebaceous glands. Cosmetics and skin contact with oils or grease can also block pores and cause acne.

There is no scientific evidence supporting the widespread belief that diet can either promote or prevent acne. The American Medical Association maintains that there is "little point in avoiding sweets such as chocolate," at least insofar as acne is concerned. Frequent washing of the face does not prevent acne, but might keep it from spreading, says the AMA.

Common treatments include topical skin ointments, antibiotics, and ultraviolet light. For very severe acne, retinoid drugs are prescribed by a medical doctor.

From Traditional Medicine

People living on the traditional human diet, composed chiefly of unprocessed whole grains, vegetables, beans, fish, and low-fat animal products, experience little or no acne. Traditional medicine has maintained that acne is the result of overly acidic blood, brought about by a wide variety of lifestyle factors, including eating refined foods, excessive amounts of dairy products, high fat and cholesterol, sugar, chocolate, and other sweet foods. Dairy products, especially when they are combined with sugar, as in ice cream, have a particularly deleterious effect on the skin because they contain sugar (lactose, plus the sugar they are often combined with), protein, and fat.

Other factors that lead to acne are poor elimination, especially from the large intestine, and weak blood-cleansing organs, particularly the kidneys.

Certain dietary deficiencies may also contribute to acne (see the supplements listed below).

REMEDIES

Foods to Eat

- Green vegetables (at least two servings per day)
- Carrots (five servings per week)
- Celery (three to five servings per week)
- Cucumber
- Onions
- Garlic
- Watercress
- Kelp
- Seaweeds
- Fish (cold-water ocean)
- Whole grains, especially brown rice and millet (daily)
- Sprouts
- Fruit
- Vegetable juices: carrot, lettuce, nettle, watercress (at least four times per week)
- Cold-pressed, unsaturated, raw oil in small amounts: make salad dressing with lemon juice

Foods to Avoid

- Sugar
- Anything fried
- Meat
- Poultry
- Dairy foods, especially dairy desserts containing sugar
- Nut butters
- Citrus, except a little lemon juice on salad
- Canned and refined foods
- Refined grains, such as white flour products
- Caffeinated drinks

Herbs for Acne

- Teas made from sassafras, dandelion, and/or burdock seed, combined or used individually
- Mix together:

  2 parts red clover
  1 part echinacea
  1 part nettles

1 part burdock root
1 part dandelion root
½ part licorice root
½ part ginger

Powder herbs and put into #00 capsules. Take two capsules three times each day, or make an infusion and drink one cup three times a day.

- Externally: make a facial using clay, avocado skins, or raw honey.

Homepathy

Homeopathic medicine regards acne as a symptom of fundamental imbalance, so treatment is long-term and constitutional; however, the remedies below may produce improvement.
Take three times daily for up to fourteen days:

- Kali bromatum 6c: for itchy pimples, fidgety feet, restless sleep, unpleasant dreams
- Sulphur 6c: for long-standing acne; rough, hard skin; condition aggravated by washing, especially if person tends not to feel the cold and is prone to diarrhea first thing in the morning
- Calcarea sulphur 6c: for blind pimples and weeping pustules that form yellow crusts, slow to heal
- Hepar sulphur 6c: for large pimples that look like boils
- Antimonium tartaricum 6c: for pus-filled pimples
- Silicea 6c: for skin that scars easily

Hydrotherapy

- Wash with warm water two times per day with mild calendula or castile soap. Alternate warm, then cold applications.
- Lemon juice diluted in water may be applied. It has an antiseptic effect.
- Ocean bathing
- Daily skin brush to entire body with loofah or soft-bristle brush

Supplements

- Beta-carotene: 15 milligrams (mg) per day
- Vitamin B_1: 1.5 mg per day
- Vitamin B_2: 1.8 mg per day
- Niacin: 20 mg per day
- Vitamin B_6: 2–10 mg per day
- Vitamin C (antibiotic, antioxidant, stress reducer): 100–500 mg per day
- Vitamin E: 100–400 IU per day
- Zinc: 15 mg per day

ALLERGIES

SYMPTOMS

Allergy symptoms commonly resemble a cold: runny nose, sore throat, mucous discharge, skin eruptions, fatigue, depression, irritated eyes, insomnia, headache, and digestive disorders, such as constipation and heartburn.

WHAT IS AN ALLERGY?

From Modern Western Medicine

A collection of disease symptoms, often affecting the skin, respiratory system, stomach, and intestines in people who are sensitive to a substance that does not affect the majority of people. Such substances, called allergens, are attacked by immune cells, causing an immune reaction that itself gives rise to the symptoms of an allergy. Most physicians state that the best remedy for an allergy is to avoid the offending allergen. Drug treatments such as immunotherapy, antihistamines, and corticosteroid drugs are frequently used.

From Traditional Medicine

Allergic reactions often stem from the inability of the liver to neutralize certain substances that build up within the body and eventually trigger an immune reaction. A substance that the immune system recognizes as foreign to the body is often referred to as an *antigen*. As these antigens accumulate within the body—in places such as the lymph, intestinal tract, liver, and spleen—the immune system is continually working to rid the system of foreign substances. Thus, the person may suffer increasingly from allergic symptoms. In addition, some holistic healers believe that there is a psychological component to allergies, including feelings of isolation, separation, arrogance, and generally toxic thinking.

WHO GETS ALLERGIES?

People of all ages and both sexes get allergies.

REMEDIES

General Recommendations

- See Part IV for foods that strengthen the liver, spleen, and intestinal tract.
- Avoid the offending allergen as much as possible.

- Follow a rotation diet that helps you identify substances in foods that may be causing the allergic reaction or contributing to it.
- Fast on vegetable juices during periods when allergies are in an acute phase.
- Soak grains, beans, and seeds. It may make them more digestible and less likely to contribute to allergies.
- Eat regular amounts of green foods, spirulina, and chlorella to strengthen the immune system and cleanse the liver and spleen.
- Avoid foods and drinks that stress the adrenal glands.

Foods to Eat

Rotation diet: Increase the variety of foods eaten and don't eat a specific food more than once every four days in order to identify food allergens. Choose additive-free whole foods from the following list:

- Limit whole grains to brown rice, millet, and amaranth (all low in gluten).
- A wide variety of fresh vegetables and fruits
- Low-fat vegetable and animal proteins
- Seaweed and microalgae, such as spirulina and chlorella
- Vegetable juices
- Seeds and nuts

Foods to Avoid

- Gluten-containing grains such as wheat, rye, barley, and oats
- Caffeine, sugar, and alcohol
- Foods containing pesticides, chemicals, or additives
- Dairy products
- Processed or denatured foods

Herbs to Treat an Allergy

- Nettles: ½ teaspoon tincture or 1–2 capsules (preferably freeze-dried) every 2–4 hours, for its antihistamine and anti-inflammatory effects
- Echinacea: ½–1 teaspoon tincture, 3–4 times daily, to stimulate the immune system

Homeopathy

- *Apis mellifica:* for swelling of the tongue or tissues of the throat, such as from a bee sting
- *Allium cepa:* for relief of runny nose and burning, watery eyes
- Combination formulas include the above single remedies in addition to euphrasia and *Histaminum.*

Chinese Medicine

- Ephedra (ma huang): one cup of tea, ½ teaspoon of tincture, or one capsule, 2–3 times daily (Important: Do not use with heart disease, diabetes, glaucoma, or overactive thyroid gland.)
- Siberian ginseng (eleuthero): ½ teaspoon tincture, 2–3 times daily to support the adrenal glands
- Citrus seed extract for allergies including hay fever
- Onions inhibit allergic reaction
- Astragalus: ½ teaspoon of tincture or 2 capsules, 3 times a day to strengthen immune function

Supplements

- Biotin: 200 micrograms (mcg) 3 times a day for candida infestation
- Comb honey (locally produced, if possible): Chew ½ tsp., once daily.
- Kelp: 2–4 tablets, three times a day
- Raw adrenal tablets: 1–2 tablets, 3 times a day
- Beta-carotene (precursor of vitamin A): 16 mg daily
- Vitamin C: 100 mg
- Vitamin E: 200–400 mg
- Zinc (as an immune booster): 15 mg daily
- Selenium (20 mcg daily) works with any chemical allergies, especially when taken with kelp.

Exercise

Daily aerobic exercise cleanses the system of antigens through sweat glands and skin.

Hydrotherapy

- Loofah brush the skin in the shower to eliminate waste and toxins through the skin
- Sauna
- Ginger compress on liver to eliminate accumulated toxins

Mind/Body

- Meditate daily, especially on positive thoughts and images.
- Self-reflect on how much self-criticism and self-recrimination you indulge in daily.
- Sing a happy song daily. Singing helps strengthen spleen, a central organ in the fight against allergies.

ANAL ITCHING

WHAT IS ANAL ITCHING?

From Modern Western Medicine

The production of mucus from the anus tends to irritate the surrounding skin and may cause pruritus ani (itching of the anus). Hemorrhoids, anal fissures, and proctitis (inflammation of the rectum) may also cause anal discharge and irritation.

From Traditional Medicine

Anal itching is caused by the inability of the liver to adequately cleanse blood. Also, the liver and spleen cannot supply the large intestine and rectum with adequate qi to maintain circulation of lymph and blood. Hence, stagnation of waste occurs, which causes mucous discharge. Anal itching is frequently associated with, or exacerbated by, the consumption of sugar and oily and spicy foods.

REMEDIES

General Recommendations

- See Part IV for methods of strengthening liver and spleen.
- Exercise tends to improve the condition because it enhances circulation of blood and lymph.

Foods to Eat

- Sour-tasting foods, such as lemon and sauerkraut, to strengthen liver function
- Two servings per day of leafy, green vegetables
- Carrot juice to strengthen liver
- Dandelion greens (for liver)
- Daikon radish (to break up fat deposits)

Foods to Avoid

- Refined white sugar, oily foods, and spices
- White wine, especially very sweet white wines and those containing sugar (injurious to spleen)

Exercise

- Aerobic exercise four to five times per week, for at least thirty minutes per session

Herbology

- Apply goldenseal ointment when itching flares
- Barberry (one of the mildest and best liver tonics known): tincture, 10–30 drops, two times per day **(contraindicated during pregnancy)**
- Dandelion (cleanses blood and strengthens the liver): tincture, 10–30 drops, three times per day
- Oregon grape (the Pacific Northwest counterpart of barberry; improves function of liver and purifies blood toxins): tincture, 10–30 drops, three times per day
- Chickweed (one of the best herbs to stop itching): infusion, 1 ounce per pint of water; drink three or more cups throughout day. If you combine chickweed with other herbs, use 6–15 g.

Chinese Medicine

- Gardenia (the "happiness herb"): decoction, 6–12 g
- Acupuncture to strengthen liver and spleen
- Acupressure to strengthen liver and spleen and to reduce tension in the pelvic muscles that may be inhibiting circulation

ANEMIA

SYMPTOMS

Pallor, fatigue, dizziness, headaches, depression, slow healing, loss of sex drive, bruising, brittle nails, nervousness, shortness of breath, and palpitations. Additional symptoms from Chinese medical diagnosis: white or coated tongue, pale tissue beneath fingernails, white tissue inside lower eyelid (pull lower eyelid down and see tissue within).

WHAT IS ANEMIA?

From Modern Western Medicine

The most common form of anemia is caused by an iron deficiency that results in reduced hemoglobin in the blood. Causes include abnormally heavy bleeding during menstrual periods, various disease states, dietary deficiency of iron-rich foods, and poor assimilation of iron. An iron-rich diet and iron tablets may be recommended.

From Traditional Medicine

Anemia is seen as a blood deficiency and is usually caused by inadequate intake of nutrients, by the inability to absorb nutrients, by the loss of blood because of gastrointestinal bleeding, by excessive menstrual flow, or by a deficient liver that is not producing adequate enzymes to metabolize iron. In addition to eating iron-rich foods, natural healers often recommend increased intake of vitamin B_{12}, vitamin C, vitamin E, and folic acid to aid in the absorption of iron and other nutrients. Interestingly, iron deficiency very often is not the cause of anemia, as indicated by blood levels of adequate iron. This usually indicates that either absorption or liver deficiency is the underlying cause.

WHO GETS ANEMIA?

People most often affected are the elderly, especially those who eat narrow or simple diets, children, and pregnant women (due to the increased need for nutrition, especially iron and other minerals, in the developing fetus).

REMEDIES

Foods to Eat

- A wide variety of unrefined vegetables, legumes, grains, nuts, and seeds provide abundant protein, copper, and the B vitamins needed for iron absorption.

- Raw or lightly steamed greens or sprouts supply the necessary folic acid to aid absorption of iron.
- Foods rich in B$_{12}$ such as fish, eggs, bitter almonds, apricots, prunes, apple seeds, grapes, miso, wheat, sunflower seeds, and spirulina aid absorption.
- Foods rich in iron such as fish, egg yolks, blackstrap molasses, dark green vegetables (such as asparagus, cabbage, broccoli, parsley, celery, kale, cucumbers, leeks, and watercress), dried fruit, berries, beets, carrots, yams, beans, grains, and grape juice
- Sautéed radish leaves, chiso leaves, and miso soup improve blood quality.
- Pounded sweet rice with mugwort, a popular Japanese blood-builder

Foods to Avoid

- All dairy products
- Coffee and tea reduce iron absorption

Herbs to Treat Anemia

- Amla: one of the most effective tonics for anemia, made with fresh Indian gooseberries. Take ½ to 1 teaspoon each morning followed by warm water or herb tea.
- Blackberry and raspberry: fruit and juice (9–15 grams (g) of the berries); blood tonic
- Grapes: 9–30 g of grapes or fruit juice for blood deficiency
- Huckleberry: 9–15 g of berries for anemia
- Teas made from dandelion, comfrey, yellow dock, raspberry, and fenugreek

Chinese Medicine

- Lycii (known as wolfberry in America) treats anemia by strengthening blood. Take 5–15 g in decoction.
- Peony nourishes the blood. Take 6–16 g in decoction.

Supplements

- Vitamin B complex: 50 mg, three times a day
- Vitamin B$_6$: 3 mg, daily
- Vitamin B$_{12}$: 4 mcg to 1 mg, daily
- Folic acid: 400 mcg to 5 mg per day
- Vitamin C: 500 mg per day (increases hemoglobin production and folic acid usage and increases iron and B$_{12}$ absorption)
- Vitamin E: 200–400 IU per day
- Calcium: 800 mg per day
- Iron chelate or ferrous gluconate: 25 mg per day (only when iron deficiency has been diagnosed)
- Copper: 3–5 mg per day or 1 mg per every 10–15 mg of zinc

ANGINA

SYMPTOMS

The main symptom of angina is mild to severe chest pain in the area of the heart. The pain, which is often accompanied by a sense of pressure in the chest, can spread to the throat, upper jaw, back, arms, and between the shoulder blades. Other symptoms may include nausea, sweating, dizziness, and shortness of breath.

WHAT IS ANGINA?

From Modern Western Medicine

Angina, literally a strangling pain in the chest, is caused by insufficient blood flow to the heart, a condition called *ischemia*. The insufficient blood flow is caused by advanced atherosclerosis, brought on by a high-fat and -cholesterol diet. (See the section on atherosclerosis.) Eventually, the atherosclerosis can result in a *myocardial infarction*, or a heart attack.

From Traditional Medicine

Angina, like many other forms of heart disease, is seen as a disorder of the fire element (see the five element theory explained in Part III), which is associated with the deficiency of blood and qi, weakness of spirit, and the absence of joy.

WHO GETS ANGINA?

More men than women suffer from angina pain, especially after men turn fifty. Women can contract angina later in life.

REMEDIES

General Recommendations

- Reduce or eliminate all animal foods to avoid saturated fat and cholesterol.
- Reduce blood cholesterol to below 180 milligrams per deciliter (mg/dL) of blood.
- Increase fiber to lower cholesterol and improve bowel function.
- Get mild but regular exercise. Walking is ideal.

Foods to Eat

- Whole grains, fresh vegetables, and fruit. Many of these are rich in vitamins C and E and beta-carotene, which reduce the incidence and severity of angina.

- White fish and salmon are rich in omega-3 polyunsaturated fat. These fish oils lower cholesterol and protect against heart disease. They also increase HDLs (high-density lipoproteins), which lower the risk of heart attack.

Foods to Avoid

- Foods rich in saturated fat, especially red meat, eggs, the skin of chicken, and whole milk products
- Refined sugar increases triglycerides (blood fat) that cause platelet adhesiveness, which increases the incidence of angina attacks.
- Coffee and alcohol interfere with calcium absorption (a factor in heart problems)
- Excess sodium (most common in table salt, pickles, and foods containing salt and sea salt)
- Partially hydrogenated vegetable oils
- Cigarettes

Exercise

- Begin with mild stretching for ten minutes, then walk for twenty to thirty minutes, starting out slowly. If angina pain surfaces, stop walking and rest.
- Avoid competitive sports.

Herbology

- Garlic lowers LDL (low-density lipoprotein) cholesterol and raises HDL (high-density lipoprotein) cholesterol, the so-called good cholesterol. Garlic inhibits blood clotting, which protects against heart attack and lowers blood pressure. Use it raw and in cooking. Garlic capsules can also be taken.

Form	Dosage
Fresh garlic bulbs	7–28 cloves daily
Dried whole garlic cloves	5–20 g daily

- *Ginkgo biloba* increases blood flow and decreases the stickiness or viscosity of blood. Dose: 40 mg three times a day; use for four to six weeks.
- Capsaicin: found in red pepper; lowers cholesterol, lowers the tendency of blood to clot
- Hawthorn (*Crataegus oxyacantha*) contains flavonoids that prevent blood vessels from constricting, thereby preventing angina pain. It lowers cholesterol and helps to reverse atherosclerosis. Dosage: 80–200 mg per day
- Gugulipid: a plant extract; lowers LDL substantially, and raises HDL. Dosage: 25 mg, three times a day
- Oat Bran: water-soluble fiber. Dosage: ½–2 cups daily
- Bitterroot: Dosage: 10–40 drops of tincture

Chinese Medicine

- Corn, amaranth, dandelion, chicory, chives, scallions, brussels sprouts, and escarole all strengthen the fire element.
- Chinese chive: 6–9 g dried or 30–60 g fresh
- Shiitake mushrooms lower cholesterol substantially and improve the immune system. Boil in water and use as a tea and use regularly in soups, stews, broths, and vegetable medleys.
- Reishi mushrooms treat heart disease, reduce cholesterol, and lower high blood pressure. Decoction, place 1–2 mushrooms in 1 ounce/pint cold water, cook over low heat reduced to ⅓ the amount started with; drink one cup three times a day; 3–6 g for less serious conditions, 9–15 for more serious conditions.

Supplements

- Vitamin E: 60–200 mg daily
- Vitamin C: 500 mg daily
- Vitamin B complex: 25–50 mg daily
- Choline: can be found in lecithin

Other

- Massage
- Daily meditation
- Hot compresses: In acute angina, apply hot, moist compress to chest or midback, then massage the muscles deeply along the spine and follow with spinal manipulation.

ANXIETY

SYMPTOMS

Anxiety is a generalized feeling of fear, danger, or dread, often resulting from an unknown source. Symptoms include stomach tension, acid stomach, muscle tension, rapid breathing and heartbeat, trembling, headaches, sweating, nausea, diarrhea, weight loss, dry mouth, difficulty swallowing, hoarseness, irritability, fatigue, insomnia, nightmares, memory problems, and sexual impotence.

WHAT IS ANXIETY?

From Modern Western Medicine

Anxiety is seen as a triggering of the fight-or-flight reaction, causing excess adrenaline to be produced by the adrenal glands, which in turn produce other hormones (catecholamines) that affect various parts of the body, such as heartbeat and respiration.

From Traditional Medicine

A certain amount of anxiety is seen as a fundamental part of life, born of humanity's sense of separation from the one or creator of the universe. Anxiety is part of what motivates humans to search for answers to life's mysteries and to establish greater faith. In health, anxiety is not experienced to any great extent and is easily overcome through a variety of natural means. High levels of anxiety are caused by an imbalance of the spleen, pancreas, and stomach, organs that comprise the earth element. These organs are destabilized by excess thinking, acid-rich foods, insufficient chewing, and excess consumption of sugar. Anxiety accelerates aging, creates muscle tension, and weakens immune response, the blood, adrenal glands, and the pancreas. Virtually all traditional systems attempt to strengthen these organs as a treatment for anxiety.

Chinese medicine also urges the person with high levels of fear to strengthen the kidneys, which are the physical organs that control or promote fear. (See Part IV for additional information on healing spleen, stomach, pancreas, and kidneys.)

WHO GETS ANXIETY?

Everyone.

REMEDIES

General Recommendations

- See Part IV for methods of strengthening spleen, pancreas, stomach, and kidneys.

- Get regular exercise.
- Avoid foods that increase nervous tension, such as sugar, soft drinks (especially those containing caffeine), coffee, and tea.
- Meditate, pray, or find some other activity that establishes greater faith.
- Try aromatherapy and essential oils.

Foods to Eat

- Whole grains, especially brown rice, barley, millet, corn, and wheat
- Seaweeds
- Kasha
- Slightly salty foods

Foods to Avoid

- Coffee
- Chocolate
- Alcohol
- Strong spices
- Sugar
- Highly acidic foods, such as tomatoes, eggplant, and peppers, which are injurious to spleen

Herbs to Treat Anxiety

The following herbs have relaxing and sedating effects and can help relieve bouts of tension and anxiety. Unless otherwise specified, take them 3–4 times a day, either ½ teaspoon of tincture or two capsules.

- Chamomile, lemon balm, and passionflower: gentle, herbal sedatives that can also relax the digestive tract and can be taken in tea form
- California poppy and skullcap: slightly stronger herbal tranquilizer
- Valerian: a powerful but safe herbal sedative, useful in cases of extreme stress

Chinese Medicine

The following tonic herbs can be used on a daily basis over a long period of time to strengthen the body and improve resistance to stress.

- Siberian ginseng: ½ teaspoon of tincture, three times daily, helps the body cope better with stress by supporting adrenal function.
- Oats: ½ teaspoon of tincture, three times daily, strengthens and relaxes the nervous system. Look for preparations that contain the oat seed along with the straw.

Ayurvedic Medicine

- Ashwaganda: one capsule or ½ teaspoon of tincture, twice daily; considered the primary strengthening tonic in Ayurvedic medicine

Homeopathy

- Ingatia: for acute emotional upset that results in fear and anxiety
- Nux vomica: for when fear or anxiety also upset the stomach
- Aconite: for anxiety caused by fear, panic, sudden shock, or upset

Supplements

- Viatmin B complex: 50 mg daily; to support nervous system
- Viatmin C plus mixed bioflavonoids: 500 mg daily
- Calcium and magnesium in a 2:1 ratio (for example, 1000 mg calcium and 500 mg magnesium); for their tranquilizing effects

Essential Oils

The most effective methods for using essential oils to help calm the mind and relax the body include massage, baths, and vaporization. Use any of the following singly or in combination:

- Lavender: sedative, tonic. Sprinkle four drops on a tissue and inhale deeply for sudden stress.
- Clary sage: sedative, tonic
- Ylang-ylang: euphoric, regulator, sedative, tonic. Use in moderation; can cause headaches in some people.

Hydrotherapy

The following blend can be used in a vaporizer, for a massage, or in a bath. If you use it for massage, add ½ fluid ounce of carrier oil.

RELAXING BLEND

2 drops geranium
2 drops lavender
2 drops sandalwood
1 drop ylang-ylang

Mind/Body

- Meditate or pray daily, preferably in the morning before or after breakfast.
- Practice surrendering the outcome of events to the great spirit, however you perceive him/her/it.
- Excessive need to control events actually increases anxiety and eventually leads to depression.

It's important to pray or meditate before the workday actually begins to reduce the excess and destructive need to control all events.

ARTHRITIS: RHEUMATOID AND OSTEOARTHRITIS

SYMPTOMS

Osteoarthritis comes on gradually, often after an injury to the bone, with worsening pain and enlargement of one or more joints. It does not migrate from one part of the body to another.

Rheumatoid arthritis comes on suddenly or gradually, with many joints involved. It is most common in the hands, feet, and arms, where it can deform joints and cause redness, extreme pain, swelling, and tenderness of joints. Rheumatoid arthritis can and often does migrate to other joints.

WHAT IS ARTHRITIS?

From Modern Western Medicine

Osteoarthritis afflicts the weight-bearing joints: the knees, hips, and spine. It causes the cartilage in the joints to degenerate. It often manifests after an injury or from repetitive physical tasks that place excess stress upon joints.

Rheumatoid arthritis is the most severe type of inflammatory joint disease. It is an autoimmune disorder in which the body's immune system attacks and damages joints and surrounding soft tissue.

From Traditional Medicine

Arthritis is marked by mineral imbalances in the affected tissue, with calcium status being a good indicator of mineralization in general. Wind and dampness, the results of a stagnant liver, prevent qi from being smoothly distributed to joints and connective tissue. Dampness is often generated by toxic, mucuslike residues from the incomplete digestion of dairy foods, meat, refined sugars, alcohol, and excessive or poor quality oil and fat. Dampness and wind obstruct the nerves and other channels of energy transport, including the acupuncture meridians. Such chronic obstruction leads to nerve, bone, and sinew pain and inflammation.

WHO GETS IT?

Arthritis affects about 34 million Americans of all ages.

REMEDIES

Foods to Eat

- Green vegetables, such as watercress, parsley, celery, kale, and okra
- Seaweeds
- Carrots
- Spirulina
- Barley and wheat grass products (anti-inflammatory and detoxifying)
- Avocados
- Pecans
- Potassium broth
- Soy products
- Whole grains, such as brown rice, millet, oats, wheat, and barley
- Cold-water fish such as salmon, sardines, or herring

Foods to Avoid

Studies have shown that all arthritis symptoms are reduced, even for those with rheumatoid arthritis, after a person adopts a vegetarian diet, free of all animal foods, including—and especially—dairy products.

CALCIUM INHIBITORS

- Reduce or eliminate red meat, dairy, eggs, and chicken
- Alcohol
- Coffee
- Refined sugar and too many sweets
- Excess salt

FOODS HIGH IN OXALIC ACID

- Rhubarb
- Cranberries
- Plums
- Chard
- Spinach

THE NIGHTSHADES

- Tomatoes
- Eggplant
- Potatoes
- Peppers
- Tobacco

FOODS THAT WILL CREATE WIND AND DAMPNESS

- Buckwheat

- Dairy foods
- All animal fat
- Nuts, oil-rich seeds, and nut butters

Herbs to Treat Arthritis

Herbal remedies will reduce inflammation and pain and stimulate circulation. Try any of the following:

- Feverfew: 2 capsules of freeze-dried herb, 3 times a day
- Devil's claw or wild yam: 1 teaspoon of tincture or 3 capsules, 3 times a day
- Hawthorn (contains flavonoids, potent antioxidants that help heal collagen): ½ teaspoon tincture, 2 capsules, or 1 cup of tea, 3–4 times a day
- White willow bark or meadowsweet (contains salicin, the same active ingredient found in aspirin): ½ teaspoon of tincture, 2 capsules, or 1 cup of tea as needed to relieve pain
- Turmeric (curcumin) (a potent antioxidant and anti-inflammatory): 2 capsules, 3 times daily

Homeopathy

Remedies are best prescribed by a homeopathic practitioner. However, the following remedies may be helpful for providing relief from joint pain.

- Rhus toxicodendron: for aching joints that are worse in the morning and better from heat and continued movement
- Colocynthis: for pain that is worse from movement but better from warmth and pressure
- Bryonia: for swollen joints and pain that is aggravated by the slightest movement
- Arnica: for a sore, bruised feeling in the joints, made worse by touch

Hydrotherapy

- Hot and cold showers to stimulate general circulation and act as a general tonic
- Hot and cold compresses, alternated (locally)
- Hot Epsom salts baths or local bath or compress
- Paraffin bath (local): 4 parts paraffin, 1 part mineral oil. Heat to 125–130°F, or let cool until thin film forms. Dip part repeatedly until ¼ inch thick, or paint on larger areas.

Chinese Medicine

Most remedies can be found in the food section, and they involve wind/dampness. This formula can be used by those with a robust constitution (strong, loud voice, and thick tongue coating):

4 parts chaparral leaf
2 parts devil's claw root
2 parts sassafras root bark
2 parts dried gingerroot
1 part black cohosh root
1 part burdock root
1 part prickly ash bark

For individuals who are weaker and more deficient (frail, pale, little or no tongue coating, introverted personality):

4 parts suma root
4 parts motherwort
4 parts prickly ash bark
4 parts osha/ligusticum root
2 parts angelica root
1½ parts Siberian ginseng
1½ parts cinnamon bark

Supplements

- Beta-carotene: 16 mg per day
- Vitamin B complex: 50 mg daily
- Niacinamide: 200–1000 mg, 2–4 times a day. Can significantly increase joint mobility when taken daily for 3–4 weeks. If nausea occurs, cut dose in half or discontinue.
- Vitamin C: 500 mg, 3–4 times daily
- Vitamin E: 60–300 IU, one to two times per day
- Calcium: 800–1000 mg per day

Essential Oils

Try any of the following singly or in combination:

- Eucalyptus
- Ginger
- Rosemary

ASTHMA

SYMPTOMS

Difficulty breathing, especially exhalation, wheezing, coughing, and a sensation of choking.

WHAT IS ASTHMA?

From Modern Western Medicine

Asthma is recurrent attacks of breathlessness accompanied by wheezing during exhalation. Severity of symptoms changes from day to day and from hour to hour. The illness frequently starts up in childhood and often clears up or becomes less severe in early adulthood.

Asthma may be caused by outside allergens that can bring on an attack or by internal causes, such as stress. For sufferers of extrinsic asthma, tests can often discover common allergens that may be responsible and thus be avoided. Prophylactic drugs are used as a means of prevention. These are frequently taken as inhalers.

From Traditional Medicine

The majority of cases fall into a general asthma syndrome. People with asthma often suffer from hypoglycemia, were weaned too early (usually before the end of the first year) and onto excessive amounts of wheat, dairy products, and sugar. The child may also have been treated for early illnesses with immune suppressive treatments (high levels of antibiotics, for example, which scientists have found to be immunosuppressive), which can trigger the onset of asthma. A history of chronic colds and bronchitis often precedes the onset of asthma. Wheat, dairy products, and sugar are common allergens for people who suffer fron asthma. Even when food intolerances are not the cause, however, they tend to play a role in the larger picture.

Traditional healers often encourage the elimination of stored toxins, mucus, and waste products. Such elimination, however, is often prevented by the use of pharmaceutical drugs, which results in increased accumulation within tissues, exacerbating the illness or acting as a cause.

Rather than focusing exclusively on the lungs and bronchial passages, Chinese medicine also treats the kidneys, which tend to be weak in asthmatics. In the Chinese five element system, the energy from the lungs should travel smoothly and efficiently into the kidneys. When the kidneys are weak or stressed, the lung energy cannot pass freely and thus becomes stagnant in the lungs, causing accumulation and the onset of asthmatic symptoms.

WHO GETS ASTHMA?

Both sexes get asthma and although it frequently begins early in life (most people have their first attack by age five), it can develop at any age.

REMEDIES

Foods to Eat

- Whole grains
- Vegetables
- Legumes
- Chlorophyll and vitamin A foods (protect the lungs and provide cell renewal): spirulina, blue-green algae, apricots (not more than two to three a day), pumpkin, carrots, and mustard greens
- Omega-3 and GLA fatty acid–rich food (exceptional for alleviating the constrictions and spasms of asthma): salmon, mackerel, sardines, herring, anchovies, rainbow trout, and tuna
- Alpha-linolenic acid is contained in the following foods and is a good source of omega-3: tofu and tempeh, flaxseed, pumpkin seed, chia seed, and dark green vegetables.

Foods to Avoid

- Dairy products, including whole and skim milk, yogurt, and ice cream
- Refined white sugar and foods that contain refined sugar
- Highly refined foods
- Foods containing artificial ingredients
- Alcohol
- Wheat
- Coffee and black tea

Herbs to Treat Asthma

- Ephedra (contains natural ephedrine, which acts as a bronchodilator): ¼ to 1 teaspoon of tincture or 1 cup of tea, 2–3 times daily. Consult a health practitioner if you suffer from heart disease, diabetes, glaucoma, or thyroid disease.
- Lobelia (antispasmodic, relaxes the bronchial muscle): ¼–½ teaspoon of tincture, 3 times a day; mix with cayenne for increased effectiveness (3 parts tincture of lobelia with 1 part tincture of capsicum).
- Capsicum desensitizes the respiratory system to irritants and is helpful in stopping an asthma attack.
- Grindelia (to ease bronchial spasms and to promote the removal of mucus from the lungs): ¼–½ teaspoon of tincture, 2–3 times daily
- Licorice (for its anti-inflammatory and antiallergenic effects): ½ teaspoon of tincture or 1 cup of tea, 2–3 times daily. Licorice should be used with caution for those who suffer with high blood pressure.

Homeopathy

- Arsenicum: for dry, wheezing asthma that comes on in the middle of the night, accompanied by anxiety and restlessness
- Ipecac: for gagging, profuse mucus that can't be coughed up, or long spasms of coughing that may end in vomiting
- Spongia: especially if asthma is accompanied by loud wheezing

Hydrotherapy

- For chronic sufferers: hot Epsom salts bath, 2 times a week; alternate hot and cold showers daily; chest packs nightly
- For acute attacks: hot chest compresses plus hot footbath
- Hot footbath with mustard and lobelia plus ice pack to back of head
- Warm bath for forty-five minutes with relaxation and diaphragmic breathing

Chinese Medicine

All the foods to eat for asthma come from the Chinese medicine recommendations. There are four basic types of asthma. The first is cold-type asthma, which is characterized by white, clear, or foamy mucus, cold extremities, pale face, and a frequent feeling of coldness. Heat-type asthma is characterized by fast, heavy breathing, red face, sensation of heat in the body, yellow mucus, dry stools, and scanty urine. Mucus-type asthma is characterized by copious mucus, the mouth is often held open, breathing is difficult when lying down, and the tongue coating is thick and greasy. Deficiency-type asthma is characterized by a weak pulse, little or no tongue coating, pale complexion, shortness of breath, head needing to be propped up in order to sleep, and breathing becoming difficult with slight body exertions.

A valuable herb/seed tea for treating cold-, mucus-, and deficiency-types of asthmas consists of equal parts of fennel seed, flaxseed, fenugreek seed, licorice root, lobelia seed and/or leaf, and mullein leaf or flower. This formula, minus the warming ingredients (fennel and fenugreek), is beneficial for heat-type asthma. For cold-type asthma, cook food moderately to well. Pressure cook and boil grains; steam and boil vegetables. Avoid raw foods.

Eat the following: garlic (for lungs and large intestine), anise (for lungs), fresh ginger (for lungs), black beans (for kidneys), and oats (for liver).

For heat-type asthma, eat daikon radish (large intestine), sprouts, apricots (a maximum of two to three daily), lemons, and tofu.

For mucus-type asthma, eat oats, brown rice, barley, black beans, nuts (especially walnuts and almonds), black beans, and buckwheat.

Supplements

- Vitamin C: 500 mg daily
- Beta-carotene: 20 IU daily

- Vitamin B_6: 3–5 mg daily
- Vitamin E: 400 IU daily
- Quercetin: 500 mg, with 250 mg bromelain, 2 times daily, for anti-inflammatory and antihistamine effects; flaxseed oil, 3 tablespoons a day, to reduce inflammation

ATHEROSCLEROSIS

See related entries for angina, circulation, and heart disease.

SYMPTOMS

There are no symptoms in the early stages of atherosclerosis. Angina pectoris, or a strangling pain in the heart and center of the chest, emerges when atherosclerosis is advanced in the coronary arteries. Atherosclerosis causes heart attack and stroke, either of which can be the first sign that advanced atherosclerosis has set in.

WHAT IS ATHEROSCLEROSIS?

From Modern Western Medicine

Atherosclerosis is the formation of cholesterol plaques that form like boils inside the arteries of the body, especially in the arteries leading to the heart and brain. It is the primary cause of most heart disease throughout the Western world. Atherosclerosis is caused by a diet rich in saturated fat and cholesterol.

From Traditional Medicine

While traditional healers accept the prevailing Western approach, they note that the liver, kidneys, and heart are all involved in the cause of the disorder. The liver processes fat and cholesterol and turns them into LDL (low-density lipoprotein, the cause of atherosclerosis). The kidneys control the heart (see the five element system explained in Part III) and directly influence blood pressure. Treatment, therefore, focuses on the liver, kidneys, and heart.

REMEDIES

General Recommendations

- Reduce or eliminate all foods high in fat and cholesterol, including red meat, the skin of chicken, eggs, and whole dairy products.
- Increase whole grains, fresh vegetables, fruit, and beans.
- Increase fiber, which lowers cholesterol.
- Enjoy mild exercise, such as walking, daily.
- Reduce blood cholesterol level to 180 mg/dL or lower.

Foods to Eat

- Whole grains, such as brown rice, barley, corn, oats, and wheat
- Fresh vegetables; a wide variety
- Beans (especially healing for kidneys)

Atherosclerosis

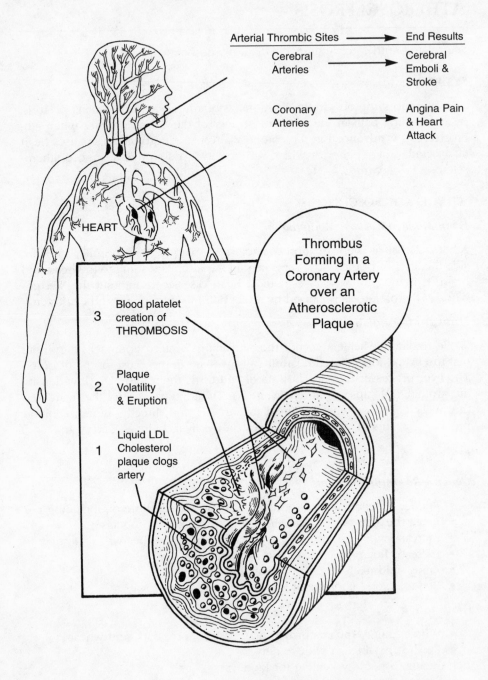

Arterial Thrombic Sites ⟶ End Results

Cerebral
Arteries ⟶ Cerebral
Emboli &
Stroke

Coronary
Arteries ⟶ Angina Pain
& Heart
Attack

HEART

Thrombus
Forming in a
Coronary Artery
over an
Atherosclerotic
Plaque

3 Blood platelet
creation of
THROMBOSIS

2 Plaque
Volatility
& Eruption

1 Liquid LDL
Cholesterol
plaque clogs
artery

- Fruit
- Low-fat white fish (See the section on healing foods, under Chinese medicine.)
- Chlorella (contains omega-3 polyunsaturated alpha-linolenic oils that lower blood cholesterol)

Foods to Avoid:

- Red meat (because of its fat and cholesterol content)
- Eggs (for fat and cholesterol content)
- Whole milk and other high-fat dairy products
- The dark meat and the skin of poultry, which is richer in fat than the white meat
- High-fat vegetable foods, such as avocados and olives
- Nut butters, such as peanut butter, tahini, and sesame butter

Herbs to Treat Atherosclerosis

- Garlic lowers cholesterol, raises HDL, and prevents blood from forming clots, which is the process by which atherosclerosis gives rise to heart attacks and strokes. Garlic capsules can also be taken.

Form	Dosage
Fresh garlic bulbs	7–28 cloves daily
Dried whole garlic cloves	5–20 grams daily

- Ginkgo biloba increases blood flow and decreases the stickiness or viscosity of blood. Dose: 40 mg, 3 times a day. Use for 4 to 6 weeks.
- Capsaicin: Found in red pepper, capsaicin lowers cholesterol and reduces the tendency of blood to clot.
- Hawthorn (*Crataegus oxyacantha*): Contains flavonoids that prevent blood vessels from constricting, thereby preventing angina pain. Lowers cholesterol and helps to reverse atherosclerosis. Dosage: 80–200 mg per day.
- Gugulipid: A plant extract that lowers LDL substantially and raises HDL. Dosage: 25 mg, 3 times a day.
- Oat bran (reduces blood cholesterol): water-soluble fiber. Dosage: ½–2 cups per day.
- Bitterroot: tincture, 10–40 drops daily
- Shiitake mushrooms
- Reishi mushrooms

Exercise

- Walking (the best exercise for all people with atherosclerosis or coronary heart disease)
- Bicycling on flat surfaces (not to be done without significant cholesterol lowering)

- Swimming (not to be done without significant dietary change and lowering of blood cholesterol)
- Water aerobics (done gently until fitness improves, and not done without significant dietary change and lowering of blood cholesterol)
- No competitive sports

Chinese Medicine

Most heart problems involve deficiency. Since the heart relies on other organs for its nourishment and energy, the majority of heart problems are caused by and treated through imbalances in other organ systems.

Supplements

- Vitamin C with bioflavonoids: 500–1000 mg, 3 times per day; helps keep plaque from forming, lowers triglycerides, strengthens capillaries, and increases HDL
- Beta-carotene: 20–100 mg per day
- Vitamin E: 60–300 mg daily

Mind/Body

- Meditation
- Relaxation and stress management techniques
- Soft, relaxing music, daily

BACK PAIN

SYMPTOMS

Pain in the lower, middle, or upper back and neck. Occasionally there is visible curvature of the spine, but usually there are no apparent external symptoms.

WHAT IS BACK PAIN?

From Modern Western Medicine

Most people suffer from back pain at some point in their lives. Multiple causes may be involved, including stress, lifting heavy objects, pregnancy, straining individual muscles, poor posture, and prolonged sitting, especially in a chair that does not adequately support the back. Rest, analgesics, and anti-inflammatory drugs are prescribed. Surgery is often used as well.

From Traditional Medicine

Back pain emerges from many causes, but the most common is from prolonged stress and fear, combined with consistent injury to the kidneys from poor dietary habits. Stress, as pioneer researcher Hans Selye pointed out, damages kidneys. Traditional medicine regards the kidneys as the source of qi that is supplied to the entire body, but especially to the muscles of the low back. As the kidneys and the related muscles of the low back weaken, the muscles go into spasm. This causes the muscles on either side of the spine to pull unequally on the spinal vertebrae. One side pulls harder than the other, causing the spine to drift in that direction. Eventually, disks and nerves become pinched from the bending of the spine to the right or left, causing acute pain.

Middle back pain is often caused by imbalances in the liver and spleen, organs that provide qi to the muscles of the middle back. Upper back pain can be caused by excess kidney energy that is transferred upward to the neck, excessive or deficient heart energy, or tension in the shoulder muscles caused by stress and liver-gallbladder imbalances.

In addition to these causes are the usual suspects: lifting heavy weight, prolonged standing, pregnancy, poor posture, lack of exercise, and kidney or reproductive problems.

REMEDIES

General Recommendations

- Review and, where possible, change the sources of the muscle tension: excess sitting; lack of exercise; jobs that require repetitive motion; stress; or repressed emotions, especially anger and fear.

Back Problems
Muscles that Support the Spine

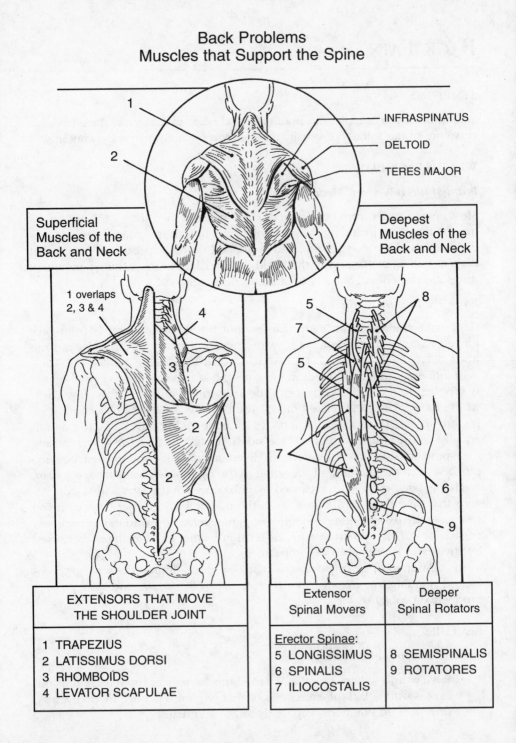

INFRASPINATUS

DELTOID

TERES MAJOR

Superficial
Muscles of the
Back and Neck

Deepest
Muscles of the
Back and Neck

1 overlaps
2, 3 & 4

EXTENSORS THAT MOVE THE SHOULDER JOINT	Extensor Spinal Movers	Deeper Spinal Rotators
1 TRAPEZIUS 2 LATISSIMUS DORSI 3 RHOMBOIDS 4 LEVATOR SCAPULAE	Erector Spinae: 5 LONGISSIMUS 6 SPINALIS 7 ILIOCOSTALIS	8 SEMISPINALIS 9 ROTATORES

- Regular aerobic exercise (see exercise section in Part III)
- Daily stretching exercise (see exercise section in Part III)
- Acupressure, therapeutic massage, and chiropractic are the most frequently successful forms of treatment. The practitioner should concentrate on relaxing and healing the muscles that support the back, rather than on forcing the spinal vertebrae back into alignment, however.
- Strengthen the kidneys, liver, gallbladder, and spleen (see Part IV).
- Avoid excess anger and stress.
- Lose weight if overweight, especially if the stomach area is enlarged. (The weight tends to pull on the low back.)

Foods to Eat

- Whole grains, especially barley (for the kidneys), brown rice, millet, corn, and oats
- A wide variety of fresh vegetables, especially leafy greens
- Beans (especially healing for the kidneys)
- Fruit

Herbs

The following herbs may be taken internally for backache. A common dosage is ½–1 teaspoon of tincture, 3–4 times daily.

- White willow bark: contains salicin, a natural aspirinlike compound that relieves pain without the harmful side effects of aspirin.
- Meadowsweet: also a natural form of salicin
- Cramp bark: relieves muscular tension and spasms

The following herbs can be used as topical applications to provide temporary relief of low back pain caused by muscular tension.

- Arnica oil or gel: Apply externally. Relieves muscular pain and inflammation; do not apply to broken skin.
- Lobelia or cramp bark: Antispasmodic herbs; add 1 tablespoon of tincture to 1 quart of hot water, soak a towel in the solution, and apply as a warm compress to the lower back.

Homeopathic Remedies

- Arnica: for backache from overexertion or for a bruised feeling
- Rhus toxicodendron: for a backache that feels better after being warmed up by continuous movement

Chinese Medicine

For backache that often results from kidney yin deficiency (or expanded kidneys):

- Millet and barley
- Tofu
- String beans
- Black beans, black soybeans, and mung beans and sprouts
- Kuzu root
- Watermelon and all other melons
- Blackberries, mulberries, blueberries, huckleberries
- Seaweeds
- Spirulina and chlorella

Foods to Avoid

- Animal products (They will stimulate the liver into a heat or stagnant condition and drain kidney yin.)
- Coffee
- Alcohol
- Tobacco
- Hot spices such as cinnamon, cloves, and garlic

Essential Oils

Essential oils can be used to help relieve backaches as a massage or compress to the painful area, or in a bath.

- Chamomile: analgesic, anti-inflammatory, antispasmodic, nervine, sedative
- Marjoram: analgesic, antispasmodic, nervine, sedative
- Lavender: analgesic, antispasmodic, nervine, sedative
- Wintergreen, camphor, and eucalyptus: help warm and relax muscles when rubbed into the back

Hydrotherapy

- Hot compresses on painful part of back increase circulation.
- Follow hot compress with cold packs to reduce swelling.
- Take hot baths, especially with mineral salts.

Exercise

- Aerobic exercise for at least thirty minutes, three to four times per week
- Stretching exercises daily

Chair exercise: Sit in chair and lean forward until pain is felt; breathe out and slowly lean farther, stretching muscles further.

Knee pulls: Sit in a straight-backed chair. Lift your right knee and clasp it in both hands and pull it as close to your chest as possible. Exhale deeply as you feel tension or mild pain in your back. Do the same with your left leg. Do several repetitions.

Do the same exercise while lying on mat placed on the floor. While lying
on the mat, pull both knees toward your chest. Breathe out as you pull
your knees toward your chest and as you feel the tension.

Reverse ankle pull. Stand at the back of a straight-backed chair. Bring your
right ankle up behind you, grasp it with your right hand, and gently but
firmly pull upward toward your back so that your thigh muscles stretch.
Exhale as you pull. Do the same with both legs.

Mind/Body

Meditate and/or pray daily. Muscle tension begins in the mind, especially with
fear. Try to release the need to control the outcomes of events but picture positive outcomes to all situations.

BLADDER PROBLEMS

SYMPTOMS

Various forms of incontinence, including *stress incontinence,* or the releasing of small amounts of urine when laughing, sneezing, coughing, or exercising; *overflow incontinence,* the inability to fully empty the bladder when urinating, with leaking of urine throughout the day; *urge incontinence,* triggered by a single glass of water or the sound of water, causing a powerful and sometimes uncontrollable urge to urinate; and *reflex incontinence,* the emptying of the bladder without perceiving the need to urinate beforehand.

WHAT ARE BLADDER PROBLEMS?

From Modern Western Medicine

Bladder problems include various forms of incontinence, swelling of the bladder or urethra, and weakness or overactivity of the sphincter muscles. These conditions can be caused by overactive or underactive bladder muscles, neurological disorders, hormone imbalances, and the side effects of medication. Another common bladder problem is cystitis (the inflammation of the urinary bladder), which is often caused by bacterial infection.

From Traditional Medicine

Bladder problems are caused by an imbalance of qi in the water element, usually brought on by highly acidic foods and drinks, spices, stimulants, and other irritants that stress the kidneys and bladder; by pregnancy; by various kinds of birth control devices, such as the IUD; and by cigarette smoking.

REMEDIES

General Recommendations

- See Part IV for ways to strengthen kidneys and bladder.
- Stop smoking.
- Lose weight. Excess weight stresses the bladder and can contribute to incontinence.

Foods to Eat

- Whole grains, especially barley, which is an herb for the kidneys, and brown rice. Cook grains with small amounts of sea salt (a pinch per pot). This small amount of salt will alkalize the grain and assist in digestion. It will also make the blood and urine slightly less acidic.

- Beans, especially black beans, long considered a traditional herb for kidneys and bladder
- Leafy greens, for their high mineral content
- White fish, which is low in fat
- Sea vegetables, such as nori, wakame, kombu, arame: mineral-rich and strengthening to kidneys and bladder. Use small amounts, such as one- or two-tablespoon-sized servings, daily.

Foods to Avoid

- Highly acidic foods, such as spices, alcohol (chronic alcohol abuse significantly weakens the bladder), sugar, tomatoes, and hot peppers
- Red meat, dairy products, and eggs, all of which raise the uric acid levels of the blood, stress the kidneys and bladder, and irritate organs
- Excess salt: Avoid adding salt or salt-rich foods at the table.
- Caffeine-containing foods and drinks, especially coffee. Also avoid tea, soda pop, and cacao-containing foods. (These act like diuretics and weaken bladder and kidneys.)

Exercise

- Kegel exercises daily: Contract pelvic muscles while urinating, causing urine flow to be halted temporarily. Then release. Stop again. Repeat the process several times while urinating. This strengthens the sphincter muscles in the bladder and provides greater control over the bladder. These exercises are especially helpful to women who have stress incontinence as a result of pregnancy. Do these exercises even when not urinating.
- Walk daily for twenty to thirty minutes to improve general fitness and lose weight. (See exercise section, Part III.)
- Aerobic exercise: twenty to thirty minutes per session, three to four times per week (See exercise section, Part III.)

Herbs

- Echinacea, especially for bacterial infections that cause cystitis: 15–30 drops, twice daily, for 3 to 5 days. Dried herb can be drunk as a decoction tea and combined with burdock root and dandelion to make a blood-cleansing and kidney-bladder-strengthening decoction or tea.
- Goldenseal: 15–30 drops, as tincture, twice daily, for 3 to 5 days
- Burdock root: strengthens kidney and bladder, cleanses blood. Can be taken as a tincture or as a dried herb in decoction tea.
- Dandelion root: dried herb can be taken as tea, along with echinacea and burdock root.
- Slippery elm: for cystitis, as a decoction tea from whole bark, 3 to 4 times per day

- Buchu: for cystitis or inflammation of the bladder; irritation of the ure-thra; high levels of uric acid; and urine retention. Use as a cold infusion. (Do not boil leaves. Rather, add three ounces of herb to water after the water has been boiled; steep for 5–15 minutes.) Drink 3 or 4 times per day.
- Uva Ursi: for bladder diseases, bed-wetting, cystitis, and kidney and bladder stones. Combines well with buchu. Use as a tincture (10–20 drops, 3 times per day), fluid extract (½–1 teaspoon, 3 times per day), or infusion (standard infusion, steep for thirty minutes), 3 cups per day.

BLOOD CHOLESTEROL

SYMPTOMS

High blood cholesterol has no symptoms, but it is the underlying cause of atherosclerosis and cardiovascular diseases, such as heart attack and stroke.

WHAT IS HIGH CHOLESTEROL LEVEL?

From Modern Western Medicine and Traditional Medicine

Blood cholesterol is measured as milligrams of cholesterol per deciliter of blood and written as mg/dL. Anything above 190 mg/dL is considered unsafe. On the other hand, research has shown that a cholesterol level of 180 mg/dL or lower is associated with very small to no risk of heart attack or stroke. An ideal cholesterol level is 160 mg/dL.

Cholesterol is carried on the backs of proteins. There are two types of proteins that are combined with cholesterol: low-density lipoprotein (LDL), which causes atherosclerosis and heart disease, and high-density lipoprotein (HDL), which promotes the elimination of cholesterol from the body and thus is protective against cardiovascular disease.

Cholesterol level is influenced by diet, heredity, and metabolic diseases such as diabetes mellitus. Contrary to what many people believe, however, the number of people who have genetically high cholesterol is minute. Thus, the overwhelming majority of high cholesterol levels—greater than 95 percent—are the result of dietary and lifestyle factors. Most cholesterol levels can be lowered significantly by diet alone.

From Traditional Medicine

High cholesterol is unheard of among people who eat a traditional diet based on whole grains, fresh vegetables, beans, fruit, and low-fat fish. The average Chinese man or woman has a cholesterol level of 154 mg/dL, and those living in the villages of China—even the elderly—have cholesterol levels far lower than the average, according to Cornell University researchers. High cholesterol is strictly a dietary and lifestyle condition that is easily remedied by adopting a diet based largely on vegetable foods.

REMEDIES

General Recommendations

- Eat whole grains, vegetables, fruits, and low-fat fish.
- Increase fiber, which lowers cholesterol.
- Eat cholesterol-lowering foods and herbs (see page 54).

- Support liver function. The liver metabolizes fat and cholesterol and turns them into LDL or HDL.

Foods to Eat

- Whole grains such as brown rice, barley, and oats
- Dried beans
- Legumes
- Fruit
- Vegetables, especially leafy greens, broccoli, and roots
- Omega-3 fatty acids, which are found in salmon, sardines, and other deep/cold-water fish
- Onions: one to two ounces per day
- Scallions
- Garlic: 7–28 fresh bulbs per day

Foods to Avoid

- Meat
- Poultry
- Eggs
- Dairy products
- All oils, even vegetable
- Cigarettes

Herbs to Treat High Cholesterol

- Garlic, dried whole: 5–20 grams (g)/day
- Garlic powder: 600–1350 mg/day
- Gugulipid: 25 mg 3 times/day
- Capsaicin: before meals as directed
- Hawthorn: leaves, 80 mg 2 times/day; standardized extract, 100–200 mg every day

Chinese Medicine

- Ginkgo biloba: 40 mg, 3 times per day
- Shiitake mushrooms
- Reishi mushrooms

Supplements

- Vitamin C: 100–500 mg per day
- Vitamin E (dry form): 60–400 IU per day
- Beta-carotene: 20 mg per day
- Charcoal powder: 1½ to 2 tablespoons (8 grams) in water, 3 times per day
- Water-soluble fiber from oats, brown rice, dried beans, legumes, and fruit

Mind/Body

Chronic stress raises cholesterol levels. Follow one of the meditation, imaging, or positive imaging regimens provided in Part IV.

BLOOD PRESSURE

SYMPTOMS

High blood pressure is referred to as the silent killer because very often there are no symptoms associated with the disorder. Severe high blood pressure, also called malignant hypertension, can cause hemorrhages of small blood vessels, headaches, vomiting, visual impairment, blindness, convulsions, paralysis, and coma. However, even mild to moderately high blood pressure is associated with an increased risk of heart attack and stroke.

WHAT IS BLOOD PRESSURE?

From Western Medicine

Blood pressure is expressed as a fraction, such as 110/70 mm Hg, which is considered an ideal blood pressure. Normal is considered 120/80 mm Hg. The measurement mm Hg stands for millimeters of mercury. The first (top) number stands for *systolic* pressure, or the pressure created when the heart contracts and pumps blood into the aorta, the body's main artery. The heart's contraction pushes blood into the arteries, causing them to expand. Once expanded, the arteries recoil, or contract, causing a secondary wave of pressure, termed *diastolic* pressure, and represented by the second (bottom) number in the blood pressure fraction.

Blood pressure is considered high, or *hypertensive,* if either the top number or the bottom is consistently above 140/90 mm Hg while the person is at rest.

WHO GETS HIGH BLOOD PRESSURE?

Forty million Americans have diastolic pressures between 90 and 100 mm Hg.

REMEDIES

General Recommendations

- Lose weight if you are overweight. Weight loss alone will lower blood pressure.
- Exercise. Mild aerobic exercise will lower blood pressure significantly.
- Don't smoke cigarettes. Cigarettes raise LDL cholesterol. One cigarette raises blood pressure for thirty minutes to an hour.
- Reduce salt intake and never use salt as a condiment, especially if you are salt-sensitive.
- Reduce fat and cholesterol in the diet. Atherosclerosis is a cause of hypertension.

- Reduce alcohol if you consume more than two drinks per day.
- Reduce protein foods, especially animal proteins, which stress the kidneys and cause mineral loss, especially calcium.
- Eat blood pressure–reducing foods and herbs (see below).

Foods to Eat

- Emphasize potassium-rich foods in your diet, such as whole grains, fresh vegetables, beans, and fruit. Low potassium is associated with high blood pressure, and studies have shown that by increasing potassium, blood pressure normalizes.
- Eat calcium-rich foods, such as leafy greens (collard greens, kale, and mustard greens) and other vegetables, tofu, seeds, nuts, and low-fat animal foods.
- Use garlic as a condiment. Garlic lowers blood pressure. Grate it raw on vegetables and salads or use it in cooking.
- Use onion, garlic, lemon, vinegars, lime, oregano, basil, and other culinary herbs to season food in place of salt.

Read labels on packaged food. "Low sodium" means that there are no more than 140 mg of salt per serving; "very low sodium" means that there are no more than 35 mg per serving. However, check serving size, which may be quite small and deceptive.

Foods to Avoid

- Red meat, eggs, fried foods, and other high-fat foods. Studies have consistently shown that vegetarians have healthier blood pressures than meat eaters.
- Reduce or eliminate salt. Use salt only sparingly in cooking (a pinch). Studies have shown that half of all hypertensives suffer from high blood pressure because of salt intake. Humans need only about 1½ teaspoons of salt per day, according to the National Academy of Sciences, which is easily obtained as a natural constituent of food.
- Reduce or avoid coffee and other drinks and foods rich in caffeine, which is associated with elevations in blood pressure.

Exercise

- Walk three to five times per week, for at least thirty minutes per walking session.
- Avoid competitive sports.
- See exercises in Part III for suggestions on healthy ways to get exercise.

Herbs for Healthy Blood Pressure

- Garlic (Research has shown that garlic significantly lowers blood pressure.)
- Shiitake mushrooms lower cholesterol.

- Reishi mushrooms lower cholesterol.

Supplements

- Potassium: 1000 mg per day (No RDA exists for potassium; it is widely available in food. Experts say 3000 mg is needed daily.)
- Calcium: 200–500 mg daily
- Fiber (Add to foods; also eat fiber-rich foods, such as whole grains, vegetables, and beans.)

Mind/Body

- Meditate, pray, do guided imagery exercises, or chant daily. Stress management has been shown to lower blood pressure significantly.
- Control hostility. Anger dramatically elevates blood pressure. When you argue, emphasize how you feel, as opposed to attacking others for their behavior or their motives; talk slowly and maintain a lower volume to your voice. (Studies have shown that the more rapid and loudly a person speaks, the higher the blood pressure goes.)

Aromatherapy

- Chamomile soothes, relaxes, refreshes, and calms the overall condition.
- Coriander warms, relaxes, deodorizes, and soothes.
- Pine promotes constancy, stability, and duration in the face of life's vicissitudes. It decongests the lungs, relaxes, and promotes confidence.

BODY ODOR

The secretion of foul-smelling perspiration.

WHAT IS BODY ODOR?

From Modern Western Medicine

Perspiration provides a supportive environment for bacteria to ground and grow on the body. The decomposing bacteria cause odor. The armpits and genital area produce ideal conditions for bacteria to flourish because of the presence of apocrine glands that, along with perspiration, also produce proteins and fatty acids. Other areas of the body produce perspiration that consists only of salt water, which does not support bacterial growth as effectively. The exception, of course, is the feet, which sweat in a warm, airless environment that supports bacteria and fungus. The most effective treatment for body odor is to wash and use a deodorant.

From Traditional Medicine

In addition to the external causes outlined above, body odor is magnified by the discharge from the body of putrifying animal foods, such as red meat and dairy products, that are decaying in the tissues. The skin is a major organ of elimination, excreting toxins from the kidneys, liver, lymph, and blood. When the blood-cleansing abilities of the kidneys and liver are exceeded by a diet that is rich in animal foods and sugar, the skin compensates by eliminating as much as possible the toxic substances that wind up in the blood, lymph, and tissues. Odor is caused by many of these products, especially since they decay and putrify rapidly inside the body.

REMEDIES

General Recommendation

Avoid antiperspirants. They contain aluminum and other questionable substances that may lead to far more serious disorders than body odor. Also, they prevent the body from eliminating waste in a normal, healthy manner.

Foods to Eat

- Vegetarian diet with no dairy products

Foods to Avoid

- Animal fats, including red meat, dairy products, eggs, and chicken
- Hydrogenated fats
- Sugar

Hydrotherapy

- Loofah brush the skin thoroughly while showering to help eliminate waste more rapidly through the skin.
- Epsom salts baths are useful for body odor due either to internal or external causes. Put 1–1½ lb. of Epsom salts into a hot tub and soak for fifteen to twenty minutes. Finish with a cold spray. Repeat daily the first week, then reduce to two to three times per week until the body odor is normal.
- Salt glow: Mix 1 lb. fine salt in enough water to make a slurry. Begin with a warm shower, then turn water off, and rub salt all over the body firmly. Finish with a cold shower. Your skin will "glow" for hours.
- Alternate hot and cold showers daily to maintain proper skin function.

Supplements

- Zinc (blood purifier): 30–50 mg, 2 or 3 times per day
- Chlorophyll (blood purifier): 2–4 tablets, 3 times a day
- Essential fatty acids (blood purifier): 4 capsules, 3 times a day
- Lecithin: 2–3 tablespoons granules, 1 or 2 times per day; or 2–4 capsules, 2 or 3 times per day

BREAST CANCER

SYMPTOMS

The most common site of a malignant breast tumor is the upper, outer part of the breast. Usually, the lump is not painful. A dark discharge frequently occurs from the nipple. The nipples can retract and frequently a dimple appears over the area of the lump. In 90 percent of the cases, only one breast is affected.

WHAT IS BREAST CANCER?

From Modern Western Medicine

Current theories on the cause of breast cancer include hormones—the incidence is higher in women who had early menstrual periods and late menopause—and diet. The disease is rare in Japan, which has a low-fat diet, but Japanese women living in the United States and eating an American diet have the same rate of breast cancer as American women. Tall, heavy women have more breast cancer than short, thin ones. Breast cancer may also be more common among women who have previously had nonmalignant cysts and tumors removed from their breasts. There is no agreement on the part played by oral birth control pills in this disease.

From Traditional Medicine

Breast cancer is due primarily to imbalances of the intestines and spleen. Intestinal health is crucial to healthy breast tissue. When constipation or diarrhea occurs, lymph vessels in the intestinal tract absorb more waste and send it up toward the shoulders, behind the clavicle bones, where two expelling lymph ducts excrete the lymph into the bloodstream to be cleansed by the liver. (These are the only lymph nodes that release lymph into the bloodstream to be cleansed by the liver in the entire body.) Along the way to those nodes, the lymph becomes stagnant in the breast tissue, where it can contribute to the environment for breast disease and cancer.

Second, breast cancer is an estrogen-dependent disease. Elevations in estrogen occur when a high-fat diet is consumed (explained above). Finally, the stomach and spleen meridians run through the breast and down to the feet, bringing qi to the breast tissue. When the stomach and spleen are weakened, breast tissue is deprived of qi, which contributes to stagnation and the likelihood of disease.

Breast Cancer

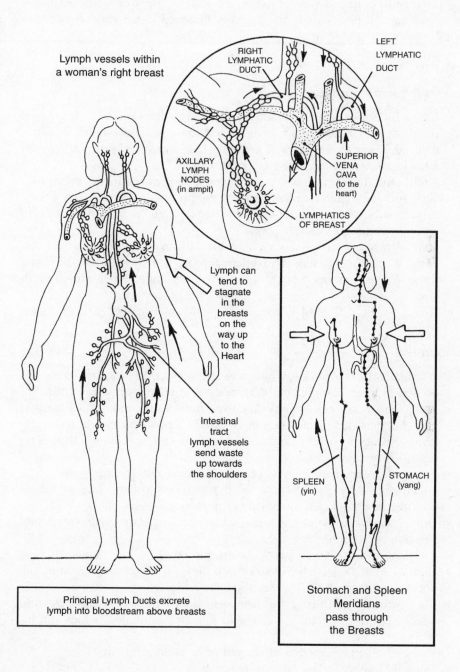

Lymph vessels within a woman's right breast

RIGHT LYMPHATIC DUCT

LEFT LYMPHATIC DUCT

AXILLARY LYMPH NODES (in armpit)

SUPERIOR VENA CAVA (to the heart)

LYMPHATICS OF BREAST

Lymph can tend to stagnate in the breasts on the way up to the Heart

Intestinal tract lymph vessels send waste up towards the shoulders

SPLEEN (yin)

STOMACH (yang)

Principal Lymph Ducts excrete lymph into bloodstream above breasts

Stomach and Spleen Meridians pass through the Breasts

WHO GETS BREAST CANCER?

This is the most common type of cancer in women: one in every nine develops breast cancer. Fewer than one in every hundred breast cancers occur in men.

REMEDIES

General Recommendations

- Increase fiber. Studies have shown that breast disease is associated with poor intestinal health, constipation, and low-fiber diets. Fiber also dramatically reduces the level of estrogen in a woman's body. Estrogen is a leading factor in the cause of breast cancer.
- Avoid saturated fat found in animal foods, such as red meat, dairy products, and eggs. High-fat diets promote the production of estrogen. Breast cancer is an estrogen-dependent disease, and is prevalent among women with high estrogen levels.
- Mild aerobic exercise is associated with a lower incidence of breast disease. Walking, bicycling, and other aerobic activities should be done three to five days per week, for at least thirty minutes per exercise session.
- Avoid alcohol. Alcohol is associated with an increased risk of breast cancer.

Foods to Eat

- Whole grains: brown rice, whole wheat, millet, corn, oats, and barley are all rich in fiber, complex carbohydrates, and vitamins and minerals.
- Miso soup promotes healthy intestinal flora and strengthens digestion and elimination. It is also rich in genistein, a powerful cancer-fighter.
- Root vegetables such as burdock, carrots, daikon, and jinenjo should be eaten every day.
- Eat round vegetables such as cabbage, onions, and squash.
- Green vegetables, especially broccoli, watercress, collard, kale, and mustard greens are all rich in anticancer nutrients.
- Dried daikon and daikon leaves, pickled with rice bran, help clean fatty substances from the blood.
- Eat small beans such as adzuki beans and lentils.
- High oleic-rich oil, such as extra virgin olive oil or unrefined sesame oil, not heated above 240°F: 1 teaspoon/day
- Chopped scallions mixed and heated with an equal volume of miso and a small portion of grated ginger help to soften hardened tissues and tumors.
- Flaxseed: 3–4 tablespoons of soaked or crushed seeds/day
- Liquid chlorophyll: 2–4 ounces, twice daily

Foods to Avoid

- All animal products, including fish
- Nuts and nut butters
- Sweets, desserts, fruit, and fruit juices
- Alcohol
- Dairy products
- Oily food
- Potatoes, yams, sweet potatoes, asparagus, tomatoes, and eggplant, because they are extremely mucus producing
- Spices and stimulants (such as coffee) because they enhance tumor growth

Exercise

- Aerobic exercise, such as walking, five times per week
- Yoga or some form of stretching exercise

Herbs to Treat Breast Cancer

- Kelp and other seaweeds (traditional Chinese medicine)
- Dandelion root is a possible preventive for breast cancer. Take a standard decoction of 3–9 g or a tincture, 10–30 drops.
- Chaparral tablets: 2 tablets, 4 times a day
- Sassafras, red clover, chickweed, and burdock tea are good teas to cleanse the blood.
- Combine clay and macerated cabbage leaves and mix together with powdered flaxseed and water. Make a thick paste, add a pinch of cayenne, and spread on a linen and apply. Leave on for a few hours.
- The Red Clover Combination carried by Nature's Way products is similar to Hoxey's formula. Take 4 tablets, 4 times a day.

Hydrotherapy

Use an albi plaster made from taro. Apply it over the affected area of the breast. It dissolves hardened tumors and lymphatic swellings, especially in breast cancer. (See Part III for instructions on how to make an albi plaster.) This will draw out poisonous waste that is stored in the cells and shrink the tumor, cancer, or swelling. The plaster should be changed every four hours, though it may be left on overnight. After this time, the poultice becomes saturated with poisons and often will turn black.

Grate taro (found in Oriental grocery stores or in powdered form in some health food stores). Add $1/10$ part grated fresh gingerroot and $1/5$ part flour. If albi cannot be found, regular potatoes can be used but are not as effective.

Homeopathy

- Pipsissewa tincture: 2–15 drops in water, as required
- Silica: (Hepar sulphuris calcareum 4X should be used first to encourage the elimination of pus.) Silica will promote the healing process. Take 5 tablets of 12X, 5 times daily.

Chinese Medicine

In Chinese medicine, foods and their preparation are matched to the condition and constitution of the individual. The traditional approach is to build up the system so that it can naturally overcome the cancer. Several regenerative diets are recommended, depending on the type of person.

- *Diet I:* Primarily grains, vegetables, seaweeds, legumes, sprouts, herbs, microalgae, omega-3 and GLA foods and oils. Most food is cooked. Whole fruits are taken but not their juice. White fish may be eaten if there is weakness. This diet reduces the toxic excess and is applicable for those who are weak, frail, anemic, cold, and deficient.
- *Diet II:* Fruits and vegetables and their juices, wheat grass juice, seaweeds, and the sprouts of seeds, grains, and legumes; also includes omega-3/GLA foods and oils and appropriate microalgae, spices, and herbs that eliminate toxins and enhance immunity. Cooked grain is eaten once a day, in addition to lightly cooked vegetables and sprouts. One ounce of wheat grass juice, three times a day. This diet is a quicker discharge diet and is appropriate for those who are strong, have strong pulses, and no signs of coldness (chills, aversion to cold, pallor, and great attraction to warmth).
- *Diet III:* Same as Diet II, except for the following: all grains are sprouted and all foods are raw except for a daily vegetable soup; purgative, highly cleansing herbs and frequent enemas are also given. Wheat grass: 2 ounces of juice, three times a day. This diet reduces stress and toxins very rapidly and is most appropriate for the strong individual who exhibits excess signs such as a thick tongue coating; loud voice, strong pulses, extroverted personality, and who also may have signs of heat such as aversion to cold; red face; great thirst; deep, red tongue; and/or yellow tongue coating.
- Acupuncture, especially for the large intestine, spleen, and liver
- Moxabustion

Mind/Body

- Daily meditation
- Join a support group. Breast cancer patients who participate in support groups live longer and have stronger immune responses than those who go it alone.
- Become a fighter. Do not accept negative pronouncements from your doctor, friends, or family. Make all medical decisions yourself after reviewing the evidence and talking openly and completely with your doctor.
- Get psychological and emotional support from a therapist or counselor.

BRONCHITIS

SYMPTOMS

Acute bronchitis causes slight fever, cough (dry or productive), mucopurulent secretions, flulike symptoms, chest pain, and reduced respiratory excursion.

Chronic bronchitis results in cough, sputum, difficulty in breathing, wheezing, asthmatic episodes, recurrences of pulmonary infection, respiratory failure, and exhaustion.

WHAT IS BRONCHITIS?

From Modern Western Medicine

Inflammation of the bronchial passages, the airways that connect the trachea to the lungs, results in a chronic cough and, very often, significant amounts of phlegm. Bronchitis can manifest in one of two forms: acute, which is the sudden onset of the illness, and which usually has a short duration; and chronic, or the persistent form of the disease that can recur over many years.

Viral infection usually causes acute bronchitis, though air pollution can also trigger the onset of the illness. Symptoms may be relieved by humidifying the lungs (through humidifier or inhaling steam) and drinking plenty of fluids.

Chronic bronchitis is defined as a cough, and the expectoration of phlegm can last as long as three consecutive months and can recur during two consecutive years. Chronic bronchitis can result in significant narrowing of the bronchial passages, causing obstruction of the airways to the lungs. Smoking is often the main cause of chronic bronchitis. The disease often coexists with emphysema.

From Traditional Medicine

Virtually all lung conditions are caused by repeated suppression of the common cold through the use of antibiotics and other forms of medication. The common cold is a normal and healthful form of cleansing of the body, and should be allowed to run its course. (See the chapter on the common cold.) Cough is one of the mechanisms by which the body eliminates mucus, airborne pollutants, and other waste products from the lungs. Thus, the bronchitis cough is a natural mechanism for cleansing the lungs, though, like the common cold, it is usually suppressed, which only makes it more chronic. Traditional forms of medicine maintain that the main causes of bronchitis are poor diet, especially excess sugar, lack of exercise (which prevents adequate movement of lymph), and the accumulation of toxins in the lungs and bronchial passages that irritate the tissues and cause inflammation.

WHO GETS BRONCHITIS?

Acute bronchitis attacks occur most often in winter, most commonly among the elderly, smokers, infants, and those who suffer from lung disease. Most of those who are afflicted with chronic bronchitis are men over the age of forty; most of these people are smokers or live in industrial cities, where they breathe highly polluted air.

REMEDIES

Foods to Eat

- Two servings daily of leafy green vegetables, especially mustard greens, watercress, kale, and collard greens
- Use gingerroot as a condiment on vegetables twice a week. (Do not overuse ginger.)
- White vegetables, such as daikon radish, turnips, and radishes (all considered traditional herbs for the lungs)

Foods to Avoid

- Refined white sugar and foods containing sugar and other artificial ingredients
- Dairy products, which weaken the lungs
- Spicy foods, such as hot peppers
- Acidic foods, such as spices, peppers, and tomatoes
- Raw foods, especially salads, which irritate the lungs and exacerbate the condition

Chinese Medicine

Bronchitis can be a result of any of the following lung conditions:

Heat congesting the lungs irritates the tissues and creates inflammation and warm phlegm. To treat, cool the heat and reduce irritation and inflammation.

- Prepare much of the diet in the form of soups.
- Eat whole grains such as millet, barley, and rice.
- Eat leafy greens, especially watercress, cabbage, and bok choy.
- Eat peaches, pears, strawberries, and citrus fruits.
- Eat seaweeds.
- Eat root vegetables, especially daikon, carrot, and pumpkin.

Phlegm in the lungs (If tongue coating is white, the phlegm is cold. If tongue is yellow, the phlegm is hot.):

- Foods that digest easily such as vegetables, fruits, sprouts, grains, beans, and almonds (small amounts)

- Watercress (cooling, for hot phlegm)
- Onions (warming, for cool phlegm)
- Turnips (neutral, for both conditions)
- Daikon radish (cooling, for hot phlegm)
- Seaweeds (cooling, for hot phlegm)

Deficient yin of the lungs (resulting from chronic lung infection, inflammation, or long-term lung disease—suggests kidney yin deficiency):

- Seaweed
- Spirulina and chlorella microalgae
- Fruits such as orange, peach, pear, apple, watermelon, and banana
- Tofu, tempeh, and soy milk
- String beans
- Rice syrup

Deficient qi of the lungs (results from long-term lung diseases, particularly those with heat signs—treatment is to tonify lung qi and improve absorption of food qi):

- Mostly cooked food
- Whole grains, especially brown rice, sweet rice, and oats
- Carrots
- Mustard greens
- Sweet potato, yam, and potato

Foods to Avoid

Chinese medicine states that the following foods either cause bronchitis or exacerbate its symptoms.

Heat congesting the lungs:

- Coffee
- Alcohol
- Animal products
- Warming fish such as trout, salmon, and anchovy
- Onion family (especially garlic)
- Ginger

Phlegm in the lungs:

- Dairy products
- Meat and poultry
- Tofu and tempeh
- Soy products such as miso and soy sauce
- Sweeteners

Deficient yin of the lungs:

- Warming foods and spices
- Bitter flavors

Deficient qi of the lungs:

- Citrus fruits
- Salt
- Dairy products
- Cereal grass products
- Seaweeds and microalgae (chlorella is okay)

Herbs to Treat Bronchitis

- Yerba santa (stimulates digestive juices and good for all types of bronchitis): Use as a tea. Steep thirty minutes, 2–3 oz., 3 times/day
- Lotus root tea or kuzu bancha tea with ginger (macrobiotic remedy for yin-type person): 3–4 times per day
- Squill (expectorant for dry cough): Tincture, 5–20 drops, 2 or 3 times per day
- Flaxseed: Decoction, 2 ounces of dried herb, 3 times per day (for hot phlegm)
- Gingerroot: Grated into cooking (for cold phlegm)
- Slippery elm bark (for yin lung deficiency): Make into a gruel by mixing powder with small amount of water. Sweeten with honey and take a tablespoonful. Teabags can also be purchased. Especially good with a little licorice.
- Elecampane (for deficient qi of lungs): 3–9 g
- Lobelia (respiratory relaxant and stimulates catarrhal secretion and expectorant): tincture, 10–15 drops, 2–4 four times/day

Homeopathy

- Ipecac (for violent, spasmodic cough): 5–15 drops tincture, 2–3 times/day
- Belladonna (for short, dry cough that is worse at night): 2 tablets, 3–5 times a day
- Pulsatilla (for a gagging cough that is dry in evening, loose in morning, and for which you must sit up in bed for relief): 2 tablets, 3–5 times a day or as directed

Physiotherapy

Add pine needles, olbas oil, eucalyptus, and elecampane to boiling water. Either the herb or oil form is okay. Make a tent covering yourself and the pot and inhale the vapors.

Supplements

- Vitamin A (excellent for lungs): 2000–20,000 IU, 2–3 times per day
- Vitamin B complex: 25–50 mg, 3 times/day
- Vitamin C: 1000 mg, 1–3 times per day

BURNS

SYMPTOMS

Damaged tissue and mucous membranes after being exposed to excessive heat, toxic chemicals, or radiation (including the sun).

WHAT IS A BURN?

From Modern Western Medicine and Traditional Medicine

Burns are classified as *first-degree, second-degree,* and *third-degree.* A first-degree burn involves the outer layer of skin, the epidermis, causing the skin to become red, tender, swollen, and sometimes feverish. The skin may blister, depending on the treatment. The more severe second-degree burn causes deeper layers of the skin to be damaged, including the dermis, with all the same symptoms as a first-degree burn, though worse. Third-degree burns affect the epidermis, dermis, subcutaneous tissues and, in severe cases, the underlying muscle. Some second-degree and all third-degree burns require special treatment to prevent scarring.

WHO GETS BURNED?

Each year, 2 million Americans are burned or scalded sufficiently to require medical treatment, with about 70,000 hospitalized. Burns are most common in children and the elderly. Most are due to preventable accidents.

REMEDIES

Foods to Eat

- Wheat or other cereal grasses

Foods to Avoid

- Animal protein (directly related to infections)

Herbs to Treat Burns

- Aloe: Apply the gelatinous inner contents of the leaves to sunburn and other minor burns.
- Aloe gel and propolis: This combines the soothing and anti-inflammatory effect of aloe with the antibiotic effects of propolis.
- Comfrey poultice: Steep comfrey leaves or boil root and apply to burn as a continuous compress.

Homeopathy

- Arnica: Used internally for shock
- Causticum: Take internally for severe cases where there is pain, restlessness, and blister formation. Removes pain in 7–10 minutes.
- Urtica urens (external remedy): ½ teaspoon of tincture in 1 cup of clean water; pat on with sterile gauze or apply compress with urtica urens lotion.
- Calendula lotion
- Hypericum lotion

Hydrotherapy

Immerse the area in cold water immediately until there is no pain. This will prevent blister formation with first-degree burns and minimize tissue damage in more severe burns. If you must go to the hospital, keep area soaking or else wrap in wet sheets and apply water at frequent intervals.

Chinese Medicine

- Wheat or other cereal grass juice applied externally
- Buckwheat flour mixed with vinegar: Make a poultice.
- Carrot juice: Apply directly.
- Cucumber and cucumber juice applied directly are especially good for sunburn.
- Squash juice: Apply directly.

Supplements

EXTERNALLY

- Vitamin E oil: Apply oil externally after soaking in water.
- Vitamin C spray: Spray on 1–3 percent solution every 2 to 4 hours, between vitamin E applications.

INTERNALLY

- Vitamin E: 400 mg per day
- Vitamin C: 80 mg daily
- Vitamin A: 400 IU a day for 2–4 weeks
- Vitamin B complex: 50 mg per day
- Zinc: 15 mg per day

BURSITIS

SYMPTOMS

Pain, tenderness, reduced mobility, swelling, redness, possible fever, and muscle weakness often in the shoulders, elbows, and knees.

WHAT IS BURSITIS?

From Modern Western Medicine

Bursitis is inflammation of a bursa, small fluid-filled sacs that act as shock absorbers between joints and at the sites where muscles and tendons join. The swollen bursa rubs against tendons and muscles, causing friction, pain, and additional swelling. Rest usually causes the pain to subside within a few days, as the excess fluid is reabsorbed into the bloodstream. Bursitis is frequently caused by trauma, such as a blow to the area; repeated shock; and overuse.

From Traditional Medicine

Traditional medicine recognizes trauma as a secondary cause of bursitis. Trauma, excessive use, or a blow does not have to result in bursitis if the underlying qi, nutrition, and flexibility are healthy. The liver is said to provide qi to the tendons and joints and thus is considered part of the diagnostic picture. Bursitis, therefore, occurs more commonly in people who have stagnation in the joints and liver imbalances.

REMEDIES

Foods to Eat

- Root vegetables, especially carrots, turnips, ginger, and rutabagas (for their immune-boosting properties and because these roots have a strengthening and tonifying effect on the body's ability to eliminate waste)
- Leafy, green vegetables (for their immune-boosting properties)
- Carrot juice (for liver)

Foods to Avoid

- Nightshades: potatoes, tomatoes, peppers, eggplant, and tobacco
- Vitamin D–fortified foods, such as milk and other dairy products, breakfast cereals, and margarine
- Potato flour as found in processed foods
- Paprika, cayenne, and Tabasco

Herbs to Treat Bursitis

- Comfrey: Use as a strong infusion, decoction, or tincture, 2 or 3 times daily for 1 to 3 months.
- Burdock root: 1 oz. root to 1½ pints water, boiled down to 1 pint, 3 or 4 times a day; or as a tincture (30–60 drops, 3 or 4 times daily)
- Chaparral: Steep 6 oz., 5–15 minutes, 3 times daily; or as tincture, 10–20 drops, 3 times daily; or as powder, 2–10 capsules (0 # capsules, 10–60 grains), 3 times a day

Chinese Medicine

- Acupuncture
- Acupressure: A therapist uses the hands in place of needles to stimulate points and deeply massage tissues.

Homeopathy

Use bryony for pain with motion. Dose: tincture, 5 drops, 2 or 3 times per day, or use as homeopathic dilution.

Hydrotherapy

- Apply an ice pack to the troubled joint to reduce swelling. Leave it on for ten minutes, several times a day.
- After swelling has disappeared, apply hot towels. Heat will increase circulation.
- Ginger bath: Make a bath full of hot water with one-third being ginger tea. Smaller quantities may be made to soak the affected part.

Supplements

- Vitamin A: 400 IU per day
- Vitamin B complex: 50 mg per day
- Vitamin B_{12}: 2–10 mcg, 1 time a week
- Vitamin C: 100 mg per day
- Vitamin E: 400 IU 2 times a day

Exercises

- Touch your elbows. Clasp your hands behind your head. Bring your elbows together in front of your face, as close as possible to one another. Then separate them as widely as you can. Repeat, gradually working up to ten repetitions. Do not try to do ten repetitions on the first few attempts, especially if pain is severe.
- Reach out. Stretch one arm straight out in front of you. Lock your elbow, and raise your arm directly over your head so that your fingers are pointing toward the ceiling. Lower the arm. Do five to ten repetitions for each arm.

- Rotate your arms. Stretch one arm out from your side so that it is parallel to the floor. Now rotate that arm in small circles forward, then in reverse. Work your way up from five to ten circles, then twenty, in both directions. Repeat with the other arm.
- Reach for the stars. Raise your arms above and behind your head as far as possible. Do not force them; just try to gradually improve the distance you can reach backward. Do five, ten, and then twenty repetitions.
- Roll your shoulders. Raise shoulders toward your ears. Then roll them back so your chest sticks out. Next, roll them down, then forward, and up. Work your way up from five repetitions to ten, then twenty.
- Do shoulder touches. Extend one arm directly out at your side, parallel to the floor. Touch your shoulder with your hand by bending at the elbow and bringing your hand back to the top of your shoulder. Work your way up from five repetitions to ten, then twenty. Repeat with the other arm.
- Lift your leg. While lying on a firm mat or on a bed, lift one leg, knee bent, and bring it toward your chest. You can use your hands to grab hold below your thigh. Do five, ten, or twenty repetitions per leg.
- Yoga

Other

- Peanut oil massage to entire area
- Green cabbage leaf poultice; apply nightly

CANCER

SYMPTOMS

The symptoms produced by cancers depend on the site of the tumor and the extent of its development. Any of the following are common: a lump, skin changes, weight loss, a sore that fails to heal, a blemish that enlarges, severe headaches, difficulty swallowing, persistent hoarseness, coughing up blood, persistent abdominal pain, change in shape or size of testes, blood in urine, change in bowel habits, change in breast shape, bleeding or discharge from nipple, or vaginal bleeding between periods.

WHAT IS CANCER?

From Modern Western Medicine

Cancer, the second most common cause of death in the United States, is a group of disease states that arise when cells reproduce without restraint and without regard for the whole body. Malignant tumors occur most commonly in major organs, such as the lungs, breasts, intestines, skin, stomach, pancreas, or bones, as well as in smaller sites, such as the nasal sinuses, the testes, ovaries, or the lips or tongue. Cancer also develops in the blood and lymph system. Surgery is the most common form of treatment, often in combination with radiation therapy and anticancer drugs (chemotherapy). Surgery, of course, is performed to remove the cancer cells or diseased organ, while radiation and chemotherapy are intended to destroy the cancer cells and arrest its development.

From Traditional Medicine

Cancer is the end result of a long-term process of degeneration. Long before a collection of cancer cells arise, the body has suffered from poor circulation of blood, lymph, and qi in that particular location. Blood brings oxygen to cells. When blood flow to cells is reduced or blocked, cells die or become deformed, sometimes becoming cancerous. When lymph is blocked, waste accumulates in the areas and contributes to the likelihood of disease. Qi is life force; without adequate qi, cells degenerate and become diseased.

The stagnation in that site has arisen out of multiple reasons that involve body, mind, and spirit. Physical influences, such as unhealthful foods, chemicals (such as pesticides and additives), lack of exercise, and physical inflexibility—especially in that part of the body—has caused poor circulation. As for the mental aspects, certain types of thoughts and fears have created muscle tension and thus contributed to the lack of circulation. Emotionally, grief and old resentments that were never resolved exist as unhealed wounds in the psyche. These emotions, and the experiences and relationships that gave rise to them, form a kind of ongoing pain that never fully heals or goes away. Like a part of us that cannot be integrated into our being or put to rest, such feelings serve as antagonists to our general sense of well-being, our immune system, and the body's detoxifying functions. Finally, cancer is related to a deeper existential feat that arises from the spirit and, specifically, out of feelings of being disconnected from others and from the universe at large. When these debilitating behaviors, thoughts, fears, and beliefs are maintained over time, they form the foundation for the illnesses known as cancer.

On the other hand, such an awareness provides the insight and guidance for treatment. The disease must be dealt with from the body/mind/spirit perspective, specifically to increase qi, blood, and lymph flow to the overall body and especially to the site of the tumor.

WHO GETS CANCER?

Cancer has affected humans since prehistoric times and is also common in domestic and farm animals, birds, and fish. Apart from childhood cancers, which may be associated with events during pregnancy, such as exposure to radiation, most cancers are a feature of aging.

REMEDIES

General Recommendations

- Eat a diet composed of whole grains, vegetables, beans, green foods, and sea vegetables.
- Eat foods and herbs that have specific anticancer properties.
- Exercise daily. Include yoga or some other meditative exercise.
- Undergo some type of energy therapy, such as acupuncture and/or the laying on of hands to promote qi flow throughout the body.
- Do whatever therapy appeals to you that will make you confront and put old emotional wounds, sadness, and unresolved conflicts to rest.
- Pray, meditate, and adopt behaviors that promote a sense of connection to the universe at large, to your sense of God, or Tao, or Great Spirit.

Foods to Eat

The choices of food and amount of cooking depend on the type of cancer and the condition of the individual. The following general recommendations will cause a slow release of toxins and can be used by anyone.

- Whole grains
- Vegetables, especially those rich in antioxidants and anticancer nutrients (See the section on nutrition in Part III for anticancer foods.)

- Seaweeds (immune-boosting and anticancer)
- Beans (anticancer)
- Sprouts (anticancer)
- Microalgae such as spirulina, chlorella, and blue-green algae (immune-boosting and anticancer)
- Flaxseed (antitumor, antiestrogenic, and antioxidant)
- Reishi and shiitake mushrooms (immune-boosting and anticancer): one mushroom per day
- Onions and garlic (immune-boosting and anticancer)
- Cruciferous vegetables such as cabbage, kale, and broccoli (immune-boosting and anticancer)
- White fish, when desired

Foods to Avoid

- Red meat
- Poultry
- Eggs
- Dairy products
- Processed or chemicalized foods
- Alcohol
- Caffeinated beverages
- Hydrogenated vegetable oils, such as margarine, shortening, or soy margarine
- Salty foods

Exercise

- Perform some aerobic exercise at least five times per week. Do not exhaust yourself. Walking is ample, but any exercise that promotes circulation and is enjoyed will be of benefit.
- Yoga, especially stretching areas of the body that are tight and inflexible

Herbs to Treat Cancer

Mix equal parts of chaparrel, bloodroot, red clover, echinacea, dandelion root, violet leaves, santicle, buckthorn bark, burdock root, ginger, and licorice root. Take two capsules four to six times a day.

Chinese Medicine

See the section on breast cancer for dietary recommendations for cancer.

Chinese medicine regards cancer as stagnation of blood, lymph, and qi. These three are the basis for health. All three must be restored to the body at large and, specifically, to the affected area for health to be reestablished.

Tissue oxygen is maximized by moderate exercise; living in a clean environment; eating freshly prepared, lightly cooked whole grains and vegetables;

eating small amounts of raw vegetables; and emphasizing chlorophyll-rich foods.

Acupuncture and an energetic exercise, such as tai chi chuan also help combat cancer.

Mind/Body

- Perform positive imaging routines daily.
- Meditate or pray.
- Identify places of tension in the body, particularly in the area of the cancer, and release the tension and emotions related to that area.

Supplements

The use of supplements in the treatment of cancer is very controversial. Many experts believe that supplements stress the liver excessively and may impair its detoxifying function; others wonder if supplements weaken immune function, especially in light of the recent report in the *American Journal of Clinical Nutrition* (62; supplement, 1995: S1427–S1430, and previously reported in *The New England Journal of Medicine*) showing that supplements of beta-carotene and vitamin E were associated with higher levels of cancer than in those cases in which people were getting beta-carotene and vitamin E from the diet alone.

The evidence suggests that supplements may be inappropriate for cancer patients and that the best way to get your vitamins and minerals is through food.

Canker Sores

SYMPTOMS

An ulcer appears in the mouth that is oval with a gray center and a surrounding red, inflamed halo. The ulcer usually lasts for one to two weeks.

WHAT IS A CANKER SORE?

From Modern Western Medicine

A small, painful sore or ulcer that appears in the mouth, on the inside of the cheek or lip or underneath the tongue. The ulcer, which usually disappears without treatment, may arise from hemolytic streptococcus bacteria, an organism that frequently appears with canker sores. Other possible causes include trauma to tissues (such as from a toothbrush or dental injection), acute stress, and allergies. They are common in women during the premenstrual period. Topical ointments may relieve the pain.

From Traditional Medicine

Sores arise as a discharge of waste that is not being cleansed by the liver and kidneys. Canker sores, therefore, indicate a depressed liver and kidney function. Treatment consists of strengthening both of these organs so that blood can be more efficiently cleansed and detoxified.

WHO GETS CANKER SORES?

Minor canker sores affect about 20 percent of the population at any given time. They are most common between the ages of ten and forty and affect women more than men. The most severely affected people have continuously recurring ulcers; others have just one or two ulcers per year.

REMEDIES

- See Part IV for methods of strengthening liver and kidneys, especially if canker sores appear chronically.

Foods to Eat

Eat foods that are easy to digest:

- Do a one- to three-day carrot-juice fast.
- Wheatgrass juice or liquid chlorophyll; drink two ounces three times a day

- Soft grains, well cooked
- Lightly cooked vegetables

Foods to Avoid

- Dairy products
- Oily foods
- Sweets such as cakes, candies, and raw fruit
- Salty foods
- Animal protein
- Less liquid

Herbs to Treat Canker Sores

- Bayberry tincture: 15–30 drops as needed. Fluid extract: ½–1 tsp. as needed. Decoction: simmer 10–15 minutes; 1 tbsp.
- Burdock: A great blood cleanser that clears kidneys of excess waste. Tincture: 30–60 drops three to four times per day. Fluid extract: ½–1 tsp. three to four times per day. Decoction: 1 oz. root to 1½ pints water, boiled down to 1 pint; 3 oz. three to four times per day. Infusion: 1 cup three to four times per day
- Goldenseal tincture: 20–90 drops three times per day. Fluid extract: ¼–½ tsp. three times per day. Infusion: steep powder until cold; 1–2 tsp. three to six times daily. Decoction: simmer 15–30 minutes; 1–2 tsp. three to six times per day
- Lobelia tincture: apply several times a day.

Hydrotherapy

- Goldenseal and myrrh: make an herb tea and gargle four to five times per day.
- Rosemary, thyme, or juniper berry oils: three drops to one cup of warm water, gargle.
- Wheatgrass juice or liquid chlorophyll: gargle.
- Black Tea: at the first inkling of a sore, apply a wet black tea bag to the ulcer; the tannin is an astringent with pain-relieving ability.

CATARACTS

SYMPTOMS

Cataracts cause an opaque blurring of vision. The condition is painless, and the onset is virtually imperceptible until vision is obscured. The person will have progressive loss of visual acuity with increased blurring.

WHAT ARE CATARACTS?

From Modern Western Medicine

Cataracts cause the lens of the eye to cloud and become hard, thus preventing adequate light from passing through the lens and interacting with the optic nerve. With time, vision becomes hazy and blurred, although complete blindness usually does not occur because the cataract does allow some light to penetrate the lens. Cataracts occur most frequently in the elderly. The disorder usually affects one eye more than the other, though both are often affected. The cause is unknown.

Treatment most often involves the surgical removal of the opaque lens and replacing it with a clear, artificial substitute. In some cases, laser surgery is used to dissolve the cataract from the lens, thus creating a hole in the lens through which light can pass.

From Traditional Medicine

The traditional approaches to cataracts emphasize prevention, rather than treatment. Alternative therapies for cataracts are not well proven, and both within and outside the medical profession, many charlatans exist who attempt to take advantage of those seeking alternatives to cataract surgery. However, it is now understood that cataracts arise among populations that subsist on a high-fat, high-protein diet, with low levels of beta-carotene and vitamin C. It is also well documented that cataracts arise from free radical formation (see the section on nutrition in Part IV); therefore, a diet rich in antioxidants protects against free radicals and the formation of cataracts. Finally, people with diabetes should make significant changes in their diet and lifestyle to protect against the loss of sight and the onset of cataracts. (See the section on diabetes.)

WHO GETS CATARACTS?

People over the age of sixty-five are most at risk. Opacification is usually minor among most elderly people and does not interfere with vision. Cataracts are considered almost normal among the elderly living in the Western world, but the condition is rare among the elderly living in traditional cultures that subsist on diets rich in grains, vegetables, and fruits.

REMEDIES

Foods to Eat

The following foods will help cleanse the body—especially the liver—of toxins. They will also encourage elimination and boost antioxidants.

- Vegetable juices (No two different juices are to be taken at one meal.)
- Whole grains
- Vegetables rich in beta-carotene such as carrots, winter squash, pumpkin, cantaloupe, apricots, collard greens, kale, and broccoli
- Vegetables and fruits rich in vitamin C
- Shiitake mushrooms

Foods to Avoid

- Animal protein, except fish
- Dairy products
- Tea
- Coffee
- Sugar
- Alcohol
- Cigarettes

Chinese Medicine

The liver meridian runs through the eyes and provides the organs with qi. Thus, the condition of the liver is reflected in the eyes. When the liver is stagnant, the eyes become inflamed and taken out of focus by the muscles that control visual acuity. The foods suggested in the list of foods to eat will stimulate, open, and remove stagnation from the liver. Eating moderate amounts of food and avoiding food late at night will also promote healing of the liver and gallbladder.

Physiotherapy

- Alternate hot and cold showers to stimulate circulation and proper hormone balance.
- Vision improvement exercises (See the section on eyes in Part IV for exercises to improve vision.)
- Local applications of cineraria maritima succus eyedrops (most tried-and-tested botanical application): 1 drop, 2 or 3 times/day

Supplements

- Beta-carotene: 20 mg per day
- Vitamin B complex: 50 mg per day
- Vitamin C: 100 mg per day
- Vitamin E: 60–400 IU, once a day

Cervical Dysplasia

SYMPTOMS

No obvious symptoms exist.

WHAT IS CERVICAL DYSPLASIA?

From Modern Western Medicine

Before any cancer appears, abnormal changes occur in cells on the surface of the cervix. These changes are referred to as varying degrees of dysplasia. The abnormal cells can be detected by a cervical smear test (Pap smear). Mild dysplasia may revert back to normal, but a woman with an abnormal cervical smear should undergo further tests, including other Pap smears. Severe dysplasia or early cancer can be treated and cured.

From Traditional Medicine

Abnormal Pap smears indicate stagnation and inadequate qi in the kidneys, bladder, and sex organs (the water element). Underlying factors that support the growth of abnormal cells or cancerous lesions may be dietary or psychological; they may indicate some form of trauma, such as one or more abortions or poorly conducted abortions or an excessive number of sex partners. They indicate a precancerous condition or the early stages of cancer, but can usually be reversed with natural therapy.

REMEDIES

Foods to Eat

- Whole grains
- Vegetables, mostly cooked, and small amounts of raw
- Beans
- Sea vegetables: Nori, wakame, kombu, and arame strengthen the water element, are mineral- and vitamin-rich, and boost immune response.
- Seeds
- Nuts
- Fish, once a week
- Carrot juice or other fresh vegetable juice combination, twice daily

Foods to Avoid

- Animal food
- Coffee

- Tea
- Sugar
- Salt
- Alcohol
- Unrefined, fried, or overcooked foods
- Foods high in fat

Exercise

- Aerobic exercise, such as walking, bicycling, swimming, or jogging, three to five times per week, for at least thirty minutes per session

Supplements

- Folic acid: 5–10 mg per day
- Beta-carotene: 20 mg per day
- Vitamin C: 100–500 mg per day

Hydrotherapy

Alternate hot and cold sitz baths are very useful if done two or three times daily to increase local circulation.

Mind/Body

The water element is associated with fear, according to the Chinese. Therefore, any disorder affecting kidneys, bladder, and sex organs suggests long-term stress, anxiety, and fear. Therefore, the following recommendations apply:

- Meditate, pray, chant, or do positive imaging exercises that promote faith and serve as an antidote to fear.
- Meditate on the tension in the pelvic region and try to discover the roots of that tension. This part of the body may be neglected by your consciousness. What is it trying to tell you? Try to satisfy the needs of your inner self who may be in fear.

CIRCULATION

SYMPTOMS

Poor circulation can manifest as cold fingers and toes, frequent bruising, infection, numbness in joints and digits, and pain. In the extreme, it can lead to claudication, gangrene, amputation, blindness, senility, heart attack, and stroke.

WHAT IS POOR CIRCULATION?

From Modern Western Medicine

Poor circulation—or insufficient blood to organs, tissues, and cells—can be caused from a high-fat, high-cholesterol diet, atherosclerosis, cigarette smoking, long periods of standing or sitting, lack of exercise, poor posture, diabetes mellitis, high blood pressure, prolonged muscle tension, injury, inflammation, and ill-fitting shoes or clothing. (See also chapters on Atherosclerosis, Blood Pressure, Diabetes, and Heart Disease.)

From Traditional Medicine

Poor circulation is caused by stagnant blood, and inadequate qi in the blood, heart, spleen, and muscles. The blood itself may be filled with toxins, such as fat and cholesterol, which prevent the blood from flowing adequately to cells via the tiny capillaries. According to the Chinese, all circulation is dependent upon a healthy spleen, which provides qi to the blood and its vessels. The spleen is also responsible for maintaining the blood in its courses; all internal bleeding and stagnation of blood is the result of a weak and overburdened spleen. Finally, the spleen maintains the elasticity of blood vessels, which sustain diastolic pressure throughout the system. Therefore, traditional Chinese medicine treats the spleen, as well as the heart, when healing all circulatory problems.

REMEDIES

General Recommendations

- See Part IV for remedies to heal the heart and spleen.
- Significantly reduce fat, cholesterol, and refined foods from the diet.
- Increase exercise.
- Maintain warmth.

Foods to Eat

These foods will increase circulation:

- Beets
- Buckwheat
- Citrus peel
- Rye
- Black soybeans
- Lentils
- Sardines
- Soybeans
- Pungent foods. These foods will move energy upward and outward to the periphery of the body. Warming pungents are more appropriate for people with cold conditions and may aggravate those who are already warm. Warming pungents include spearmint, rosemary, scallions, garlic, all onion family members, cloves, cinnamon bark and branch, fennel, anise, cayenne, dill, mustard greens, horseradish, basil, and nutmeg.

    Cooling pungents are more appropriate for warm conditions and may aggravate those who are already cold. They include peppermint, marjoram, elder flowers, white pepper, and radish. Neutral pungents are taro, turnip, and kohlrabi.

    Warm conditions are marked by aversion to heat, feeling hot, flushed face, bloodshot eyes, deep red tongue and possible yellow coating, and great thirst—can also include signs of deficient yin such as tidal fevers, hot palms and soles, fresh red cheeks and tongue, frequent light thirst and night sweats.

Foods to Avoid

- Cold foods
- Sweets
- Meat
- Dairy products
- Eggs
- Ice cream

Herbs to Treat Circulatory Problems

- Michael Tierra's Planetary Herbs Formula 42 (for yin, cold conditions) promotes circulation, digestion, and warms the whole body; dose is ⅛–¼ teaspoon, one to three times daily.
- Tree Peony promotes blood circulation and helps dissolve masses; dose is 6–12 gm per day.

- Goldenseal sustains circulation and is useful where extremities are cold and lips bluish. To strengthen weakened condition, take with 1 part each capsicum, skullcap to 1 part goldenseal. Dose is 10–30 grains powder; tincture: follow directions on bottle.

Chinese Medicine

See above, all of which is from Chinese medicine.

Supplements

- Vitamin E: 60–300 IU daily

Exercise

- Walk

See also

Claudication
Diabetes
Blood Pressure

COLD SORES

SYMPTOMS

A small skin blister occurs anywhere around the mouth. Usually several such blisters appear together in a cluster. An outbreak is often preceded by a tingling in the lips. The blisters are small at first but soon enlarge, causing itching, irritation, and soreness. Within a few days, they burst and become encrusted, and they usually disappear within a week.

WHAT IS A COLD SORE?

From Modern Western Medicine

The strain of the virus most often responsible for cold sores is called HSV1 (herpes simplex virus 1). The first attack may pass unnoticed or may cause an illness resembling influenza and painful ulcers in the mouth and on the lips—a condition called gingivostomatitis. Subsequently, the virus lies dormant in nerve cells, but in some people it is occasionally reactivated when the person is exposed to hot sunshine or a cold wind, has a cold or other infection, or is feeling run down. Women seem more likely to develop cold sores at the time of their periods, and some people are afflicted regularly throughout the year. No effective preventive treatment is available, although some people find that applying a lip salve before sun exposure does help prevent outbreaks. If cold sores are particularly troublesome, a physician may prescribe idoxuridine paint or the antiviral drug acyclovir to sooth them.

From Traditional Medicine

Cold sores arise from acid-rich blood, which itself is caused by a diet rich in acidic foods and spices. Acidic foods weaken the spleen, liver, and stomach. They also drain the body of minerals and weaken the immune system. Once the immune function is depressed, and the blood is richer in acid, the virus can take hold in the system. Stress also plays a role in the onset of the condition, especially since it contributes to acidity. The primary form of treatment, therefore, is to eat more alkalizing and mineral-rich foods, and reduce stress.

WHO GETS COLD SORES?

Most people—perhaps as many as 90 percent worldwide—are infected at some point during their lives.

REMEDIES

Foods to Eat

- Beta-carotene–rich foods, such as squash, carrots, collard greens, kale, mustard greens, and broccoli are all immune boosters.
- Mineral-rich foods, such as leafy greens, roots, and sea vegetables are immune boosters.
- Shiitake mushrooms are immune boosters, antiviral, and antifungal.
- Garlic is an immune booster, antiviral, and antifungal.
- Whole grains are rich in vitamin E, fiber, and complex carbohydrates.
- Miso soup is alkalizing, especially to digestion.

Foods to Avoid

- Red meat and other high-protein foods (Protein is converted to uric acid in the blood and increases the likelihood of infection.)
- Spices
- Tomatoes

Herbs to Treat Cold Sores

- Black Walnut: tincture, 10–20 drops, 3 times daily; fluid extract, 1–2 teaspoons, 3 or 4 times/day; infusion, 6 ounces, applied 1–4 times daily
- Goldenseal ointment applied topically; alternate with aloe vera.
- Goldenseal: tincture, 15–30 drops per cup of water, 2 times daily

Physiotherapy

Apply ice at first sign of tingling for 15–20 minutes; repeat frequently throughout the day. Apply vitamin E between applications.

Supplements

- Zinc ointment (topical)
- Beta-carotene, 15–20 mg per day
- Vitamin B complex, 50 mg, once daily
- Pantothenic acid, 250 mg per day
- Zinc, 15 mg, once per day

COLIC (INFANTILE)

SYMPTOMS

Abdominal pain, distention, restlessness, insomnia, and crying in infants are all signs of colic. Babies are said to be suffering from colic when they are crying (even screaming), irritable, and drawing up their legs, suggesting pain in the abdomen. The baby may be red in the face and may pass gas. Symptoms usually worsen at night.

WHAT IS INFANTILE COLIC?

From Modern Western Medicine

Infant colic usually begins around the third or fourth week of life and clears up spontaneously by the twelfth week. It is thought to be due to spasm in the intestines, although there is no proof of this, and the cause of the spasm is unknown.

From Traditional Medicine

Infant colic occurs when an infant's digestive system is not able to fully assimilate and eliminate the food being fed to the baby, whether it is mother's milk or formula. In the case of breast-fed babies, the mother's diet is the most important factor. (See foods to eat and avoid below.)

Formula-fed babies may be allergic to milk, wheat, soy, or sugar. In such cases, vitamin- and mineral-enriched goat's milk may be a better alternative. Carefully monitor all foods being fed to the baby or the foods consumed by the mother. After weaning, examine the foods being fed to the baby in the same way. Certain foods promote intestinal disorders more than others. (See below.)

WHO GETS COLIC?

Infantile colic is common, occurring in approximately one in ten babies.

REMEDIES

Foods to Eat

- Breast-feed whenever possible; mothers should monitor their diets.
- When breast-feeding is not possible, enriched goat's milk should be the choice.
- After weaning, introduce new foods one at a time.

For babies who have been weaned (after six months):

- Feed very wet (watery), soft grain that has been ground up and had the fiber removed by a food mill (such as the Fowley food mill).
- Sweet vegetable broths, such as carrots, squash, parsnips, and sweet potato, milled to be made soft
- Cooked fruit, milled to be soft

Foods to Avoid (for Baby and Mother)

- Cabbage
- Onions
- Garlic
- Wheat
- Yeast
- Brussels sprouts
- Broccoli
- Fried foods
- Refined foods, such as sugar, white flour products, and foods containing artificial colors, flavors, and preservatives
- Cow's milk and other dairy products
- Formula containing milk, wheat, soy, or sugar
- Wheat
- Harsh and hot spices
- Carbonated beverages

Herbs to Treat Colic

The best way to treat nursing babies with herbs is to treat the mother. Any herb consumed by the mother will go directly to her milk and on to the baby. The mother should drink the herb as a tea for rapid assimilation into her blood and breast milk.

Make a tea with a combination of equal parts chamomile, fennel, and lemon balm. If the mother is not nursing, a plastic eyedropper can be used to administer mild herbal tea. Squeeze a dropperful of the tea into the baby's mouth several times throughout the day.

Wild yam root (as an herbal tincture) works rapidly in acute infant colic. The dose is 7 to 14 drops of tincture in water every ½ hour for 1 to 2 hours.

Other

- Take the baby for a ride in the car.
- Place a warm washcloth on the baby's stomach.
- Place the baby on his or her stomach and rub his or her back.
- Rock the baby in a rocking chair.
- Carry your baby in a front sling.

COLITIS

SYMPTOMS

Ulcerative colitis causes attacks of bloody diarrhea, cramps, blood in stools, and mucus. Spastic colitis causes abdominal pain, abdominal distention, cramps, gas, constipation, diarrhea, but no blood in stools. In both cases, symptoms may disappear between episodes.

WHAT IS COLITIS?

From Modern Western Medicine

Literally, inflammation of the colon, colitis arises from unknown causes. It usually begins in young adulthood and may be due to viral infection or a bacterium that produces poisons that irritate the intestinal lining. Colitis may also be caused by antibiotics that are taken for two weeks or more. Antibiotics kill friendly bacteria, which are replaced by hostile flora (usually *Clostridium difficile*), which produce toxins that can injure the intestinal wall. Often, the infections that give rise to symptoms of colitis are defeated by the body without treatment.

Antibiotics are the most common form of treatment. Corticosteroid drugs are also prescribed for both ulcerative colitis and Crohn's disease; occasionally, special diets and supplements are recommended.

From Traditional Medicine

Colitis, like other so-called civilized diseases, is rare in countries that subsist on the traditional human diet and avoid pharmaceutical drugs. Traditional healers regard diet as the central cause of the illness, especially the consumption of animal proteins and refined foods, both of which give rise to constipation and an unhealthy bacterial environment. Another cause is the lack of exercise.

Animal foods cause poor intestinal health in several ways. They are difficult to digest and eliminate and thus promote constipation. The caliber of a chewed piece of meat is small and requires the intestine to contract significantly in order to move the meat through the colon. The degree of contraction causes pockets to form within the intestine (diverticula) that become storage areas for waste and toxins. These toxins can produce fissures and sores within the intestinal lining that eventually become ulcers, cysts, or polyps. Red meat also encourages the growth of unfriendly bacteria that produce toxins that further exacerbate the unhealthy environment and can even injure the intestinal lining. Finally, meat products increase the levels of bile acids within the intestine, which can further damage the organ.

Refined foods lack fiber, which makes elimination difficult and encourages the accumulation of waste products within the intestine. Such waste products ferment, irritate, and eventually can cause inflammation and ulcers on the organ's lining. The repeated use of harsh laxatives and antibiotics contribute to the disorder. Laxatives force the colon to function temporarily, but the long-term effect of laxatives is to weaken the organ.

REMEDIES

General Recommendations

- A high-fiber, low-protein diet is the best prevention and cure. However, initially the person's colon may be so irritated that fiber can further exacerbate the symptoms. Thus, fibrous foods must be introduced slowly.
- Mix whole grains with refined ones, such as brown rice with white or whole wheat noodles with white noodles, to reduce the fiber content of the food and make it easier for the intestines to adapt to the new diet.
- Boil or pressure cook grains with plenty of water so that the grain dish is wet, with the consistency of a soupy porridge.
- Eat alkalizing fermented foods, such as miso soup and tamari- and shoyu-based broths, with vegetables.

Foods to Eat

- Brown rice, boiled and served soupy, mixed with white rice to reduce fiber
- Whole-grain noodles mixed with white noodles
- Basmati rice
- Wild rice
- Squash, boiled or baked until soft, 2–3 times per week
- Sweet potatoes and yams
- Boiled carrots, served soft
- Root stews, composed of rutabagas, parsnips, carrots, and onions, boiled till soft
- Onions, baked and boiled
- Miso, shoyu, tamari, and tempeh (only the highest quality, organic fermented soybean products to replace friendly bacteria that have been destroyed by antibiotics)
- High-quality (preferably organic) sauerkraut
- Carrot juice
- Apple juice

Also include the following fruits:

- Stewed or baked apples
- Applesauce, warmed slightly before eating

Chinese Medicine

Meat and other animal proteins, which cause an overproduction of acid in the intestines, are a primary cause of the inflammation, along with stagnation of the liver, which may be caused in part by repressed emotions. Lifestyle changes that include a significant reduction in all animal foods; an increase of whole grains, vegetables, and alkalizing foods; deep relaxation; regular exercise; and some form of therapy to release inhibited emotional stress are all strongly recommended. All food must be chewed thoroughly (thirty-five to fifty times per mouthful) to make the food less irritating to the intestines. Chewing also enhances secretion of pancreatic enzymes and provides the initial step in digesting the complex carbohydrates found in whole grains, vegetables, and fruits. Finally, chewing increases the saliva content of the food; saliva is highly alkaline and acts as a healing salve on the intestinal wall.

Use soothing, mucilaginous foods and preparations:

- Waters, soups, or congees of oats, barley, or rice
- Honey water
- Tofu
- Soy milk
- Cabbage
- Cereal grass, microalgae, and liquid chlorophyll

Foods to Avoid

- Dairy products
- Fried foods
- Heated or poor-quality vegetable oils
- Red meats
- Coffee
- Hot spices
- Excessive salt
- Vinegar
- Citrus
- Tobacco

Herbs to Treat Colitis

- Comfrey root decoction: Drink two ounces, four times a day.
- Psyllium: Powder or soaked seeds will assist easy evacuation during colitis. Take a teaspoon of powder or ground, soaked seeds in warm water, three times a day. For children, take ½ teaspoon.

- Kelp: Sprinkle on food, 1 tsp. one to two times daily; or take 3–5 #0 capsules 1 or 2 times a day.
- Comfrey tablets: When the condition clears, take 10–20 daily with meals.
- Slippery elm tea (warm, not hot)
- Comfrey tea (warm, not hot)

Hydrotherapy

- Cold compress: Apply over abdomen to reduce inflammation.
- Warm fomentations over the lower spine and stomach
- Warm, full-body baths

Supplements

- Beta-carotene, 500 IU per day
- Vitamin B complex: Liquid B is best, taken once daily.
- Vitamin C (buffered): Take in powdered form diluted in water, 100 mg per day.
- Calcium, 800–1000 mg per day
- Spirulina, 1 tsp. daily

Probiotics

- Acidophilus
- Bifidobacteria (including *B. bifidum, B. infantis,* and *B. longum*)
- *Lactobacillus bulgaricus*
- Chlorella

COLON (OR LARGE INTESTINE) CANCER

SYMPTOMS

Symptoms of colorectal cancer are inexplicable change in bowel movements, often accompanied by blood in the feces and tenderness in the abdomen.

WHAT IS COLON CANCER?

From Modern Western Medicine

The second most common form of cancer, colorectal cancer is responsible for about 20 percent of all cancer-related deaths in the United States annually. The types of tumors found in the colon (also referred to as large intestine) include carcinoid tumors (slow-growing and usually symptomless) and lymphomas. Colon cancer is far more prevalent in the Western world, where animal foods, such as red meat, dairy products, and eggs are consumed in high quantities; the disease has a much lower incidence in countries that subsist on a diet rich in grains, vegetables, fruits, and low-fat animal products, such as fish. Studies have shown that a diet rich in meat and fat and low in fiber has a high association with colon cancer, and the National Academy of Sciences has stated unequivocally that animal fats have "causal" relation to the disease.

In most cases, treatment includes the surgical removal of part of the colon, including much of the tissue surrounding the tumors. Approaches other than surgery, such as drugs or radiation, are not considered curative.

From Traditional Medicine

The cause of colon cancer, according to numerous traditional healing systems, is an overconsumption of high-fat foods; animal foods, especially red meats; a lack of dietary fiber, whole grains, vegetables, and fruits, all of which are rich in anticancer nutrients, such as antioxidants and phytoestrogens; estrogens produced by anaerobic bacteria, which flourish in the colon on low-fiber diets; chronic constipation; stress; and, very often, unresolved emotional issues, especially grief. According to Chinese medicine, the colon (large intestine) and lungs are the organs within which the body holds its sadness or grief. Long-standing grief weakens the immune system and, specifically, the large intestine. When the other disease-causing conditions are present, grief encourages the onset of malignancy.

REMEDIES

General Recommendations

- See also the sections on breast cancer and cancer.
- Increase fiber. Animal studies show that an increase in dietary fiber reduces the size and number of cancerous polyps in the intestinal tract.
- Eat pungent foods. According to traditional Chinese medicine, pungent tastes strengthen the large intestine and lungs.
- Increase whole grains, fresh vegetables, and fruits.
- See Part IV for methods of strengthening the large intestine function.

Foods to Eat

- Eat whole grains, especially brown rice. According to traditional Chinese medicine, brown rice is an herb for the large intestine.
- Consume a wide variety of leafy greens, especially the cruciferous vegetables, such as kale, collard greens, mustard greens, watercress, cauliflower, and broccoli. Scientific studies have shown that these vegetables have powerful anticancer properties; the section on nutrition in Part III.
- Eat onion family foods, especially garlic. These are specific for strengthening the large intestine and have strong anticancer properties.
- Turnips
- Ginger
- Horseradish
- Cabbage (cooling)
- Radishes, including daikon (cooling)
- White peppercorns
- Seaweeds
- Flaxseed
- Beta-carotene–rich foods, such as carrots, winter squash, pumpkin, broccoli, kale, turnip, mustard greens, watercress, and microalgae such as blue-green algae.
- Eat high-fiber foods, such as all whole grains, fresh vegetables, and beans; bran of grains; and pulp of fruits.

Foods to Avoid

- Foods rich in fat
- Refined foods, especially those devoid of fiber and sugar
- Red meats
- Dairy products
- Eggs
- Spicy foods

Mind/Body

- Meditate to experience and release the sadness and grief that may be related to the onset and encouragement of the disease. (See Part III for
meditation routines related to emotions.)
- Use positive imaging exercises, stress reduction, and relaxation response
to deal effectively with stress, which can weaken immune response and
support the illness.
- Yoga and stretching exercises promote the release of tension and toxins
that are trapped in the pelvis and intestinal tract. Gentle yoga routines
can be done daily, but should be practiced anywhere from three to five
times per week.

COMMON COLD

SYMPTOMS

Any or all of the following symptoms may be present with a cold: nasal mucous discharge, blocked nasal passages, sore throat, cough, chills, fever, headache, joint aches, irritability, frequent urination, diarrhea, skin rash, swollen glands, and fatigue.

WHAT IS THE COMMON COLD?

From Modern Western Medicine

Orthodox medicine defines a cold as a viral infection of the upper respiratory tract, causing inflammation of the mucous membranes that line the bronchial passages, throat, eustachian tubes, and nose. The result is a mucous discharge from the nose, blocked or stuffed nasal passages, and occasionally, headache and fever. A cold is caused by any one of two hundred viruses, the most common being *rhinoviruses* and *coronaviruses,* which are usually airborne on droplets that have been coughed or sneezed by someone nearby.

From Traditional Medicine

All forms of traditional medicine view the common cold as the body's attempt at internal cleansing and detoxification. The common cold eliminates accumulated waste from the cells, organs, and tissue fluids. These waste products weaken the immune system and create the conditions for cold viruses to gain a foothold within the body and flourish. Suppression of cold symptoms, which is routinely accomplished by pharmaceutical drugs, drives these waste products deeper into the body, creating greater stagnation and forming the basis for more serious illness later on. The symptoms of the common cold indicate the organs that are detoxifying. Cough and sore throat are the body's way of eliminating mucus and waste from the lungs and large intestine. When the large intestine is unable to fully eliminate (such as from chronic constipation), waste infiltrates the lymph system, causing swollen glands, sore throat, and cough. On the other hand, diarrhea occurs when the body is attempting to rapidly eliminate accumulated waste, a pathogen, or some other toxin. Frequent urination suggests cleansing of the kidneys, bladder, and blood. Fever is the body's effort to create a hostile condition for bacteria or a virus that may live in the blood, tissues, liver, or spleen. Sweating cleanses the tissue fluids, lymph, and blood, and takes the burden off the kidneys. In short, a cold is an efficient, rapid form of internal cleansing.

WHO GETS COLDS?

People of all ages and both sexes contract colds.

REMEDIES

General Recommendations

- See related entries for constipation, cough, fever, headaches.
- Do not overmedicate a cold, even with holistic methods.
- Respect the demands of your body while you have a cold. This short period of bed rest and cleansing establish a basis for your long-term good health.
- Get plenty of rest, sleep, low light, keep warm, and sweat.

Foods to Eat

Do not overeat when you have a cold to avoid stressing your digestive tract. Lighter foods are better than heavy ones; soups are easier on digestion, enhancing both assimilation of nutrients and elimination of waste. (See the section on nutrition in Part III for more information on healthful eating, as well as the food sources of important vitamins and minerals.)

- Soupy vegetable broths that contain root vegetables, cabbage, leafy greens, or shiitake mushrooms
- Miso soup with land and sea vegetables, including shiitake mushrooms and wakame
- Soupy grains, such as boiled brown rice, with finely chopped vegetables, such as carrots, onions, and celery, and a small amount of freshly grated gingerroot
- Steamed or boiled leafy greens, including collard greens, kale, mustard greens, broccoli, brussels sprouts, and watercress
- Cooked fruit (compote or baked apple)
- Small amounts of citrus fruits for vitamin C
- Herbal teas, such as chamomile, hibiscus (rich in vitamin C), kukicha

Foods to Avoid

- Foods containing sugar, artificial ingredients, and refined flours
- Dairy products
- Red meat
- Raw foods, except for small amounts of fruit
- Cold foods and drinks
- Foods rich in fat, especially animal fats
- Fried foods

- Highly acidic foods, such as spices, tomatoes, eggplant, coffee, and alcohol
- Cigarettes and other tobacco products

Herbs to Treat a Cold

- Ginger in hot tea (either freshly grated or in teabags), with honey, to induce sweating and elimination. Hot ginger tea also supports and tonifies stomach, spleen, and large intestine; and improves bowel function.
- Echinacea, as tincture (15–30 drops, 2 or 3 times per day) in water or juice or as infusion boosts immune function and fights infection. Bring water to a boil, turn off flame, add 1 teaspoon of dried herb per cup of water, steep up to 20 minutes, and drink as tea. For children, use 10–15 drops, once or twice a day, or 1–2 cups of tea made from the dried herb.
- Goldenseal, in tincture (15–30 drops, 2 or 3 times per day); or as an infusion in water that has been previously boiled: Steep for 10–20 minutes; drink as tea. (If used with echinacea, dried herbs can be combined in water and boiled: 1 teaspoon of each herb in 2 cups of water. Goldenseal and echinacea are often sold together in tincture form, already mixed in the same tincture bottle.) Goldenseal boosts the immune system, cleanses mucous membranes, reduces inflammation, fights bacterial infection, cleanses blood, and promotes healing. For sore throat, swab with goldenseal or gargle with goldenseal and water.
- Use slippery elm as tea for sore throat, cough, lung congestion, nausea, and digestive disorders. Can be purchased as teabags or the dried herb can be boiled in water. Add a small amount of honey and cinnamon for children.
- Garlic is antibacterial, antiviral, immune-boosting, and liver-cleansing. Use it freshly grated or eaten as a raw vegetable. Add chopped parsley ro reduce odor.

Homeopathy

- Aconite is taken only in the earliest stages of a cold, when symptoms are first experienced, or when a person is exposed to wind. Otherwise, the treatment has little effect.
- Allium cepa is used for sneezing, watery eyes, runny nose, raw and sore upper lip, and painful cough.
- Arsenicum treats thin, watery mucous discharge and cold symptoms in the chest, with dry cough that worsens after midnight.

Hydrotherapy

- Take hot Epsom salts and/or mineral baths. They improve circulation, open pores, cause sweating and elimination, increase relaxation, and improve sleep. After the bath, dry the body thoroughly, get into bed under plenty of warm blankets, drink tea, and sweat. Keep warm.

- For lung congestion, create a vaporizer by boiling eucalyptus leaves, cloves, and pine needles. Take the pot off the stove, place it in a comfortable location or next to your bed, and hold your head over the vapors. Drape a towel over your head, creating a tentlike effect, to capture and hold vapors within. Breathe in and exhale deeply. Or, place these herbs in a vaporizer and allow the steam to permeate your bedroom; breathe in deeply.
- See the entry for fever.

Chinese Medicine

- Astragalus can be used as a vegetable (purchase in most Chinese food stores or by mail order). As food, place it in soup and boil it along with vegetables. Add miso. As tincture, 15–30 drops in water or apple juice. (For children, 10–15 drops, once or twice a day.) Strengthens immune system, improves digestion, and promotes healing.
- Herbal cold formula: lonicera, forsythia, arctium, platycodon, mint, soja seed, licorice, lophatherum, schizonepeta. Mix equal portions (one teaspoon, for example) of each dried herb and boil in water for 20 minutes. Allow to steep for 10–30 minutes; drink. Can be reheated. Treats all common cold symptoms.

Supplements

- Vitamin C, 100–500 mg/day, strengthens immune function; stops free radical formation; promotes production of T cells, and encourages phagocytosis.
- A low-dose multivitamin and mineral supplement (See the section on nutrition in Part III for recommended vitamins and minerals, their sources, and information on the RDAs and safe dosages that exceed the RDA.)

CONSIDERATIONS IF COLDS ARE CHRONIC

See Part IV for treatments and lifestyle habits that will strengthen the following organs: lungs, large intestine, liver, spleen, and the immune system.

CONSTIPATION

Infrequent and/or difficult bowel movements, headaches, coated tongue, tiredness, bad breath, mental depression, and mental dullness are all possible symptoms of constipation.

WHAT IS CONSTIPATION?

From Modern Western Medicine

Regularity and comfort of bowel movements are more important than frequency. Constipation is usually not considered harmful unless it appears suddenly and persists in an adult over forty. The most common cause is insufficient fiber in the diet. Lack of regular bowel moving habits is another cause. This may be the result of inadequate toilet training in childhood or of repeatedly ignoring the urge to move the bowels. In elderly people, there may be a weakness in the muscles of the abdomen and pelvic floor. In many cases, constipation can be cured by establishing a regular routine for using the toilet, acting on any urge to move the bowels, avoiding the use of laxatives and purgatives, increasing the amount of fiber in the diet, and drinking more liquids.

From Traditional Medicine

Intestinal health is fundamental to the overall good health of the body. Ideally, people should have an adequate bowel movement once a day, but many years on the highly refined Western diet may have made that goal impossible for many. In that case, ample and regular bowel movements every other day should be the norm.

If the main cause of constipation is a fiber-deficient diet, then both prevention and cure must lie in an unrefined, high-fiber diet. If constipation is habitual and of long duration, the weakened bowels must first be strengthened and reeducated, even before a high-fiber diet will stimulate regularity. Often, specific short cleansing fasts or mono diets (see below) with herbal aids, and hydropathic applications will rectify intestinal action.

Many people with intestinal disorders suffer from spleen imbalances. Chinese medicine maintains that the spleen provides qi to the large intestine, and thus is considered the "mother" of the colon. Chinese physicians, therefore, treat both the spleen and the large intestines when treating chronic constipation.

REMEDIES

Foods to Eat

- High-fiber diet consisting of whole grains, leafy greens, beans, and fruit
- Apple mono diet (3 days): This consists of four to five meals of raw apples with apple juice between meals. On the evening of the third day, the patient takes 2 tablespoons of raw, unrefined olive oil. Take no enemas or laxatives. Take twenty-five drops of cascara sagrada tincture diluted in water, four times a day. When taken regularly in low doses, cascara acts as a tonic, not a laxative. Continue taking cascara for two weeks, then gradually reduce.
- Eat plenty of raw fruit and vegetables.
- Bran: 1–2 tablespoons with water at mealtimes
- Prune, raisin, and fig tea: Cut up 10–12 figs and place in a saucepan together with 10–12 cut-up prunes and about 2 tablespoons raisins. Cover with 2 pints of water and simmer for 30 minutes.
- Olive oil
- Four to eight glasses of water per day
- Black sesame seeds (Chinese medicine)
- Fruit juice fast (3 days) with nightly enemas
- Miso, tamari, and shoyu, preferably organic: All are fermented foods, rich in friendly bacteria to restore the health of the colon.

Chinese Medicine

The large intestine is dependent upon a healthy spleen. Chinese medicine regards the spleen as the governor of digestion, passing life force, or qi, from the small intestine to the large, and thus ensuring healing assimilation and elimination. Among the foods that injure the spleen are refined white sugar and foods containing sugar. Such foods weaken the spleen and prevent it from passing adequate qi to the large intestine. For many people, sugar sometimes can act as a laxative, but over time, it causes constipation. The intestine itself may be constitutionally strong but conditionally weak, due in large measure to the fact that the spleen is being weakened constantly by the intake of sugar.

Foods that lubricate intestines are sesame seeds and oil, honey, pears, prunes, peaches, apples, apricots, walnuts, pine nuts, almonds, alfalfa sprouts, soy products, carrots, cauliflower, beets, okra, and seaweed.

Foods that promote bowel movement are cabbage, peas, black sesame seeds, sweet potatoes, asparagus, figs, bran from oats, and wheat or rice.

Flora-enhancing foods are miso, sauerkraut, wheat grass, and microalgae.

Other helpful therapies are regular acupressure massage, shiatsu massage, and acupuncture.

Foods to Avoid

- Meat
- Fats and other rich foods
- Spicy foods
- Coffee
- Refined foods
- Sugar
- Alcohol

Herbs to Treat Constipation

- Cascara bark
- Rhubarb root
- Barberry bark
- Dandelion root
- Senna
- Flax: Soak and eat, or consume after using in tea.
- Fenugreek (as above)
- Psyllium (as above)

The above three herbs are most effective when equal parts are taken, but any one will be helpful alone. Take 3 tablespoons of the combination or any single seed once or twice a day.

- According to Michael Tierra's *Planetary Herbology*: Rhubarb root (3–6 g) (substitute cascara if liver stagnation is present); gingerroot (1–2 g); licorice root (1–2 g)

Homeopathy

- Nux vomica: If you are hooked on laxatives, this will break the habit. Take a dose a few hours before bedtime. You can take a daily dose for a few days.
- Use sulfur when it's painful to pass stools due to a rectal fissure (a crack in the lining of the rectum), or if feces are hard, dark, and dry and there is a tendency to have hemorrhoids.
- Alumina may help when there is difficult passage of soft, sticky stools. (Aluminum can cause this problem, so don't use aluminum cookware.)
- Use bryonia for a large, dark stool that is difficult to pass, often looking burnt. It is also used if a person is irritable and ill-tempered. It is frequently used for children.
- Use graphites when there is no urge to defecate and when the stool comes, it takes the form of round balls stuck together with mucus and is difficult to pass. Other symptoms are fissures or cracks and hemorrhoids that burn and itch.

- Use silica for a bashful stool that starts out and goes back. There is soreness and often oozing of mucus.

Hydrotherapy

- Hot compress to abdomen
- Hot sitz baths
- Warm enemas of chamomile tea

Probiotics

- Acidophilus
- Bifidobacteria (including *B. bifidum, B. infantis,* and *B. longum)*
- *Lactobacillus bulgaricus*

Exercise

- Walking daily stimulates and strengthens abdominal muscles and promotes healthy intestinal function.
- Yoga or stretching exercises promote the flow of qi through the large intestine and spleen meridians.

COUGH

WHAT IS A COUGH?

From Modern Western Medicine

A cough is a reflex reaction to try to clear the airways of mucus, phlegm, a foreign body, or other irritants or blockages. Most coughs are due to irritation of the airways by dust, smoke, or mucus dripping from the back of the nose. A cough is said to be productive when it brings up mucus or phlegm, and unproductive, or dry, when it does not.

In some cases, a dry cough may be relieved by sucking on throat lozenges or by drinking warm, soothing drinks, such as honey and water. If this is ineffective, narcotic cough remedies afford symptomatic relief, particularly at bedtime to permit sleep. When there is productive coughing, suppressants should be avoided since they can do more harm than good. An expectorant medication or drinking lots of fluids can help loosen mucus or phlegm if there is difficulty coughing up. A physician should be consulted if any cough persists for more than two or three days, is severe, or is accompanied by symptoms such as chest pain, green phlegm, coughed-up blood, or breathing difficulty.

From Traditional Medicine

In the most simple terms, a cough is one of the body's mechanisms for elimination of mucus, cigarette tar and other toxins, air pollutants, viruses, and bacteria. Often, coughs arise when the lung energy is inadequate or deficient, causing inefficient elimination of waste. This results in stagnation of waste products within the lungs that eventually leads to a chronic cough.

Lungs are weakened by excessive consumption of dairy products, high-fat foods, and inadequate intake of leafy greens and other foods that strengthen lung energy (placed collectively under the metal element; see the section on Chinese medicine in Part III). Other substances that injure the lungs are, of course, cigarettes, drugs, and highly processed foods. The Chinese regard the lungs as the repository of unresolved and unexpressed grief, emotions that can also injure the health and vitality of the lungs.

REMEDIES

Foods to Eat

See the bronchitis entry and the section on lungs in Part IV.

Foods to Avoid

See the bronchitis entry and the section on lungs in Part IV.

Herbs to Treat a Cough

There are two main groups of herbs: expectorant or phlegm-dissolving herbs and antitussive or cough-relieving herbs. In general, however, most expectorant herbs have cough-relieving properties and most cough-relieving herbs tend to aid in the elimination of mucus. The expectorants are in turn divided into two groups, according to whether their nature is cooling or warming. Clear or white phlegm means that the condition is caused by cold, whereas yellow or blood-tinged phlegm is more reflective of heat and stagnation.

Cooling expectorants are for hot phlegm (dry cough, difficult expectoration, bleeding from the lungs): Many possess moistening properties.

- Kelp: 3–15 g (contraindicated for people with weak, cold digestion)
- Comfrey moistens lungs and helps dissolve mucus: 3–9 g; tincture, 10–30 drops.
- Bamboo is used for lung inflammation and phlegm that is difficult to expectorate. Bamboo is especially useful for treating children's coughs: 3–12 g.

Warming expectorants (herbs that warm and dissolve cold phlegm) are used for a cold condition, which is indicated by clear, whitish phlegm, coldness, and a pale complexion. These herbs also will eliminate the accumulation of mucus by improving digestion. They are contraindicated for dry cough and inflammatory conditions.

- Yerba santa is an excellent expectorant, especially when combined with grindelia. Dosage is 3–9 g; tincture is 10–30 drops.
- Grindelia should be used with other herbs: 3–6 g; tincture, 5–30 drops.

Antitussive Herbs relieve coughs, regardless of a person's condition. These can be combined with herbs from the previous categories that treat the underlying causes.

- Wild cherry bark: 3–9 g; tincture, 10–15 drops
- Apricot seed (contraindicated for diarrhea): 3–9 g of crushed seeds (Higher doses could be poisonous.)
- Mulberry acts as an anti-inflammatory to the lungs and quiets a cough. Dose is 6–15 g in decoction.
- Lungwort: 3–9 g; tincture, 10–30 drops

Homeopathy

- Use aconite for a cough that comes on after exposure to cold, dry wind or if a constant, short, dry cough wakens the patient from sleep, and the patient awakens feeling anxious. Use also for a cough that becomes worse when entering a warm room.

- Use belladonna if the person is red-faced, burning hot, with dilated pupils, for the sudden onset of a dry, teasing cough.
- Bryonia treats a hard, dry cough that hurts the chest, necessitates sitting up in bed, and is worse when entering a warm room.
- Pulsatilla treats a dry cough in the evening or a loose cough in the morning; coughing with gagging and yellowish mucus; the person feels better in open air, and he or she may feel as though there is weight on the chest.
- Nux vomica treats a dry, teasing cough, sore larynx and chest, a cough that occurs in spells and ends with retching, one that is more apt to occur in cold, dry weather, and it is for a person who is oversensitive.
- Phosphorus is often indicated when a head cold has gone into the chest; a dry, tickling, and exhausting cough; a cough that is induced by talking or by being in the open air, and a person who is thirsty for ice-cold drinks and fruit juices.

Chinese Medicine

Please see the section on bronchitis and the list of foods to eat.

- Elecampane brings up and dissolves phlegm, and stops coughs and wheezing. Dose: tincture, 10–30 drops; infusion, 3–9 g
- Acupuncture
- Acupressure
- Moxabustion

CROHN'S DISEASE

SYMPTOMS

Spasms of pain in the abdomen, diarrhea, loss of appetite, anemia, and weight loss are the most common symptoms occurring in young people. In the elderly, the disease more commonly affects the rectum and results in bleeding. Both groups may suffer from anal disorders, such as chronic abscesses, deep fissures (cracks), and fistulas (openings in the organ).

WHAT IS CROHN'S DISEASE?

From Modern Western Medicine

Crohn's disease is an inflammatory illness most commonly afflicting the small intestine (especially where it joins with the large intestine), but it can affect any part of the gastrointestinal tract, from the mouth to the anus. In addition to the inflammation of the intestinal wall, which can become quite thick, deep ulcers may also form. The cause of the disease is unknown. Corticosteroid drugs and sulfasalazine are often prescribed to combat the inflammation. Some patients benefit from a high-vitamin, low-fiber diet. The severity of the illness varies, but it tends to be chronic among all people afflicted with the disease. Surgery may be required to treat the complications arising from the illness.

From Traditional Medicine

Inflammation of the small intestine is associated with an excess of acid in the gastrointestinal tract, created as a by-product of high animal food consumption. There may be an acute sensitivity among people who contract Crohn's disease or colitis to animal foods and the acids they give rise to.

Chewing food very well (thirty-five to fifty times per mouthful) is essential to emulsify the food and alkalize it with saliva salts, thereby making it soothing and healing to the intestine. Chewing also enhances production of pancreatic enzymes, which encourage proper digestion.

According to Chinese medicine, the stomach and spleen-pancreas work together as an organ pair. The stomach receives the food mass, churns it into chyme, and prepares it for absorption by the small intestine. The Chinese healers describe the stomach's function as extracting a "pure essence" (or qi), which is sent to the spleen. The spleen distributes the qi to the intestinal tract and the blood; it is said that the spleen oversees digestion and controls the blood and the health of all blood vessels. The spleen works in harmony with the pancreas, which produces enzymes and insulin to make assimilation of nutrition and energy usage possible. Therefore, virtually all problems associated with the small intestine are also seen as imbalances of the spleen and pancreas.

WHO GETS IT?

The incidence of Crohn's disease varies between three and six new cases per year per 100,000 population in most developed countries; the incidence seems to have increased over the last thirty years. A person may be affected at any age, but the peak ages are in adolescence and early adulthood and after sixty.

REMEDIES

Foods to Eat

- All foods should be well-cooked, soft (even pureed), and easy to digest. After the acute phase, one or more of the remedies can continue to be taken at every meal.
- Fiber is essential, but too much fiber may be irritating to the small intestine. Therefore, combine whole grains with refined grains to reduce the fiber content of the food.
- To heal the inflamed lining of the stomach, use soothing, mucilaginous foods and preparations.
- See the section on colitis and ways of healing the small intestine in Part IV.

Foods to Eat

- Whole grains, made soft and soupy
- Soups
- Oats, barley, or rice congee
- Honey-water
- Avocados
- Tofu
- Soy milk
- Cabbage
- Potatoes

Chlorophyll-rich products are the only foods that can be taken raw.

- Cereal grass
- Microalgae, such as spirulina and chlorella
- Liquid chlorophyll
- Raw cabbage juice on an empty stomach and immediately after juicing
- Black or green tea, four times a day
- Flaxseed tea: highly effective European folk remedy for general gastrointestinal ulceration, inflammation, and bleeding; counteracts the in-

flammatory influence of excessive arachidonic acid. (Place ¼ cup of flaxseed in 1 quart of warm, purified water for eight hours, then strain.)
- Fresh figs (or dried, soaked in water): several each day

Foods to Avoid

- Meat
- Eggs
- Dairy
- Sugar
- Oily food and poor quality oil in general
- Intoxicants
- Spicy foods
- Vinegar
- Additives, chemicals, pesticides, and preservatives

Herbal Teas to Treat Crohn's Disease

- Licorice root
- Slippery elm
- Marshmallow root
- Red raspberry leaf
- Chamomile
- Flaxseed (See foods to eat, above.)

Probiotics

- Acidophilus
- Bifidobacteria (including *B. bifidum, B. infantis,* and *B. longum*)

CUTS

Most cuts can be successfully treated at home, but those that bleed excessively, are dirty, or infected may require medical attention. Clean dirt from minor cuts and scrapes by rinsing under cold running water and washing with a mild soap and clean washcloth. Dry with a sterile gauze or a clean cloth, and apply a healing remedy.

REMEDIES

Herbs to Treat a Cut

Use the following herbs to help stop bleeding. Sprinkle directly onto the wound or apply the herbal tincture to gauze and cover the affected area.

- Yarrow has powerful astringent properties.
- Goldenseal is an astringent and an antibacterial.

Apply one of the following antibacterial herbs in tincture form (dilute in five parts water) after the bleeding has stopped, to prevent infection.

- Echinacea
- Usnea
- Calendula

Soak a sterile cotton pad in the dilute tincture and apply to the wound, securing with a bandage, or spray 3 to 4 times daily directly on cuts and abrasions that are not covered by a bandage.

Use either of the following herbs in ointment form to encourage healing of a cut or scrape. Both contain allantoin, which has been proven to prevent scar formation.

- Comfrey
- Plantain

The following herbs can be taken internally for up to a week to boost immunity and promote recovery:

- Usnea: ½ teaspoon of tincture, 2–3 times daily
- Echinacea: ½ teaspoon of tincture, 3–4 times daily

Homeopathy

Homeopathic lotions or tinctures can be applied to minor cuts and abrasions by moistening the dressing and then covering it with sterile gauze. Use either of the following remedies:

- Calendula: for a superficial laceration or incision, or minor abrasion
- Hypericum: when the injury is causing nerve pain

To aid recovery, take tablets of the following internal remedies:

- Phosphorus: for small wounds that bleed a lot
- Ledum: for penetrating or puncture wounds
- Aconite: for severe bleeding or if the injured person is turning pale and faint

Chinese Medicine

Yunnan paiyao promotes blood coagulation. Break open a capsule and spread the powder on the bleeding cut, or take it internally when a cut is severe: one capsule 2–3 times per day. Pregnant women should not take yunnan paiyao internally.

Supplements

- Vitamin A (as beta-carotene): 15–30 mg per day to stimulate healing
- Zinc: 15 mg to accelerate healing
- Vitamin E: Apply topically after a scab has formed to prevent scarring.

CYSTITIS AND URETHRITIS

SYMPTOMS

Frequency and burning during urination; tenderness and pain in bladder area; intense desire to pass urine even after bladder has been emptied; cloudy urine that may have a strong odor.

WHAT IS CYSTITIS AND URETHRITIS?

From Modern Western Medicine

Cystitis and Urethritis are characterized by inflammation of the inner lining of the bladder, which is caused by a bacterial infection. People with such symptoms should drink plenty of fluids, especially cranberry juice, which promotes acidity of the urine that in turn fights the infection. Often, antibiotics are prescribed to destroy the bacteria and prevent the infection from spreading, which is usually accomplished within twenty-four hours. Occasionally, the infection spreads to the kidneys and may cause swelling and some damage (pyelonephritis).

When symptoms of cystitis are present but there is no evidence of infection, the disease may be urethritis (inflammation of the urethra).

From Traditional Medicine

Although bacteria may indeed be present in the bladder, they are not the real cause of the disease; otherwise everyone would likely suffer from cystitis. In health, the body's immune system is able to destroy bacterial invasion, thus preventing the bacteria from ever gaining a foothold. Therefore, the traditional approach is twofold: address the immediate symptoms, meanwhile boosting the overall health of the immune response through diet, exercise, and appropriate lifestyle considerations.

WHO GETS CYSTITIS AND URETHRITIS?

Women are far more susceptible to cystitis than men because the urethra in women is short and in close proximity to the anus, which makes it easier for bacteria and infectious agents to migrate to the bladder. Most women have cystitis at some time. Men contract cystitis on rare occasions when there is an obstruction present in the urethra or the prostate becomes enlarged, causing a buildup of bacteria in the urethra and bladder. Children may suffer from cystitis if there is a structural abnormality in the ureters (the tubes that carry urine from the kidneys to the bladder), causing reflux of urine back into the ureters where bacteria can develop.

REMEDIES

General Recommendations

- See the section on ways to boost the immune system in Part IV.
- See the section on ways to improve the health of the bladder and kidneys in Part IV.

Foods to Eat

According to Chinese medicine, the most effective foods are cooling foods with some bitterness. Less food is recommended, also.

- Lightly cooked, organic vegetables
- Salads
- The most cooling vegetables are celery, carrots, winter squash, potatoes with skins, asparagus, and mushrooms.
- Whole grains
- Vegetables that are high in protein, such as beans, especially adzuki beans (effective against damp heat), and lima beans
- Fish containing essential fatty acids, such as salmon and sardines
- Fresh fruit in small amounts (except citrus)
- Cranberry juice slightly acidifies urine, increases urine flow, and reduces the adherence of bacteria to the mucous membrane walls; drink four glasses per day.
- Apple cider vinegar, water, and honey: 1 cup, three times/day
- Carrots and carrot juice
- Lemon juice
- Pure spring water: eight or more glasses per day

Foods to Avoid

- Meat
- Eggs
- Dairy food
- Citrus fruits
- Refined sugar and other concentrated sweeteners
- Refined white flour products
- Greasy, oily foods

Herbs to Treat Cystitis

- Uva ursi: tincture, 10–20 drops, three or more times daily; fluid extract, ½–1 tsp., three times daily; infusion, steep thirty minutes, 3 oz. as needed, up to 3 cups/day
- Slippery elm as decoction (whole bark): simmer 5–15 minutes, 3 oz. three to four times daily

- Chaparral (one of nature's best antibiotics): add to formulas in kidney and bladder infections. As infusion, steep 5–15 minutes, 6 oz., three times daily; tincture, 10–20 drops, three times daily; powder, 2–10 #0 (10–60 grains) three times daily

Homeopathy

- Aconite treats sudden retention of urine from chill or fright.
- Cantharis treats persistent and violent urging, passing a few drops at a time. These symptoms may be accompanied by aching in the small of the back.
- Mercurius carrosivus (mercury chloride) treats persistent urging with intense burning, unfulfilled need to urinate, with constant urging and straining. Urine may be mixed with a little blood.
- Nux vomica treats frequent and painful urging with little result.

Chinese Medicine

This is a result of a damp condition in the bladder that has combined with heat. Infections thrive in damp environments caused by too many acid-forming foods (see foods to eat and foods to avoid).

Supplements

- Beta-carotene: 15–30 mg per day
- Vitamin C: 100–500 mg per day
- Niacin: 20 mg per day
- Vitamin E: 100–400 IU per day

DANDRUFF

SYMPTOMS

Symptoms of dandruff are flaking and scaling of scalp, often accompanied by itching. Occasionally, a rash or broken skin will also appear.

WHAT IS DANDRUFF?

From Modern Western Medicine

Dandruff is the flaking and shedding of dead skin from the scalp. Dandruff may be accompanied by an itchy, scaly rash, *seborrheic dermatitis,* which can occur on the face, chest, and back, as well. The primary treatment is the use of an anti-dandruff shampoo. Physicians may prescribe a corticosteroid cream or lotion, or an anti-fungal cream, if the shampoo fails. Whatever the treatment, dandruff usually requires constant control.

From Traditional Medicine

Dandruff is the body's way of eliminating excess proteins and fats that are accumulating in the system and cannot be assimilated. These proteins and fats prevent healthful circulation of oils and water in the scalp. Dandruff is also a symptom of liver and kidney imbalances, organs that detoxify the body and eliminate waste from the blood. Highly acidic foods, such as spices and tomatoes, also play a roll. Treatment includes a sharp reduction in animal foods and the promotion of liver and kidney health, along with a more alkalizing diet.

REMEDIES

General Recommendations

- Reduce or eliminate animal proteins until condition subsides.
- Increase exercise to promote better circulation and elimination of fats and oils.

Foods to Eat

- A diet composed primarily of whole grains, fresh vegetables, beans, and fruit
- Most of the vegetables should be cooked, though raw vegetables can be eaten regularly, but in smaller amounts than those that are cooked
- Low-fat animal products, such as white fish
- Fruit—berries, apples, and pears; avoid citrus until dandruff clears
- Raw vegetable juices

- Sunflower seeds and pumpkin seeds
- Salads
- Tofu
- Seaweed
- Microalgae, such as spirulina and chlorella

Foods to Avoid

- Foods rich in saturated fats, especially red meat, eggs, and dairy products
- Citrus
- Excess salt
- Sugar
- Alcohol

Herbs to Treat Dandruff

- Wahoo: Dose is ½ tsp. (5–10 drops) two or three times daily (contraindicated if there is a cold condition, fluid deficiency, emaciation, and weak digestion).
- Ginger Sesame Oil: Rub on scalp and leave it overnight. Shower it out in the morning. Repeat two to three times per week. (To make this, use a mixture of equal amounts of sesame oil and fresh ginger juice. To extract the ginger juice, grate the ginger and express the juice by squeezing it through a cheesecloth.)
- Citrus seed extract: use externally. (It is available as liquid extract, spray, ointment, and in a variety of other forms.)

Physiotherapy

- Scalp massage: To 4 oz. pure distilled water add 20 drops of 85% grain alcohol and 2–6 drops of oil of pine. Massage into scalp and then follow this by massaging a small amount of white vaseline into the scalp.
- Shampoo with pine tar shampoo or alternate with olive oil shampoo.
- Crude oil scalp massage, 2 times per week: Massage unrefined, undiluted Pennsylvania grade crude oil (Crudoleum, Cayce product) into the scalp vigorously with the fingertips and then massage the entire scalp for 30 minutes with an electric vibrator.

Supplements

- Beta carotene: 16 mg per day
- Zinc: 15 mg per day
- Calcium: 500 mg per day

Exercise

- Walking, jogging, bicycle riding or any aerobic sport performed regularly.

DENTAL FILLINGS (MERCURY AMALGAMS)

SYMPTOMS

A host of mysterious physical symptoms may occur from toxic reactions to mercury in dental fillings, especially among those who may have an acute sensitivity to mercury. Some people, including some dentists, maintain that mercury fillings can cause dizziness, arthritis, colitis, multiple sclerosis, loss of mental acuity, and psychosis in highly sensitive people. There is small but existing evidence to support a possible link to immune disorders, Alzheimer's disease, Parkinson's, and other degenerative illnesses of the nervous system. Mercury is one of the most toxic substances on earth. It is well established that mercury fillings do outgas mercury vapors every time one chews food, drinks fluids, or brushes one's teeth.

WHAT IS THE MERCURY AMALGAM STORY?

From Conventional Dentistry

Half of the standard silver filling, known as an amalgam, is composed of mercury. The rest is made up of silver, copper, zinc, and tin. Fillings containing mercury have been in use for 150 years, a fact the American Dental Association sees as proof that such amalgams are safe. More than 85 percent of the American public has amalgam fillings, and each year more than 200 million restorations are performed, the vast majority of which contain mercury. Nevertheless, there is a small but growing body of evidence that suggests that mercury poisoning may occur in some people. The Food and Drug Administration has called for more research, stating that nothing to this point has been proven.

Alternatives

A growing number of dentists in the United States have expressed concern over the use of mercury, but only 3,000 out of 150,000 dentists in the United States have stopped using amalgams entirely. Several thousand more dentists now offer alternatives to amalgams made of plastic composites, porcelain, and gold.

Taking an active stand against amalgams or recommending that existing amalgam fillings be removed for health reasons places a dentist at risk of having his or her license revoked by the ADA. For this reason, many dentists are reluctant to reveal their concerns about amalgam fillings.

There is some concern that mercury might be replaced with other metals that are equally toxic. Most mercury-free dentists are selective about the qual-

Dental Fillings

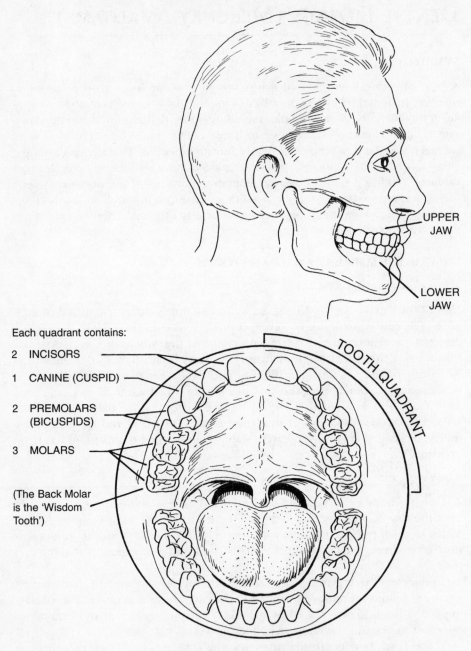

UPPER JAW

LOWER JAW

Each quadrant contains:

2   INCISORS

1   CANINE (CUSPID)

2   PREMOLARS
     (BICUSPIDS)

3   MOLARS

(The Back Molar
is the 'Wisdom
Tooth')

TOOTH QUADRANT

There are 32 permanent adult teeth.
Each upper and lower jaw contains 16 (2 quadrants of 8).

ity of the composites that they choose, but patients should always ask for composites that do not contain aluminum, barium, or other metals, to avoid the possible toxic effects of these metals.

Dr. Michael Ziff, an Orlando, Florida–based dentist and a leading proponent of alternatives to mercury fillings, points out that composite fillings (generally made of plastics) are made of long chains of molecules that are too big to be absorbed by cells in the mouth and digestive tract. Studies have shown that the body eliminates through the feces any pieces that come off the composite filling. In any case, Ziff says, the composites do not remotely compare with the potential toxicity of mercury. Research has also shown that composites hold up as well as mercury fillings if the composite is placed correctly. For this reason, composites, which are termed *technique sensitive,* require an experienced dentist to fit them properly. In the meantime, new composites are being developed each year that are stronger, more durable, and easier to work with.

HOW TO FIND A MERCURY-FREE DENTIST

Even if a dentist claims to be mercury-free or holistic, you should interview your dentist about his methods and techniques. Dr. David Kennedy, a San Diego–based dentist and nationally known expert on placing composites, says that most composite fillings fail because they shrink after being installed. The plastic's shrinkage causes the filling to move away from the borders of the cavity, allowing the filling to fall out. Sometimes the filling is not fitted into the tooth properly, causing the filling to break up or decay at the edges of the tooth.

All these things have to do with placement and not durability of the materials. Therefore, the following standardized procedure has been designed to insure successful fillings. You can interview your dentist and make sure he is aware of these techniques.

- The tooth must be kept free of moisture and isolated with a rubber dam. The dam makes the tooth sit up and helps keep it dry so that the bonding agents adhere better to the surface.
- High-speed suction is used to keep the tooth dry while the work is being done.
- The tooth must be thoroughly cleaned and free of bacteria.
- The area where the filling will be placed must be etched, usually with phosphoric acid, to create a better bonding surface.
- Two forms of bonding agents, one made of dentin, the other of enamel, should be used to secure the filling. Unlike an amalgam filling, which is sealed to the tooth with a corrosion technique, composite fillings are bonded to the tooth surface. Unless these bonds are established properly, the composite can come loose, especially when it begins to shrink.

- The composite should be cured, or placed under high heat, to prevent it from shrinking and withdrawing from the tooth surface. Dentists should not just use a heat lamp but should cure or bake the composite in a laboratory before installing it in the tooth. This requires the dentist to take a mold of the tooth and then create a filling to fit the mold.

Having a composite filling placed and having an existing amalgam removed are very different issues. Few dentists are willing to advocate removing existing amalgams, and the ADA has made it a violation of its code of ethics for any dentist to recommend that amalgam fillings be removed for health reasons. Dentists who have urged the replacement of amalgams have lost their licenses. Removing amalgams will release mercury into the bloodstream and may well have a greater toxic effect than if your fillings were left alone.

The following are organizations that can help you find a qualified dentist to provide mercury-free services.

The International Academy of Oral Medicine and Technology
Dr. Michael Ziff, Executive Director
Box 808010
Orlando, FL 32860-5831

DAMS Newsletter
(Defense Against Mercury Syndrome)
725-9 Tramway Lane NE
Albuquerque, NM 87122

Queen and Company
Health Communications, Inc.
Box 49308
Colorado Springs, CO 80949-9308

DEPRESSION

SYMPTOMS

Depression is characterized by withdrawal from the daily activities of life, accompanied by a reduced sense of well-being and feelings of sadness, hopelessness, pessimism.

WHAT IS DEPRESSION?

From Modern Western Medicine

Everyone experiences some degree of depression now and then, and for the vast majority of people, the condition rights itself without intervention of any kind. For many, however, depression persists and deepens, requiring psychological and medical assistance.

Depression may have some physical or organic origins; for instance, hormonal imbalances, such as those resulting from childbirth. Numerous drugs can also cause depression. Many mood-altering and psychotherapeutic drugs, birth control, and sleeping pills can bring on the condition.

From Traditional Medicine

Depression is often the result of inadequate levels of serotonin, the brain neurotransmitter responsible for feelings of well-being, confidence, positive outlook, and restful sleep. Serotonin is increased in the brain by high consumption of carbohydrate-rich foods, such as whole grains, beans, and vegetables. The Chinese regard many cases of depression as a deficiency of nutrition (see below), a stagnant liver, weak spleen, and hypoglycemia.

Studies have shown that exercise relieves depression. So, too, does reducing the amount of sleep from eight hours to five or six hours per night.

WHO GETS DEPRESSED?

While everyone is prone to occasional bouts of depression, more women than men seek treatment for the condition (one in six women, as opposed to one in nine men, seek help). This may indicate a greater willingness to confront and deal with depression, rather than a greater susceptibility. More than 15 percent of Americans suffer from clinical depression, while severe depression affects 5 to 10 percent of the population. Depression tends to increase with age.

REMEDIES

General Recommendations

- Foods rich in complex carbohydrates should dominate your diet. These include whole grains, vegetables, beans, and fruits. These foods will boost serotonin and promote feelings of well-being, security, and inner peace.
- Mild aerobic exercise, at least five days per week
- Yoga
- Journal writing: Spend ten to twenty minutes per day writing down your feelings in your diary. Studies have shown that writing relieves depression and other mild psychological disorders.

Foods to Eat

- Whole grains rich in complex carbohydrates, such as brown rice, barley, corn, millet, oats, and whole wheat (Eat these foods at least twice per day.)
- Vegetables
- Beans
- Cucumbers
- Apples
- Fresh wheat germ
- Kuzu root
- Wild blue-green microalgae (¼ g one to three times daily)

Foods to Avoid

Avoid the following foods, which obstruct and/or damage the liver.

- Meat
- Dairy
- Eggs
- Hydrogenated and poor-quality fats (such as shortening, margarine, and refined and rancid oils)
- Nuts and seeds
- Chemicalized food and water
- Intoxicants
- Highly processed, refined foods
- Drugs (even prescription, if possible)

Chinese Medicine

When the liver is not functioning properly, myriad emotional problems can occur. Many liver conditions involve excess of one kind or another. The most frequent kind occurs when too much food is eaten—especially rich and greasy food—and the liver becomes swollen and sluggish in its attempt to circulate qi energy smoothly through the body. The qi then stagnates in the liver.

The following foods stimulate a stagnant liver. The first remedy is to eat less of all foods.

- Moderately pungent foods, spices, and herbs
- Sprouted grains, beans, and seeds
- Watercress
- Onion family
- Mustard greens
- Sweet brown rice
- Beets
- Amasake
- Strawberries
- Peaches
- Cherries
- Chestnuts
- Cabbage, turnips, kohlrabi, cauliflower, broccoli, and brussels sprouts
- Apple cider vinegar (1 teaspoon in a little water up to three times/day)

Herbs to Treat Depression

- Lemon balm: ½ to 6 g moves liver and spleen qi.
- Gardenia (sometimes called *the happiness herb* because it relieves liver congestion and blocked emotions): 6–12 g
- Pulsatilla: Prepare from the fresh herb. Macerate 2 pounds in 4 pints of strong alcohol. Two to three drops of the tincture are taken three or four times a day in a spoonful of water. Use within a year of preparation.
- Ginkgo biloba: available in pills and capsules
- Gotu kola: available in pills and capsules
- Slippery elm: available as a tea

Supplements

- Vitamin B_1: 1.5 mg per day
- Vitamin B_6: 2–10 mg per day, especially if there is edema or if depression is related to the menstrual cycle
- Vitamin B_{12}: 2–10 mcg per day
- Vitamin B complex: 50 mg per day
- Vitamin C: 100–500 mg per day
- Calcium/magnesium: in a 2:1 ratio (500 mg of calcium; 250 mg of magnesium) per day

Sleep Management

Studies have shown that people who reduce the amount of sleep they are getting from eight or more hours per night to five or six hours experience dramatic improvements in mood.

Mind/Body

- Daily meditation, prayer, and guided imagery routines
- Support groups
- Chanting and singing
- Writing in a journal daily
- Write in a personal journal about the most traumatic and/or shameful experience you have had for four days, at least 20 minutes per writing session. This method, developed by Southern Methodist University psychologist James Pennybaker, Ph.D., has been proven effective in alleviating many kinds of psychological disorders, including depression.

Aromatherapy

- Lavender

Exercise

- Walking daily
- Yoga and stretching exercises specifically boost brain levels of serotonin, the neurotransmitter that promotes feelings of well-being, positive outlook, deeper sleep, and higher self-esteem.
- Bicycling, jogging, swimming, and any aerobic activity or sport

DIABETES (TYPE I AND TYPE II)

SYMPTOMS

People with diabetes may experience chronic thirst, excessive urination, excess hunger, muscle wasting, weight loss, weakness, dry skin, itching, rashes, numbness, tingling of hands and feet, neuropathy with severe pains, vascular degeneration, atherosclerosis, heart disease, retinopathy, loss of sight, kidney disease, gangrene in dependent limbs due to poor circulation (diabetes is the number-one cause of amputation). Tests reveal elevated blood sugar levels and sugar in the urine.

Diabetes doubles the risk of suffering a heart attack or a stroke. It dramatically increases the risk of kidney disease, blindness (from retinopathy), amputations (due to lack of circulation to limbs), infections, and complications from childbearing. The reason diabetics have such high rates of these disorders is because the illness is associated with exceedingly high blood cholesterol levels, which prevent the circulation of blood and oxygen to organs and limbs.

WHAT IS DIABETES?

From Modern Western Medicine

There are two kinds of diabetes, type I, known as *juvenile diabetes,* and type II, also called *adult-onset diabetes.* Type I, or juvenile diabetes, occurs when the pancreas fails to produce adequate insulin, the hormone used by the body to make blood sugar (glucose) available to cells. Many theories exist as to why the pancreas is unable to produce insulin, but recent evidence reported by Johns Hopkins University suggests that consumption of dairy products by sensitive children causes the immune cells to respond with excessive aggressiveness to antigens in cow's milk. These antigens may attach themselves to cells in the pancreas. Once attached, the antigens are attacked by immune cells that, in the process, destroy both the antigens and the pancreatic cells that produce insulin. All of this occurs in childhood (hence the name of this type of diabetes). Without regular injections of insulin, the sufferer lapses into a coma and dies.

Type II, the most common form of diabetes, occurs in adulthood (usually in people older than forty). For most adult-onset diabetics, the pancreas actually produces more insulin than is necessary, at least in the early stages of the illness. The problem is that dietary fat and cholesterol infiltrate the blood and block insulin from making glucose available to cells. As the disorder continues, the pancreas weakens, and production of insulin diminishes until insulin injections may be necessary. Most type II diabetics do not need insulin, at least in the early or middle stages of the disease.

Because the glucose is not consumed by cells, blood sugar becomes abnormally high, causing excessive urination and constant thirst and hunger. But more dangerously, cells cannot obtain fuel to function, causing fatigue and eventually the death of cells and the body itself.

From Traditional Medicine

Diabetes is clearly a disease of civilization. In population groups where little animal fat and no refined sugars are consumed, diabetes is rare to nonexistent.

In addition to the causes already described, traditional medicine points to stress, adrenal exhaustion, and prolonged demands on the pancreas and liver as secondary causes of the disease. Coffee, nicotine, alcohol, and recreational drugs all cause the adrenals to be overstimulated and eventually unable to function.

The possibility of curing diabetes depends on the type a person suffers from, the severity of the illness, and the length of insulin dependency. Type I (juvenile) cannot be cured, but many of the related problems associated with diabetes—such as heart disease, claudication, amputation, and blindness—can be avoided if the person adopts a diet low in fat and rich in complex carbohydrates. He or she should also get regular exercise. Type II diabetes can be controlled and even cured by an appropriate diet and lifestyle. (The Pritikin Longevity Center in Santa Monica, California, restores to normal function more than 75 percent of type II diabetics who arrive at the center taking diabetic medication.)

WHO GETS IT?

Thirteen million Americans suffer from diabetes, with the majority (90 percent) suffering from type II, or adult-onset diabetes.

REMEDIES

General Recommendations

- Reduce dietary fat and cholesterol to lower blood cholesterol, which reduces or eliminates the need for medication for type II diabetes.
- Reduce dietary fat and cholesterol to lower blood cholesterol and thereby avoid related circulatory problems, including heart disease, stroke, claudication, retinopathy, and amputation.
- Increase fiber and complex carbohydrates to lower cholesterol. Fiber binds with cholesterol and helps eliminate it from the system. It also lowers blood insulin levels.
- Exercise daily.

Foods to Eat

Chew everything very well to improve nutrient assimilation and make it less likely you will overeat. The following foods are helpful for all types of diabetes.

- Whole grains, especially millet, rice, sweet rice, and wheat
- Chlorophyll-rich foods, especially wheat or barley grass, spirulina, and chlorella
- Vegetables
- Beans
- Whole and cooked fruit

The following foods have an insulinlike action and should be included regularly.

- Brussels sprouts
- Cucumbers
- Green beans
- Garlic
- Oatmeal or oat flour products
- Soybeans and tofu
- Avocados
- Raw, green vegetables
- Wheat germ
- Buckwheat
- Fresh flaxseed oil (high in linoleic fatty acid, which enables insulin to be more effective)
- GLA oils (available in evening primrose, black currant seed oil, and spirulina)

Dietary Recommendations from Chinese Medicine

- Cooked vegetables and fruit
- Carbohydrate-rich vegetables: winter squash, carrots, rutabagas, parsnips, garbanzo beans, black beans, peas, sweet potatoes, yams, and pumpkin
- Pungent vegetables and spices: onions, leeks, black pepper, ginger, cinnamon, fennel, garlic, and nutmeg
- Small amounts of certain sweeteners and cooked fruits: rice syrup, barley malt, molasses, cherries, and dates.

For excess-type diabetes, typified by a robust person who is overweight and constipated, with signs of excess such as ruddy complexion, thick (possibly yellow) tongue coating, strong pulses, and an outward-oriented personality:

- All of the above
- Raw vegetables and fruit (Fruit should be either acid or subacid, because the acidic, sour flavor lowers the blood sugar; for example, lemons and grapefruit.)

Foods to Avoid

- Foods rich in fat, especially animal foods, such as red meat, eggs, and dairy products
- Sugar
- White flour
- White rice

Herbs to Treat Diabetes

- Cinnamon (triples insulin's efficiency)
- Hawthorn (for heart and cholesterol)
- For all pancreatic problems:

  1 part uva ursi
  1 part goldenseal
  1 part elecampane
  2 parts dandelion root
  2 parts cedar berries
  1 part fennel
  ½ part ginger

Mix the powdered herbs and put them in #00 capsules. Take them after every meal.

- Huckleberry leaf tea: drink 1 cup, 3 times a day.
- Barberry: one of the mildest and best liver tonics known: tincture, 10–30 drops; standard decoction or 3–9 g
- Fenugreek seeds (one of the oldest known herbs; used by Hippocrates—good for regulating insulin). Dosage is 3–9 g.

Hydrotherapy

Hot and cold packs over the pancreas and kidneys will help insulin production and kidney elimination.

Supplements

- Beta-carotene: 15–30 mg per day
- Vitamin B complex: 50 mg per day
- Vitamin C: 100–500 mg per day
- Vitamin E: 200–400 IU once a day

- Vitamin B_6: 250 mg per day (especially useful in pregnancy-onset diabetes)
- Zinc: 15 mg per day (essential for insulin secretion)

Exercise

- Walk and stretch four to five times a week for at least thirty minutes per session, or as much as can be accomplished. Vigorous exercise will also lower blood sugar levels and reduce the need for insulin. Exercise also improves circulation, which tends to be poor in diabetics.
- Avoid competitive sports. Diabetes is associated with high blood cholesterol and heart disease. Competitive sports can easily bring on a heart attack or stroke.
- Avoid contact sports to prevent bruising. Diabetics often suffer from poor circulation. Bruising can create pools of blood in tissues and give rise to infection and gangrene.

Diarrhea

SYMPTOMS

Diarrhea is characterized by greater than usual fluidity, frequency, or volume of bowel movements, as compared to the normal pattern for a particular person. Diarrhea is not considered a disease of itself but a symptom of an underlying disorder.

WHAT IS DIARRHEA?

From Modern Western Medicine

Acute diarrhea, which starts suddenly and, for most people, usually lasts only two or three days, is often the result of consuming contaminated food or drink. The condition normally subsides without treatment. Chronic diarrhea may be due to a serious intestinal disorder and requires medical attention. Diarrhea in infants and the elderly can be a more serious disorder because of its potential to cause dehydration.

Common causes of acute diarrhea include anxiety, flu, food allergy, food poisoning, side effects of drugs and drug toxicity, and food intolerance. In addition, Crohn's disease, ulcerative colitis, diverticular disease, cancer, thyrotoxicosis, and irritable bowel syndrome can cause chronic diarrhea.

Treatment involves replacing the lost water and electrolytes (salts) to prevent dehydration, usually by drinking water in which salt and sugar have been added. The formula for salt-and-sugar water is one teaspoon of salt and four teaspoons of sugar in one quart of water. Electrolyte mixtures are also available from pharmacies.

Diarrhea in infants, recurring diarrhea that persists for more than a week, and diarrhea that contains blood in the stools requires medical attention.

From Traditional Medicine

Acute diarrhea is the body's normal reaction to the presence of a toxic agent. It is an efficient way of eliminating toxic foods, viruses, or bacteria from the system. Chronic diarrhea, in most cases, is due to weakness in the digestive system, which includes the spleen, stomach, pancreas, liver, gallbladder, and small and large intestines.

In the view of Chinese medicine, diarrhea is most frequently caused by deficient spleen-pancreas qi or deficient fire element (heart and small intestine). Finally, healers using Chinese medicine also point out that diarrhea can manifest as a result of excessive heat and cold influences. (See Part III for an explanation of heat and cold conditions.)

The first set of foods recommended below are for general causes and can be used for any type of diarrhea. The second and third set are for cold and hot conditions, respectively.

REMEDIES

General Foods to Eat

According to Chinese medicine, the basic diet should consist of small meals that are well chewed. Healing foods include the following:

- Water (to replace lost fluid)
- White rice or white bread
- Rice or barley broth
- Blackberry juice
- Garlic (especially when there is bacterial contamination)
- Leeks
- String beans
- Eggplant
- Sunflower seeds
- Umeboshi plums
- Crab apples
- Olives
- Adzuki beans
- Sweet rice
- Yams
- Carrots
- Buckwheat

Diarrhea may manifest as a result of hot or cold influences on the body. Symptoms of cold conditions include watery stools; copious, clear urine; chills; and a white, wet tongue coating. Symptoms of excess heat include stools causing burning sensation in anus, yellow coating of the tongue, yellow urine, aversion to heat, and a desire for cold drinks.

For Cold Diarrhea

- Red, black, or cayenne pepper
- Cinnamon bark
- Dried ginger
- Nutmeg
- Chestnuts
- Chicken eggs (organic and fertilized)

For Hot Diarrhea

- Millet congee
- Tofu
- Mung beans
- Persimmons
- Pineapple

Foods to Avoid No Matter What Kind of Diarrhea You May Have

- Honey
- Spinach
- Cow's milk
- Apricots
- Plums (umeboshi plums are helpful)
- Sesame seeds
- Oils
- Any food difficult to digest

Herbs to Treat Diarrhea

- Blackberry tea: 3–4 cups per day
- Peppermint essence: 3–15 drops, every 2–3 hours
- Cranesbill (one of the safest and most effective astringent herbs for gastrointestinal problems): root powder, 20–30 grains; tincture, 2–30 drops
- Rose hips: 3–12 g
- Nettles: 9–30 g

Homeopathy

The following remedies will help relieve the miseries of diarrhea without interfering with its cleansing action.

- Arsenicum: if stomach feels heavy, there is nausea, vomiting, and weakness, which come from spoiled food or excessive fruit
- Cuprum arsenicosum for burning, cramping, colicky pain in lower bowels, vomiting, and a sensation of collapse
- Gersemium: for diarrhea caused by anticipation of even an enjoyable social engagement or from fear
- Sulfur for changeable stools that are sometimes yellow and watery and sometimes slimy, or for an urgent need to defecate early in the morning
- Veratrum album: treats similar symptoms to arsenicum, but the patient experiences a cold sweat and feels on the verge of collapse

For children, be alert if diarrhea continues for any length of time and watch for signs of dehydration.

- Aconite: Use after exposure to cold wind.
- Arsenicum album: for diarrhea from spoiled food or too much fruit, to treat frequent, dark, offensive stools; restlessness; or thirst for small sips of water.
- Chamomilla treats greenish, slimy stools during teething.
- Nux vomica: for diarrhea resulting from overfeeding; usually, small quantity is passed each time.

Diverticulitis and Diverticulosis (Diverticular Disease)

SYMPTOMS

Only 20 percent of those with diverticulosis experience symptoms, which can include intestinal cramps, pain, sensitivity, and irregular bowel movements. Some may experience symptoms of irritable bowel, such as alternating diarrhea and constipation. The disease can lead to complications, however, including the development of a stricture (narrowing of the intestine) at the site of the inflammation or a fistula (narrow channel) connecting one part of the intestine to another).

WHAT IS DIVERTICULAR DISEASE?

From Modern Western Medicine

Diverticulosis is a condition in which pockets, called diverticula, form in the large intestine. Diverticulitis is a more advanced condition in which inflammation and, in some cases, perforation of the pockets or sacs occurs, along with tenderness, hardness, and rigidity of the abdomen; pain; infection; and fever. In rare cases, the infection can lead to an abscess in the lining of the colon, eventually causing peritonitis (inflammation of the lining of the abdomen).

The main cause of the disorder is the consumption of meats and the absence of fibrous foods. Red meat passes into the large intestine as a small-caliber wad. The large intestine is lined with muscle. In order to move waste through the intestine, these muscles expand and contract (an action called peristalsis). The small caliber of the meat requires the intestine to contract significantly to move the mass through the intestinal system. This contrasts with fibrous foods, which fill up with water and become a wide mass that is easily moved through the intestinal tract. Diverticulosis is also associated with herniations of the intestinal wall and can lead to diverticulitis, a condition characterized by inflammation (often due to obstruction) and, occasionally, perforation (the formation of a hole) in one or more diverticula.

When patients with diverticulosis have muscle spasms that cause cramps, a high-fiber diet, fiber supplements, and antispasmodic drugs may eliminate the symptoms. A high-fiber diet has also been shown to reduce the incidence of complications.

Diverticulitis, the more severe condition, usually subsides with bed rest and antibiotics. If the symptoms are severe, treatment may also include a liquid diet or intravenous fluids. Surgical treatment may be needed if perforation

Diverticulosis/-litis

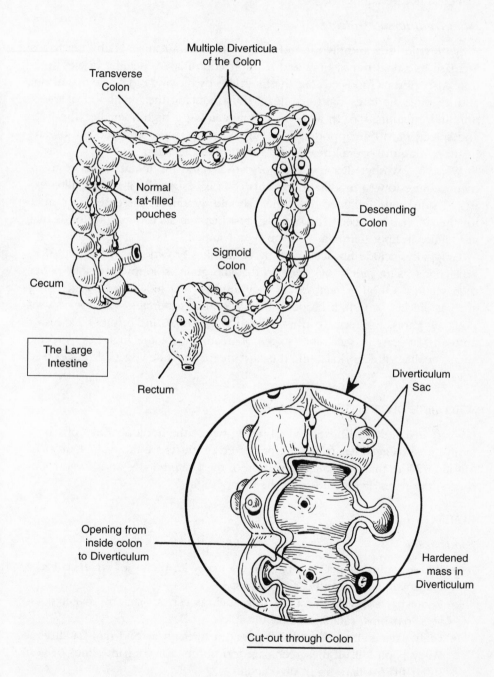

Multiple Diverticula
of the Colon

Transverse
Colon

Normal
fat-filled
pouches

Descending
Colon

Cecum

Sigmoid
Colon

The Large
Intestine

Rectum

Diverticulum
Sac

Opening from
inside colon
to Diverticulum

Hardened
mass in
Diverticulum

Cut-out through Colon

causes a large abscess or peritonitis, if a tight stricture develops, or if hemorrhage cannot be controlled.

From Traditional Medicine

A diet low in fiber and high in red meat is the central cause. High-fiber foods increase intestinal transit time and support coordinated, healthy bowel function. Also, fibrous foods cleanse the intestines by moving old waste matter out and keeping the intestinal tract clean, thus reducing the likelihood of infection and inflammation. In addition to maintaining a high-fiber diet, the liver and spleen must be supported (see Part IV), since these are essential organs in supporting the overall health and function of digestion.

While a low-fiber diet is the major cause, often the initial stages of treatment require low to moderate amounts of fiber, especially if diverticulitis exists. Those with inflamed intestines should gradually increase fiber after inflammation is reduced. The bowels must become accustomed to foods that are higher in fiber than was previously consumed.

Gradually include fibrous foods by combining brown rice with white rice; boil grains using plenty of water so that the grain is soupy and soft, rather than glutinous; boil vegetables till they are soft; eat less fibrous vegetables, such as onions, squash, broccoli, brussels sprouts, watercress, potatoes, sweet potatoes, yams, and roots (carrots, rutabagas, parsnips, and turnips). Eat lesser amounts, at least in the initial stages of treatment, of the high-fiber greens, such as collard greens, kale, and mustard greens. Include vegetable juices (see below).

WHO GETS DIVERTICULAR DISEASE?

It is rare in Third World nations and Japan, where the traditional diet of whole grains, fresh vegetables, fruit, and fermented products are the main sources of nutrition. More than half the population of the United States and Western Europe suffer from diverticulosis by the age of eighty.

REMEDIES

Foods to Eat

- Whole grains, boiled or pressure cooked with plenty of water to make grain wet, soupy, and easy to digest
- Root vegetables, boiled until soft, such as carrots, onions, sweet potatoes, parsnips, rutabagas, and turnips
- Leafy greens, boiled until soft and run through a food mill (such as a Foley Food Mill) if the greens are too fibrous for your intestines or you suffer from a flare-up of diverticulitis

Choose any of the following during the acute stage, consuming only one type of liquid at any single meal.

- Water (6–8 glasses)
- Carrot juice
- Carrot and lettuce juice
- Celery and lettuce juice
- Beet root juice
- Watercress juice
- Grape juice
- Apple juice
- Chlorophyll liquid
- Spirulina liquid drinks

After all painful symptoms have subsided, add semisolids slowly and carefully, watching for a reaction.

- Papaya
- Mashed banana
- Steamed carrots
- Baked yams or sweet potatoes

If the above can be tolerated, begin to add more high-fiber foods.

- Raw, grated apple
- Raw, grated carrot
- Brown rice, well cooked and masticated
- Tofu
- Steamed fish

After about six weeks, continue with a high-fiber diet. This will help heal the intestinal walls and prevent further severe attacks of diverticulosis.

Foods to Avoid

- Fruit skins and fruit
- Fruit and vegetables with small, hard seeds, such as tomatoes, cucumbers, figs, strawberries, raspberries, and guavas

For the regeneration of the liver, be sure to avoid:

- Intoxicants
- Stimulants
- Oily foods, especially poor-quality oils
- Meat

- Dairy products
- Eggs
- Poultry
- Spicy foods

Herbs to Treat Diverticular Disease

- Slippery elm tea
- Comfrey tea
- Marshmallow tea
- Fenugreek and comfrey tablets, 2 tablets every 2 hours
- Myrrh/goldenseal capsules, 2 capsules every 2 hours, when there is inflammation
- Follow the herbal treatment for colitis

Hydrotherapy

- Alternate hot and cold sitz baths
- Hot, moist compress for pain relief
- Hot sitz bath for pain relief

Supplements

- Beta carotene: 15–30 mg per day
- Vitamin B complex: 25–50 mg per day
- Vitamin E: 100–400 IU per day
- Vitamin C: 100–500 mg per day

DIZZINESS

SYMPTOMS

Loss of equilibrium, with light-headedness, a sensation of spinning, often accompanied by nausea, vomiting, sweating, or fainting.

WHAT IS DIZZINESS?

From Modern Western Medicine

Harmless in most cases, dizziness usually is caused by a momentary decline in the blood pressure of the brain brought on when one gets up quickly from a sitting or lying position. Such sudden drops in brain blood pressure, called postural hypotension, is most common among the elderly and in people taking medication for high blood pressure. Similar symptoms may come from temporary or partial blockages in the blood supply to the brain, known as a TIA (transient ischemic attack).

Other causes include fatigue, fever, stress, anemia, disorders of the heart, and hypoglycemia. Chronic loss of equilibrium is usually due to a disorder of the inner ear, acoustic nerve, or brain stem.

Brief episodes of mild dizziness usually clear up after taking a few deep breaths or resting for a short time. Severe, prolonged, or recurrent dizziness requires medical attention.

From Traditional Medicine

In Chinese medicine, dizziness is thought to be brought on by an imbalance in the liver meridian and the condition known as wind. Wind is described in Chinese classics as an environmental force that enters the body, often in combination with heat, cold, dampness, or dry conditions. The general signs of excess wind are instability or turbulence of one's physical, emotional, and psychological condition, manifesting as sudden changes in physical health or onsets of anger, for example. Fat- and cholesterol-rich foods raise blood pressure and heat within the body. As heat rises, a turbulent condition (wind) develops in the liver meridian, blood vessels, and brain, causing dizziness. The person with turbulent wind and dizziness needs yin fluids—fluids that create relaxation—to cool, calm, and nurture the liver, all of which will inhibit wind and heat. (See page 144.)

REMEDIES

General Recommendations

- Rest and get plenty of sleep to calm the liver and liver meridian.
- Drink vegetable juices, especially celery and carrot juice.

- Avoid anger, stress, and emotional upset.
- Take warm baths for short periods (no more than twenty minutes).
- Spend time in relaxing environments, such as in nature.

Foods to Eat

The following foods stimulate the liver out of a stagnant condition and overcome dizziness.

- Sour and pungent foods
- Watercress
- Onion family
- Mustard greens
- Raw foods, herbs, and spices
- Honey mixed with lemon, lime, or grapefruit juice: 1 teaspoon honey per cup of juice
- Turmeric
- Basil
- Cumin
- Dill
- Ginger
- Black pepper
- Sauerkraut: 1–2 teaspoons, 3 or 4 times per week
- Vegetable juices, especially carrot and celery

Foods for building liver yin and blood:

- Mung beans and sprouts
- Chlorophyll-rich foods
- Cucumber
- Tofu
- Millet
- Fresh, cold-pressed flaxseed oil
- Dark grapes
- Blackberries and raspberries
- Blackstrap molasses

The following specifically reduce liver wind.

- Celery
- Oats
- Black soybeans
- Black sesame seeds
- Kuzu
- Coconut

Foods to Avoid

According to Chinese medicine, the following foods obstruct and damage the liver.

- Meat
- Cheese
- Eggs
- Hydrogenated and poor-quality fats
- Nuts and seeds (in excess)
- Chemicals (as found in food and water)
- Intoxicants
- Processed and refined foods
- Crabmeat
- Buckwheat

Herbs to Treat Dizziness

- Catnip: infusion, steep 5–15 minutes, 1 oz to 1 cup as needed. (Do not boil herb.)
- Chamomile: tincture, 30–60 drops, 3 times/day; infusion, steep ten to thirty minutes (do not boil flowers), 6 oz., 2 or 3 times daily
- Peppermint: infusion, steep 5–15 minutes, 6 oz., 3 times daily; fluid extract: ½–2 tsp., 3 times daily
- Chinese herbs: Dong quai, rehmannia, and peony can be used singly but are even more effective when taken together in equal parts. Good when liver blood is excessively tight from stress, alcohol, high fat, and deficiency.

Hydrotherapy

- Ginger compress on liver

DYSPEPSIA

SYMPTOMS

Heartburn, nausea, reflux, stomachache, cramps, belching, and flatulence are all listed under the general rubric known as dyspepsia.

WHAT IS DYSPEPSIA?

From Modern Western Medicine

Dyspepsia is the medical term for indigestion and is usually caused by eating spicy foods, fatty foods, eating too rapidly, or overeating. Eating when under stress, when angry, or when suffering from some other acute emotional condition can also cause dyspepsia. Chronic indigestion can also be caused by peptic ulcer, gallstones, or esophagitis (inflammation of the esophagus).

The best remedy is to avoid overeating, eating too quickly, and to avoid foods that cause indigestion. Antacids and milk may help symptoms subside.

From Traditional Medicine

Indigestion is caused by numerous factors, among which are poor food combinations, failure to chew adequately, emotional upset, eating too rapidly, and from excessively cold foods or excessively spicy ones.

Food combining is an important element in establishing healthy digestion, although individuals may have to decide for themselves which combinations of foods work best. Different types of foods require different digestive enzymes. Some foods may inhibit the production of enzymes needed to digest others. When many different types of foods are eaten in the same meal, or when food is eaten chaotically, the body is unable to manufacture all of the necessary enzymes simultaneously. Digestion still takes place, but partially through bacterial action, which always results in fermentation and the associated problem of indigestion. The general recommendations below are useful guides to proper food combining.

REMEDIES

Foods to Eat

The following are techniques for successful food combining.

- Eat simpler meals.
- Eat protein and starchy foods in separate meals.
- Proteins, fats, and starches combine best with green and nonstarchy vegetables.

- Salty foods should be eaten first.
- Fruits and sweetened foods should be eaten alone.
- Melons are eaten alone since they digest very quickly.
- Celery and lettuce are the only two vegetables that can be eaten with fruit.
- Don't drink fruit juice between meals unless two hours have passed since a starch meal or four hours after a meal containing concentrated proteins.

Specific foods to aid indigestion are:

- Apples inhibit growth of ferments and disease-producing bacteria in the intestines.
- Barley treats indigestion from starchy food stagnation or poorly tolerated mother's milk in infants.
- Grapefruit peel moves and regulates spleen-pancreas digestive energy and is good for getting rid of gas.
- Lemons and limes are especially helpful for those who eat a high-fat, high-protein diet. They alleviate flatulence and indigestion.
- Umeboshi plums (sometimes called Japanese Alka-Seltzer): Take 1 plum or ½ teaspoon of umeboshi paste. Will cure most dyspepsia in ten minutes.
- Carrots treat indigestion, excess stomach acid, and heartburn.

Foods to Avoid

- Poor food combinations
- Meat
- Dairy products
- Eggs
- Poor-quality oils
- Sugar
- Spicy foods
- Fried foods
- Intoxicants

Herbs to Treat Dyspepsia

- Make an infusion of the following:

  2 parts angelica
  ¼ part fennel seed
  ¼ part anise seed
  ½ part ginger

Make an infusion of a teaspoon of herb to one cup of boiling water. Drink one-half cup four times daily between meals.

- According to Michael Tierra, author of *Planetary Herbology,* make an extract in any white wine using:

1 part dandelion root
1 part calamus root
1 part gentian
1 part angelica
1 part valerian
½ part gingerroot

Use two ounces of herbs to one pint of wine and let sit for two weeks. Take one teaspoon before and after meals.

Homeopathy

- Bryonia: if your stomach feels heavy after eating and is sensitive to touch; moving makes you feel worse; or if you have bitter risings and may vomit
- Carbo vegetabilis: if even the plainest food causes gas and belching about one-half hour after eating; if any indulgence causes a headache; or if there is craving for fresh air
- Chamomilla: if indigestion follows a fit of anger and irritability; if stomach is distended with gas and cramping; if your mouth has bitter taste; if your cheeks are flushed; or if you have an aversion to warm drinks
- Ignatia: if you are tense and nervous and crave food that doesn't agree with you; for rumbling in the bowels and sour belching; or for a tendency to take deep breaths or sigh frequently
- Nux vomica: for the hard-driven type who overindulges; for heartburn, belching, and bloating of the abdomen a few hours after eating; and for possible constipation

Chinese Medicine

Congee is a simple rice soup that harmonizes digestion. It is eaten throughout China as a breakfast food and is made by cooking rice with plenty of water. Different foods are added, which makes them more therapeutic and more easily assimilated because of being cooked with the rice. Try the following combinations:

- Rice with carrot as a digestive aid
- Rice with fennel harmonizes the stomach and expels gas
- Rice with ginger for deficient, cold digestive weakness, vomiting, and indigestion
- Sweet rice for vomiting and indigestion

EARACHE AND EAR INFECTION

SYMPTOMS

Two types of earaches are most common: *otitis externa,* a severe and stabbing pain that is sometimes accompanied by fever and loss of hearing; the second, *otitis media,* is associated with irritation, itching, discharge (such as a boil or abscess), and temporary, mild loss of hearing.

WHAT IS AN EARACHE AND/OR EAR INFECTION?

From Modern Western Medicine

The most common form of earache, otitis media, is caused by an infection of the middle ear and is what most young children suffer from when they have an earache. Bacteria or viral infections cause inflammation and blockage in the eustachian tubes, which results in pain. Such earaches account for nearly one-third of all doctor's visits for children up to age five.

Otitis externa (inflammation of the outer ear canal) is often caused by infection from bacteria growing in the ear, caused most commonly by water infiltrating the ear canal while swimming or showering (swimmer's ear). Infection may be localized or affect the whole canal.

A much rarer cause of earache is herpes zoster infection, which causes blisters in the ear canal and may persist for weeks or months after the infection has cleared.

Dental problems, tonsilitis, throat cancer, pain in the lower jaw or neck muscles, and other disorders affecting areas near the ear may cause occasional earaches, as well.

Analgesics for pain and antibiotics for infection are often prescribed. Pus in the outer ear may need to be aspirated, which requires a visit to your doctor. Pus in the middle ear may require draining through a hole made in the eardrum.

From Traditional Medicine

Many chronic or recurrent middle ear infections have a nutritional basis. A diet rich in mucus-forming foods, such as fatty foods, refined grains, artificial ingredients, dairy products, sugar, wheat, and excessively cold drinks will all bring on ear infections in children. This diet and the lack of vegetables and mineral-rich foods are usually the primary cause. Such a diet can be immune-depressing and increase the likelihood of infection. The body is then susceptible to colds, flu, tonsilitis, and other diseases that may affect the ear. Once an infection damages the tissues of the inner ear or canal, recurrent infections

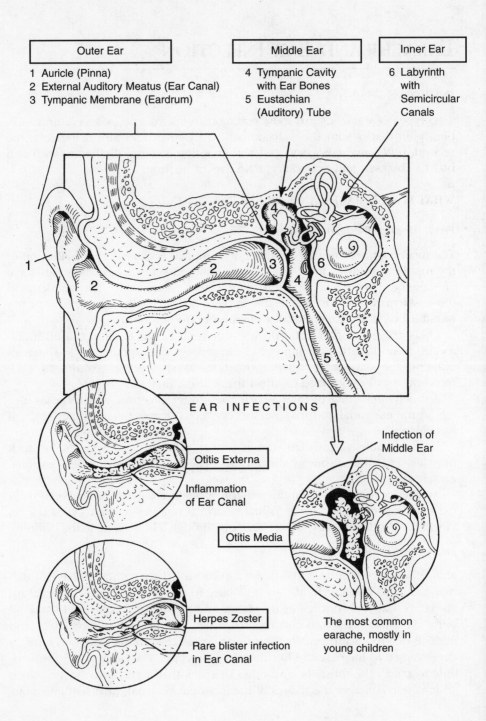

Outer Ear

1 Auricle (Pinna)
2 External Auditory Meatus (Ear Canal)
3 Tympanic Membrane (Eardrum)

Middle Ear

4 Tympanic Cavity
  with Ear Bones
5 Eustachian
  (Auditory) Tube

Inner Ear

6 Labyrinth
  with
  Semicircular
  Canals

EAR INFECTIONS

Otitis Externa

Inflammation
of Ear Canal

Herpes Zoster

Rare blister infection
in Ear Canal

Infection of
Middle Ear

Otitis Media

The most common
earache, mostly in
young children

are far more likely. In addition, a diet rich in saturated fats encourages the excess production of earwax, which can contribute to infection and earache.

External ear infections have more to do with the environment and the infiltration of water (i.e., swimmer's ear).

It is possible to treat many of these infections at the early stages using natural means; however, if the infection has progressed to acute pain, antibiotics may be necessary.

REMEDIES

Foods to Eat

- Juice, vegetable, and water fast
- Carrots and carrot juice (The beta-carotene/vitamin A is anti-inflammatory and protects against ear infections.)
- Parsley
- Citrus
- Steamed onions
- Honey/onion syrup: Slice a large onion thinly, place in a bowl, and cover with one to two tablespoons of honey. Cover container tightly and allow to sit for eight hours. Mash, strain, and take in one-teaspoon doses, four to eight times per day.
- Potassium broth: Take a quarter inch of outer peelings of potatoes (including skin), fresh parsley, unpeeled carrots, beet greens, onions, garlic, and any other organically grown green vegetables. Prepare broth by washing and chopping the vegetables and then simmering in a large, covered pot of water for thirty to forty minutes. Strain and drink the broth, discarding the veggies. Excess may be stored in glass containers in the refrigerator up to two days.
- Raw green apples

Foods to Avoid

- Wheat
- Dairy products
- Meat
- Hydrogenated oils
- Sweets
- Refined foods
- Additives
- Stimulants
- Alcohol

Herbs to Treat Earache and Ear Infection

- Mullein (antibacterial)—most effective application: 4–6 drops, 4 times a day in the ear
- Citrus seed extract is an extremely potent natural antibiotic. According to Chinese medicine, because of its bitter properties, it dries damp conditions, as in the case of severe ear infections.
- Garlic oil: Place in the ear canal once a day to help clear infections. Safe for children. To prepare the oil, crush several garlic cloves and soak in three ounces of olive oil for at least three days. Then strain the oil through a cloth.
- Echinacea in tincture form, both as eardrops and taken internally: ½–1 teaspoon, three or four times per day

Homeopathy

- Pulsatilla: for an earache that comes on after a cold, or in a child who tends to whine rather than cry loudly
- Chamomilla: for the child who is extremely irritable and cries loudly; for soreness and severe pain; or if ears feel stopped
- Aconite: for the external ear when it is red, hot, painful, or swollen
- Belladonna: for earaches with a sudden onset, especially when earache is in right ear; for severe pain in the middle and external ear; and for throbbing pain deep in the ear, which is at the tempo of the heartbeat
- Magnesia phosphorica: for earaches without respiratory infection; for sharp, aching, jerking or tearing pain; or for intermittent pain

Essential Oils

Massage these oils around the outer ear and neck.

- Chamomile: analgesic, antiseptic, antibacterial
- Lavender: analgesic, antimicrobial, sedative
- Tea tree: anti-infectious, anti-inflammatory, immunostimulant

ECZEMA

SYMPTOMS

Chronic skin eruptions occur, often inflamed and red, accompanied by scaling, blisters, and itching.

WHAT IS ECZEMA?

From Modern Western Medicine

Sometimes called dermatitis, eczema is caused by an allergy but often occurs for no known reason. There are several types. *Atopic* eczema, which occurs in people who have an inherited tendency to the disorder, is a chronic, superficial inflammation. Common in infants between the ages of two months and eighteen months, atopic eczema occurs as a mild but very itchy rash, consisting of small red pimples that usually appear on the face, in the inner creases of the elbow, and behind the knees. The rash spreads as the baby scratches the irritation. Atopic eczema often clears up by itself, but emollients, such as petroleum jelly, are usually effective in providing some comfort and reducing the irritation. Doctors prescribe corticosteroid ointments and antibiotic drugs in severe cases.

Nummular eczema usually occurs in adults as an itchy, scaly rash that often appears in circular patches. Cortiscosteroid ointments are often prescribed, but the disorder does not respond well to treatment.

Hand eczema is caused by irritating substances, such as detergents, that come in contact with the skin. The hands and palms may be covered with itchy blisters, scales, and cracks. Protective gloves can prevent exposure to irritants. To further protect the hands, thoroughly dry after washing and cover with an unscented hand cream.

People with varicose veins can suffer from *stasis* dermatitis, a condition in which areas of the legs can become inflamed, irritated, and discolored. The legs can be wrapped with compression bandages or special stockings to reduce swelling. Mild corticosteroid ointments are prescribed by doctors.

In order to reduce irritation of the skin, absorbent cotton fabrics should be worn.

From Traditional Medicine

The skin is one of the ways the body eliminates waste products. When the blood-cleansing and eliminative organs—especially the liver and kidneys—function properly, the demands on the skin to eliminate waste is small, and can be handled easily without causing any skin irritation or eruption. However, when waste products accumulate and exceed the capacity of the blood-cleansing organs, the skin is utilized by the body to eliminate waste. Such elimination can manifest as skin eruptions, scaling, pimples, and rashes, such as eczema.

Most skin diseases, including eczema, are caused by an excess of saturated fats. Omega-3 polyunsaturated fats, such as fish oils, improve overall fat metabolism when they are eaten as food, rather than taken in capsules or added to foods.

REMEDIES

Foods to Eat

- Whole grains
- Vegetables, especially beta-carotene–rich ones such as carrots, winter squash, and leafy greens
- Beans
- Seaweeds (to detoxify)
- Sprouts, especially alfalfa and soy
- Microalgae
- Whole fruits, in moderation
- Sesame seeds, which are rich in oleic fatty acids
- Unrefined sesame oil

Foods to Avoid

- Animal products
- Fruit juices
- Spicy foods
- Fatty foods
- Sweets
- Citrus fruits

Herbs to Treat Eczema

The following herbs are used to induce sweating, which is a good way to eliminate the toxins that are trying to come out.

- Sarsaparilla root
- Burdock seed
- Yarrow leaves and flowers

The following herbs are all potent blood cleansers (use any one).

- Dandelion root
- Goldenseal
- Chaparral leaves

- Echinacea root
- Yellow dock root
- Burdock root
- Red clover blossoms
- Horehound leaves
- Poke root, which is a traditional Western tea for chronic skin conditions. (Use no more than one tablespoon of poke tea twice daily.)
- Equal parts of sarsaparilla root, yellow dock, sassafras root bark, marshmallow root, and red clover blossoms

Hydrotherapy (apply to surface of the skin)

- Raw honey
- Goldenseal or poke root tea
- Slices of fresh papaya
- Grated crushed daikon radish or raw potato (squeeze out juice)
- Sliced cucumber, dabbed with vinegar

Chinese Medicine

The above dietary suggestions are consistent with Chinese medicine. Chronic eczema is frequently caused by inadequate yin, or the capacity to withhold energy in the kidneys and other organs. Symptoms of deficient yin that manifest as eczema include frequent thirst, weight loss, insomnia, night sweats, and hot palms and soles. Other symptoms may include anxiety, surface energy, irritation. Any one of these symptoms may suggest inadequate yin, in which case the following foods and herbs are recommended: millet, barley, wheat germ, wheat, rice, seaweeds, microalgae (especially spirulina and chlorella), tofu, black beans, kidney beans, mung beans and their sprouts, beets, string beans, kuzu, persimmon, grapes, blackberry, and watermelon. Herbs that strengthen yin are marshmallow root, prepared rehmannia root, mandarin, asparagus root, and aloe vera gel.

EDEMA

SYMPTOMS

Swelling of hands, ankles, feet, face, abdomen, or other areas of the body. Edema is often a secondary symptom associated with normal changes in one's physical condition, such as pregnancy or the menstrual cycle, as well as with a wide array of more serious disorders, such as injury or kidney, liver, and heart disease. It can also be a side effect of any one of several drugs.

WHAT IS EDEMA?

From Modern Western Medicine

Edema is an abnormal accumulation of fluid in the body tissues. The swelling can be local (at the site of an injury, for example) or general (such as from kidney or heart disease). The kidneys maintain the balance of liquid in the tissues. Illnesses affecting the kidneys, such as nephrotic syndrome (in which the kidneys excrete an abnormal amount of protein from the blood) or renal failure (in which salt is prevented from being excreted from the body) can upset the liquid balance of the body. Disorders involving other organs, such as the liver (in the case of cirrhosis) and heart (such as heart failure) can also give rise to edema. Finally, corticosteroid and androgen drugs, high-estrogen contraceptives, and antidiuretic hormones all can throw off the fluid balance in the body and cause edema.

Usually, edema does not result in weight gain until after the fluid in the tissues increases by more than about 15 percent. Then, the ankles usually begin to swell, but in some severe cases, body cavities can fill with fluid. Edema usually causes the swollen area to respond slowly to pressure from your finger. If you press the swollen area with your finger and the tissue remains indented, you have edema.

Treatment is directed at the primary disorder that may be causing the edema, but if the underlying cause is intractable, excess fluid may be removed from the body by restricting sodium intake and taking diuretic drugs.

From Traditional Medicine

Edema can be a sign of a serious underlying disease—such as congestive heart failure, kidney disease, or cirrhosis—and warrants a physician's examination before you engage in any self-treatment. Once the possible serious disorders have been ruled out, the milder issues, such as menstrual cycle, pregnancy, and diet can be dealt with. Excessive consumption of salt or sodium-containing foods is one of the most common causes of edema. Weak kidneys are also a common cause of excess fluid retention.

REMEDIES

General Recommendations

- Have serious illnesses ruled out by a physician before self-treating.
- Strengthen kidneys and bladder (See Part IV).
- Eat moderate amounts of low-fat protein foods, such as fish and beans, which stimulate kidney function (a healthful guideline: fish once or twice a week; beans daily).
- Avoid excess protein. If you are eating a relatively high-protein diet, significantly reduce protein. (Guideline: A daily consumption of an animal food, such as fish, poultry, eggs, dairy products, and meat can be considered a high-protein diet.) Excess protein weakens the kidneys and will lead to a reduction in their overall strength and efficiency. High-protein consumption also contributes to bone loss such as osteoporosis, kidney disorders, and is associated with numerous types of cancer.

Foods to Eat

The following foods help reduce swelling.

- Fish
- Adzuki beans
- Barley
- Grapes
- Kidney beans
- Kombu/kelp seaweed
- Lettuce
- Nuts and seeds
- Peas
- Pineapple
- Pumpkin
- Soybeans
- Zucchini
- Watermelon

Foods to Avoid

- Processed foods
- Animal products
- Salty foods

Herbs to Treat Edema

- Blue cohosh: tincture, ½–1 tsp., 3 or 4 times daily; fluid extract, 10–30 drops (⅙ to ½ tsp.), 3 or 4 times/day
- Cleavers: fluid extract, ½–1 tsp., 3 or 4 times daily; infusion, 3 oz.–2 pints cold water, let stand 3–4 hours, drink 3 oz. (cold), 3 or 4 times daily, or

1½ oz.–1 pint of warm water, steep two hours, take 1 cup 3 or 4 times daily
- Corn silk (good when weak heart is the cause): infusion, steep 5–15 minutes, take 3 oz. as needed
- Gravel root or queen of the meadow: tincture, 30–60 drops (½–1 tsp.), 3 times daily; fluid extract, ½–1 tsp., 3 times/day
- Hawthorn berries (for edema of heart origin): tincture, 10–20 drops
- Watermelon seed: Use infusion of dried seeds.

Hydrotherapy

- Hot and cold sitz baths

Supplements

- Beta-carotene: 15–30 IU per day
- Vitamin B complex: 25–50 mg, once a day
- Vitamin C: 100–500 mg
- Vitamin E: 100–400 IU, 1 or 2 times per day
- Potassium: 500 mg per day (No RDA for potassium exists. It is widely available in fruits and vegetables. Experts recommend 3000 mg per day, which is easily obtainable from food alone.)

EMPHYSEMA

SYMPTOMS

Difficulty inhaling and exhaling, accompanied by wheezing, chronic cough, expectoration, shortness of breath, and sometimes by foul breath.

WHAT IS EMPHYSEMA?

From Modern Western Medicine

Emphysema is a condition in which the air sacs in the lungs, called alveoli, become damaged and eventually burst open, thus reducing the number of alveoli. In effect, the lungs get smaller, the blood receives less oxygen, and more carbon dioxide is retained within the lungs and blood. A chemical within the lungs, called alpha-antitrypsin, prevents some of this damage, but its protective effects are inadequate against the main cause of ephysema, which is cigarette smoking. In time, the lungs lose their size, functional capacity, and elasticity, causing ever-increasing difficulty breathing.

A host of secondary illnesses usually set in, including chronic bronchitis, pulmonary hypertension (elevated blood pressure in the pulmonary artery), cor pulmonale (enlargement and strain on the right side of the heart), and edema (accumulation of fluid in the tissues), especially in the lower legs. People with advanced stages of the illness sometimes turn blue or purple.

By far, the most common cause of emphysema is cigarette smoking, though air pollution can be a contributing factor. In rare cases, an inherited deficiency of alpha-antitrypsin may give a person a predisposition to the illness.

Treatment can only control the disease. The person must stop smoking and then work on improving the efficiency of the remaining lung tissue with bronchodilator drugs, which widen the bronchi and bronchioles. Corticosteroid drugs may be used to reduce inflammation in the lungs. To treat edema, diuretic drugs will be given. Sometimes, if the level of oxygen has dropped significantly, the patient can use a mask or cannula to take in more.

From Traditional Medicine

Emphysema is the result of many years of abuse. Optimal lung conditions cannot be restored, but with proper care, a reduction in the severity of the symptoms can be accomplished.

REMEDIES

Foods to Eat

- Whole grains
- Vegetables, especially cooked leafy greens, such as kale, collards, and mustard greens, twice daily (Steaming leafy green vegetables is an ideal preparation.)
- Legumes
- Chorophyll and Vitamin A foods (protect the lungs and provide cell renewal)
- Cereal grasses, such as wheat grass
- Apricot (not more than two or three a day)
- Pumpkin
- Carrots and carrot juice
- Daikon radishes
- Onions
- Garlic
- Citrus with pulp (high in vitamin C and bioflavonoids)

Foods to Avoid

- Dairy products
- Refined foods
- Alcohol
- Wheat

Herbs to Treat Emphysema

- Ephedra: tincture, ¼–1 teaspoon; tea, 1 cup, 2–3 times daily. Contains natural ephedrine, which acts as a bronchodilator. Consult your health practitioner if you suffer from heart disease, diabetes, glaucoma, or thyroid disease.
- Quebracho blanco (respiratory stimulant): tincture, 5–25 drops, three times/day
- Comfrey: decoction, simmer root thirty minutes, take 3 oz. frequently

Physiotherapy

- Postural drainage with percussion: Hang from the waist over the edge of a bed with a bowl placed at the head for easy expectoration. Apply a hot, moist compress to the back repeatedly for five to ten minutes, and then have a friend pound vigorously on the back with open palms. As mucus is loosened, it should be expectorated. Repeat one to three times per day.
- Alternate hot and cold chest packs to stimulate circulation, respiration, and mucus elimination.
- Alternate hot and cold showers.

- Stationary bicycling has been shown to be helpful. Increase amount and speed of any exercise. Best done in a warm, moist environment so as not to dry out the mucous membranes.
- Inhalations of various herbal steam mixtures help heal the lungs:

Mixture 1: Eucalyptus oil
Fir balsam
Tolu
Benzoin

Mixture 2: Sage
Thyme
Rosemary
Cloves

Supplements

- Beta-carotene: 15–30 mg per day
- Vitamin B complex: 50 mg per day
- Vitamin C: 100–500 mg per day
- Vitamin E: 100–500 mg per day

ENURESIS OR BED-WETTING

SYMPTOMS

Uncontrolled urination during sleep that occurs more than once a month. Enuresis is not considered a significant problem in children six years or younger.

WHAT IS ENURESIS OR BED-WETTING?

From Modern Western Medicine

In most cases, bed-wetting is due to the slow maturing of the nerves that control bladder function. In a minority of cases, there is an organic or physical disorder that causes the problem.

Treatment usually consists of reminding the child to urinate regularly during the day in order to help him or her recognize that his or her bladder is full. Sometimes a nighttime alarm system can be used to remind the child to get up and urinate. Restricting the intake of liquids two to three hours before bedtime reduces the need to urinate during the night. Making the child urinate before bed also helps, as well as waking him or her up two to three hours after falling asleep to go to the bathroom.

From Traditional Medicine

Eating excessive amounts of sugar and/or drinking too many soft drinks can expand the bladder or weaken control over it. A related problem is hypoglycemia, or low blood sugar, which tends to increase urination and can contribute to bed-wetting among children who have trouble controlling their bladders. Excessively cold conditions cause frequent urination in children, which may contribute to the problem.

Psychological reasons may be why a child of five years or older, who has gained control of his bladder, suddenly loses it. Among the most common of such problems are the birth of a second child, the separation of parents, or a reluctance to enter school. Check to see if the child has dreams or nightmares that trigger the bed-wetting. (See homeopathy on pages 163 and 164.)

Spinal lesions, caused by a trauma at birth or from a fall, are the most important physical reasons for bed-wetting. The lesions interfere with the normal flow of both nerve impulses and circulation to the bladder. This is so common that all children suffering from enuresis should receive a spinal exam.

Finally, some children who wet the bed have no other problem but that their bladders are small. These children should avoid drinking too many liquids, should be encouraged to urinate before bed, and should be wakened in the middle of the night, if necessary.

WHO GETS ENURESIS?

About 10 percent of children older than five suffer from enuresis, with a slightly greater number of boys having the problem than girls.

REMEDIES

General Recommendations

The remedies listed below are all designed to strengthen the bladder or improve control over the bladder, or both. See Part IV for ways to strengthen the kidneys and bladder.

Foods to Eat

- Brown rice and other grains
- Small amounts of nori seaweed to increase minerals and strengthen kidneys and bladder (Flavored or spicy nori is available and widely enjoyed by children.)
- White fish
- Beans, especially black beans
- Parsley
- Wheat berry, as bread, whole berries, or herb tea
- Sweet rice
- Squash
- Onions (especially baked onion)

Food to Avoid

- Anything suspected of being an allergen
- Strong spices
- Salt
- Sugar
- Non-organic foods containing pesticides
- Refined white sugar
- Excessive intake of soft drinks

Herbs to Treat Enuresis

- Parsley: standard dosage or 3–9 g
- Dioscorea (qi tonic): 6–15 g
- Rose hips (good for all complaints of deficient kidney yin): 3–12 g

Homeopathy

Choose the most appropriate remedy and take two tablets, three times a day. Reduce frequency as child improves and discontinue when improvement is established.

- Belladonna: for the child who sleeps so deeply he cannot wake up or who is sensitive to jarring, the cold, and changes in the weather
- Causticum: for the child who wets the bed in the first few hours of sleep and tends to wet the bed more frequently in dry, clear weather or who has weakness and spasms in various parts of the body
- Equisetum: for children who have dreams or nightmares that trigger bed-wetting
- Pulsatilla: for the child who is shy, sensitive, weepy, and affectionate
- Sepia: for children who wet in their first few hours of sleep; especially good for children who enjoy vigorous activity but are sensitive to cold air

Hydrotherapy

Cold sitz baths are essential to tone the bladder and associated organs. They stimulate both circulation of blood and lymph as well as nervous flow to these areas. Cold sitz baths strengthen both voluntary and involuntary muscles in the pelvic region. Begin the bath with just cool water and add colder water progressively until the temperature is as cold as the child will bear without undue complaint. The object is to stay immersed from hips to mid-thigh in very cold water for up to five minutes. The duration of the sitz bath should begin with short immersions, gradually increasing the treatment time to the maximum of five minutes. If the child is willing, it is more therapeutic to immerse directly into very cold water rather than decrease the temperature gradually.

Repeat this cold sitz bath one or two times daily for several months or longer, as needed. Follow the bath by vigorously drying with a rough towel until the child feels warm. If the cold sitz bath is too cold for your child, try the alternate hot and cold bath, remaining in the hot water one minute and the cold water for two to three minutes. Repeat three times, ending with the cold water.

Chinese Medicine

Enuresis indicates that the kidneys lack sufficient qi or energy to control the urine, and they therefore need to be strengthened. Recommended foods to strengthen the kidneys are listed above. Other things that are helpful are crushed or whole oyster shell and clam shell. They can be purchased at Chinese herb stores. They should be crushed and decocted into a tea. Oyster-shell calcium supplements can also be taken. Raspberry and blackberry leaves are helpful in the form of herbal teas.

Supplements

- Beta-carotene: 15–30 mg per day
- Vitamin B complex: 25 mg per day
- Vitamin E: 100–200 IU, one time per day

EPILEPSY

SYMPTOMS:

Transient neurological abnormalities or seizures provoked by aberrant electrical activity in the brain are known as epilepsy.

WHAT IS EPILEPSY?

From Modern Western Medicine

Epilepsy is associated with recurrent seizures of the central nervous system that cause temporary changes in brain function. Usually, there are no apparent causes for the onset of the seizures, though they have been known to be set off by trauma, shock, and flashing lights. Epilepsy may be caused by any of a wide variety of conditions, including head injury, birth trauma, brain infection, brain tumor, stroke, drug intoxication, drug or alcohol withdrawal states, or metabolic imbalances in the body.

Epileptic seizures are classified in two categories: generalized and partial seizures, depending on how rapidly the seizure spreads to other parts of the brain, which determines how severe the seizure is and how much of the body is involved. Generalized seizures affect the entire body and may involve a large part of the brain. The two main types of generalized seizures are *grand mal* and *petit mal* (absence seizures).

A grand mal seizure causes unconsciousness and uncontrollable jerking and twitching of the entire body. Once the seizure has passed, muscles relax, but bowel and bladder control may be lost temporarily. The person is often disoriented. Petit mal seizures occur in children with epilepsy. They cause a momentary loss of consciousness that can last for a few seconds to half a minute, but no abnormal movements take place during the seizure.

Partial seizures are categorized as *simple seizures,* in which consciousness is sustained, and *complex seizures,* in which it is lost. Simple partial seizures cause abnormal twitching movements, tingling sensations, or hallucinations involving smell, vision, or taste. They last several minutes and can occur without warning. During complex partial seizures, the person is dazed, unresponsive, and may suffer from jerking or twitching movements.

The frequency of seizures can be controlled through anticonvulsive drugs and by avoiding stress and fatigue. One-third of those who get epilepsy eventually outgrow the disorder; another third are able to control the frequency of the seizures with drug therapy.

From Traditional Medicine

Some research points to vitamin and mineral deficiencies as possible causes of epilepsy. The key nutrients that appear deficient in epileptics are vitamin B$_6$, vitamin A, folic acid, vitamin D, zinc, taurine, magnesium, and calcium. Both calcium and magnesium supplements have been shown to control seizure activity.

On the other hand, toxic metals such as lead, copper, mercury, and aluminum have also been known to cause seizures. Children are especially sensitive to such metals, and exposure is common through aluminum cookware, auto exhaust, industrial pollution, and copper water pipes. Hypoglycemia, which brings on feelings of fatigue and stress, may be a secondary factor in triggering the onset of convulsions. Scientists have estimated that between 50 and 90 percent of all epileptics suffer from low blood sugar, and 70 percent have abnormal glucose tolerance levels. Case studies have suggested that a wide array of chemicals—including pesticides, food additives, and even foods such as peanuts and tea—have brought on seizures.

WHO GETS EPILEPSY?

About one person in two hundred suffers from epilepsy. About one million U.S. citizens have epilepsy. It usually starts in childhood or adolescence. Many outgrow it and do not require medication.

REMEDIES

Chinese Medicine

Mucus, or what Chinese healers call *mucus-foam,* and internal heat combine to obstruct the nervous system and trigger a variety of disorders, including epilepsy. Heat is often seen as yang, or outgoing energy (see Part III), that, when it is excessive, can destabilize the nervous system. The combination of heat and mucus combine to create symptoms associated with epilepsy: yellow tongue coating, fast pulse, and sudden, forceful, or violent movement. Most cases of excessive mucus and heat improve if certain foods (see opposite) are reduced or totally eliminated.

Foods to Eat

- Whole grains
- Vegetables: A wide variety must be eaten, including leafy greens, round vegetables, tubers, and roots.
- Beans
- Sea vegetables are rich in minerals, which are essential to healthy nervous system function.
- Miso soup

Foods to Avoid

In addition to the following foods, avoid eating late at night, overeating, and eating an excessive number of ingredients within a single dish or single meal.

- Meat
- Dairy products
- Eggs
- Sugar
- Refined foods
- Cigarettes
- Cold liquids
- Coffee
- Alcohol
- Nuts and seeds (especially peanuts)
- Simple sugars from sweeteners and fruit

Herbs to Treat Epilepsy

All the herbs below are contraindicated for deficient nervous conditions and neurasthenia.

- Valerian is sedating, but it is warming, so people with warm conditions may not benefit (see the section on herbology in Part III). Infusion, 3–9 g; tincture, 10–30 drops
- Lady's slipper: decoction, 3–9 g; tincture, 10–30 drops; 3 or 4 times daily
- Skullcap: Take with valerian or lady's slipper. Make sure you get the genuine herb and not germander. Infusion, 3–9 g; tincture, 10–30 drops
- Passionflower: infusion, 3–9 g; tincture, 10–30 drops

Supplements

- Beta-carotene: 15–30 mg per day
- Vitamin B complex (essential to proper nervous system functioning): 50 mg per day
- Vitamin B_6: 2–10 mg per day
- Vitamin C: 100 mg per day
- Folic acid: 1 mg per day
- Vitamin E: 100–400 IU per day
- Calcium: 800–1000 mg per day
- Magnesium: 400–500 mg per day

FATIGUE

SYMPTOMS

Fatigue is the experience of lack of energy, mental and physical weakness, lethargy, and depression, all of which combine to make performance of ordinary daily activities difficult or impossible.

WHAT IS FATIGUE?

From Modern Western Medicine

Perhaps the most common complaint among people today, fatigue is related to a number of factors that are taken for granted in modern life: sleep deprivation, stress, and bouts of depression. Fatigue is also a symptom of a more serious illness, such as a degenerative disease. A physical examination by a medical doctor can help to determine the cause of the fatigue.

From Traditional Medicine

Fatigue is a symptom that suggests that the body is out of balance. Ideally, our lives should be a balanced blend of work, play, rest, and intimacy with ourselves and our loved ones. Intimacy with self, of course, includes whatever spiritual practices and emotional pleasures one feels nourished by. Modern life tends to emphasize work above all other considerations, causing increasing mental, physical, and emotional tension. Such tension may be utilizing the available energy on one hand, and preventing energy from flowing smoothly throughout the body on the other. Without the free flow of energy throughout the body, individual organs become fatigued, elimination of waste is hampered, accumulation of toxins takes place, and one or another illness manifests. Fatigue, therefore, is the body's way of communicating that an imbalance exists that must be addressed and corrected.

Many different functions within the body may be responsible for creating fatigue. The first to be considered is nutrition. The primary and preferred source of energy for the human body is complex carbohydrates, found in whole grains, fresh vegetables, and fruits. Complex carbohydrates are composed of long chains that are digested slowly, providing long-lasting energy and endurance.

A diet composed of refined foods and simple sugars, on the other hand, can give rise to low blood sugar (hypoglycemia), one of the most common causes of fatigue. Typically, hypoglycemia causes feelings of weakness in the middle of the morning and the late afternoon, when the blood sugar supply from breakfast and lunch have been burned and glucose levels are low, often below fasting levels. At that point, sugar cravings arise. Consumption of sugar usually gives an initial burst of energy that is quickly burned off, leaving the person once again exhausted and feeling stressed, irritable, and weak. For those who suffer from hypoglycemia, the pancreas and adrenals are usually debilitated, making all stressful situations exceedingly difficult to deal with. Worry, anxiety, and fear arise easily when blood sugar levels fall and the adrenal glands are taxed beyond their limits.

Vitamin and mineral deficiencies can also cause fatigue. A lack of iron or vitamin B$_{12}$ can cause anemia. Other common deficiencies among people who eat a highly refined diet and suffer from fatigue include a lack of B vitamins, vitamins C and E, folic acid, zinc, and copper.

Caffeine often plays a major role in the onset of hypoglycemia and chronic fatigue. Caffeine overworks and eventually weakens the kidneys and adrenal glands. In Chinese medicine, kidney qi is regarded as the root of life energy and the basis for long-standing vitality and endurance. When the kidneys become depleted, the person experiences a deep sense of weakness, lack of willpower, and fatigue, as if the life force had been sapped from his or her tissues. (See Part IV for strengthening kidneys and bladder.)

Both an excess and a deficiency of protein can cause fatigue, as well. Excess protein causes the production of uric acid, which must be removed by the kidneys. In time, protein's acid by-products weaken and damage the kidneys, causing, among other things, fatigue. People with weak kidneys should sharply limit dietary protein. On the other hand, a protein deficiency prevents production of dopamine, a neurotransmitter that is essential for coordinated muscle action, physical alertness, aggression, and the utilization of energy.

Poor intestinal health can cause or contribute to lethargy and fatigue, as anyone who's ever suffered from constipation or diarrhea can attest to. Finally, lack of exercise causes poor circulation of blood and lymph, resulting in accumulation and stagnation of waste products throughout the body, which can cause fatigue.

REMEDIES

General Recommendations

- Get adequate sleep.
- Eat whole grains, fresh vegetables, and fruits.
- Avoid refined foods, especially simple sugars.
- Consider a multivitamin and mineral supplement while you are improving your diet.
- Exercise aerobically at least three or four times a week.

Foods to Eat

Iron-rich foods:

- Whole grains
- Legumes

- Fish
- Eggs
- Blackstrap molasses
- Green vegetables, such as parsley, collards, cabbage, kale, and watercress
- Dried fruit
- Apples
- Beets
- Carrots
- Yams
- Grape juice

Foods rich in vitamin B_{12}:

- Fish
- Eggs (fertilized and organic)
- Bitter almonds
- Apple seeds
- Apricots
- Prunes
- Miso
- Wheat
- Sunflower seeds
- Seaweed
- Spirulina

Foods rich in folic acid:

- Dark green, leafy vegetables
- Lentils
- Grains
- Spirulina

Foods to Avoid

- Refined foods
- Processed and devitalized foods
- Caffeinated beverages
- Meat
- Dairy products
- Excess oils, especially hydrogenated oils
- Sugar

Herbs to Treat Fatigue

- Siberian ginseng or eleuthero (strengthens adrenal glands): ½ teaspoon, 2 or 3 times/day
- Ginseng (strengthens adaptability to stress, energizes): tincture, ½ teaspoon; tea, 1 cup; capsules, two, 2 or 3 times daily
- Oats (counters exhaustion and depression): tincture, ½–1 teaspoon, 3 times/day; look for preparations that contain oat seed along with the straw.

Homeopathy

- Arnica: for fatigue from overwork
- Arsenicum: for anxiety and restlessness

Chinese Medicine

Fatigue is often a sign of weak spleen-pancreas qi. This qi, often called the middle qi, animates the periphery of the body. The strength of the arms and legs depends on this qi. To strengthen, use warming foods such as most complex carbohydrates, especially brown rice. Also good are oats, sweet rice, and pounded sweet rice. Carbohydrate-rich vegetables such as carrots, rutabagas, winter squash, parsnips, turnips, black beans, and pumpkin are excellent along with onions, leeks, black pepper, ginger, fennel, and garlic. Food must be chewed well and taken in small and frequent meals.

Physiotherapy

- Deep breathing exercises
- Outdoor exercise
- Morning walks on wet grass
- Meditation
- Massage: therapeutic, acupressure, or deep-tissue

Supplements

- Beta-carotene: 15–30 mg per day
- Vitamin B complex: 50 mg per day
- Vitamin C: 100 mg per day
- Vitamin E: 100–400 IU per day
- Calcium: 800 mg per day
- Magnesium: 400 mg per day
- Royal jelly: 1–3 capsules or 100–400 mg daily

Exercise

- Daily walking or some other form of light aerobic activity to boost circulation and promote increased oxygen intake
- Yoga and stretching exercises

Body/Mind/Spirit

- Meditate on why your life may be imbalanced, and take steps to correct that imbalance.
- Spend at least thirty minutes daily doing what you enjoy that does not include eating or watching television or any job-related activity.
- Maintain or restore a positive attitude toward your life through prayer, chanting, meditation, and play.

Fever

SYMPTOMS

A sudden and significant increase in body temperature, as measured by touch or with a thermometer. Fever is often accompanied by other symptoms, including pale, dry skin, sweating, cold chills, weakness, malaise, headache, and changes in breathing. There can be alternating conditions of dry, cold shivering and feelings of heat and sweating or combinations of both, such as cold and sweating.

WHAT IS FEVER?

From Modern Western Medicine

A fever is defined as a body temperature above 98.6° F when measured orally, and 99.8° F when measured from the rectum.

Most fevers are caused by bacterial or viral infections. Fevers are triggered by the body's immune system, specifically by macrophage and CD4 cells. These cells produce cytokins, which are chemical messengers that signal the brain to raise the body temperature in an effort to destroy the invading microorganism.

Fever may also accompany other conditions, such as dehydration, heart attack, and tumors of the lymphatic system. Its function is not understood in these cases.

From Traditional Medicine

Fever is not of itself a disease, but a response initiated by the body to cure an underlying disease. In short, a fever is part of the solution to illness and therefore should not be repressed unless it gets above 103° F. Brain damage can occur if a fever is allowed to reach 106° F. Most fevers never go above 102°F, and most last only a few days. In the meantime, they do much to assist the body in its attempts to destroy and eliminate from the system the causes of the underlying disease. Hippocrates once said, "Give me fever and I will cure all disease."

The exception is in the case of an infant. Children are far more sensitive to changes in temperature and therefore all fevers warrant consultation and supervision by a medical doctor.

REMEDIES

Foods to Eat

Liquids are most beneficial for a fever. Take liquids for three to five days.

- Water
- Diluted fruit juices (if fever dominates over chills)

- Hot water and lemon juice
- Hot teas (to induce sweating)
- Vegetable or grain soup (if chills dominate over fever)

After the fever has subsided, eat easily digested foods.

- Cooked fruit
- Sprouts

Foods to Avoid

Avoid all food until the acute stage has passed. After the acute phase, avoid:

- Animal foods
- Dairy products
- Flour products

Herbs to Treat Fever

- When there is sweating, make a tea using:

  2 parts cinnamon
  2 parts peony root
  2 parts gingerroot
  1 part licorice

Simmer one ounce of the herbs in a quart of water along with four dates for twenty minutes. Take three or four cups a day, and one-half hour after taking the tea, eat a small bowl of watery brown rice.

- Boneset: infusion, steep 3 oz., 5–15 minutes, 3 times daily; tincture, 10–40 drops, 3 times daily; fluid extract, ½–1 tsp., 3 times daily
- Lemon Balm (good for children): infusion, steep 5–15 minutes, take 6 oz. as needed frequently, and add honey.
- Pleurisy root tea (to induce sweating): infusion, steep 30 minutes, take 1–2 cups daily; for children, 1–5 drops in hot water every 1 or 2 hours
- Peppermint: infusion, steep 5–15 minutes, take 6 oz., 3 times daily. Do not allow leaves to boil because they contain volatile medicinal properties. Good when combined with lemon balm.

Physiotherapy

- Tepid thirty-minute bath
- Baths followed by intense towel rubs when patient's vitality is high
- Hot compresses, used with sweating teas

Homeopathy

- Aconite: for sudden onset of symptoms, when patient is nervous, restless, or anxious, and for hot and dry skin
- Arsenicum: for a patient who is fearful and restless and has burning pains relieved by warmth, is very thirsty for frequent sips of water, and if the fever is worse after midnight
- Belladonna: for sudden onset of symptoms, flushed face and high temperature, strong and fast pulse, or for a patient who does not experience much thirst
- Bryonia: for a patient who prefers to lie still, is worse from movement, is very thirsty, and who is usually pale and quiet
- Ferrum phosphoricum: for gradual onset of symptoms; red cheeks and throbbing head; if there are symptoms for which belladonna would be prescribed, but milder; if pulse is fast but not strong; and if the patient feels better from cold applications on the head
- Gelsemium: for a patient who feels chilly, aches all over, and doesn't want to move, who has a dull headache, droopy eyes, heavy limbs, chills up and down back, and who has no thirst

Chinese Medicine

In Chinese medicine, fever is a sign of an exterior condition, which means that the body surfaces that are exposed directly to the environment are affected first. The most common conditions considered external are fevers, chill, colds, and flu. To balance such conditions, we must choose herbs that are more expansive and reach toward the periphery of the body and those that open the sweat glands to sweat out the exterior disease factor lodged near the surface. This is not the time to take in strengthening, salty, or building foods as these will only trap pathogens inside the body. Allow the person to sweat, but not to the point of exhaustion. If there is weakness with the fever and not much improvement, use herbal preparations that build the protective qi such as fresh gingerroot or cinnamon twig tea.

Supplements

- Beta-carotene: 15–30 mg per day
- Vitamin B complex
    Thiamine: 1.5 mg per day
    Riboflavin: 1.8 mg per day
    Vitamin B_6: 2–10 mg per day
    Vitamin B_{12}: 2–10 mg per day
    Niacin: 20 mg per day
- Vitamin C: 100 mg per day

Fibrocystic Breast Disease

SYMPTOMS

Breast tenderness and the presence of cysts within the breast tissue, often manifesting just before and during the menstrual cycle. Eventually, the cysts remain in place, making the breasts nodular, with some cysts deep within the breast and others free-moving near its surface.

WHAT IS FIBROCYSTIC DISEASE?

From Modern Western Medicine

Cysts are fluid-filled sacs that appear in the breast or milk glands within the breast that may become closed off and thick. One or both breasts become tender and lumpy a week or so before a menstrual period starts. Many women experience an increase in the number of cysts and tenderness until menopause, when estrogen levels fall and cysts often disappear. Studies have shown that estrogen is a major factor in the onset of both cysts and malignant breast tumors. Recent evidence has also shown that foods and drinks containing methylxanthines (see the section below on foods to avoid) can aggravate this condition.

About 80 percent of breast lumps are benign; however, all possible breast lumps need assessment. There is a three- to sevenfold increase in the chance of cancer for women with fibrocystic disease.

Traditional Medicine

The cause of fibrocystic breast disease is the standard high-fat, Western diet, which increases the female hormone estrogen, a hormone that in turn deforms breast tissue and triggers the onset of cysts. Fat cells produce estrogen. In fact, in an obese postmenopausal woman, fat cells produce more estrogen than any other source. Estrogen acts like growth hormone on breast tissues, deforming the tissues and preventing healthy circulation of blood and lymph and the elimination of waste products. Another cause of fibrocystic breast disease is food that is devoid of fiber. Fiber binds with estrogen in the intestines and brings it out of the body. Studies have shown that when estrogen levels are lowered in women with breast disease, the lumps often disappear.

WHO GETS FIBROCYSTIC DISEASE?

Women between the ages of thirty and sixty are most prone to this condition.

REMEDIES

General Recommendations

- Significantly lower blood cholesterol levels (preferably to 170 mg or lower) by reducing foods that contain all forms of fat, especially saturated fats and cholesterol.
- Increase fiber, which binds with estrogen in the intestine and eliminates it from the body.
- Consider stopping birth control pills, which increase estrogen levels and raise the likelihood of breast disease.
- Have estrogen levels checked and reduce them.

Foods to Eat

- Whole grains
- Fresh, organic vegetables
- Vegetable protein such as beans, tofu, and tempeh
- Sea vegetables
- Carrot juice

Foods to Avoid

Significantly reduce or avoid all high-fat foods, including:

- Red meat
- Dairy products
- Eggs
- The fatty part of chicken, turkey, and other fowl
- Fried foods

The following foods contain methylxanthines:

- Coffee
- Tea
- Cola
- Chocolate

Herb to Treat Fibrocystic Disease

Dandelion cleanses the liver; drink as a tea.

Chinese Medicine

Breast lumps are associated with stagnation and irregularity of liver qi. Bupleurum is used by the Chinese as a primary herb for moving liver qi. It is the major herb in several harmonizing formulas that have been in use for nearly two thousand years.

The following formula may be used for regulating stagnant qi.

7 parts poria cocos

4 parts bupleurum root

4 parts atractylodes

4 parts chaste berries

4 parts dong quai

3 parts peony root

3 parts cyperus rhizome

3 parts black haw bark

3 parts wild yam

3 parts magnolia bark

3 parts ginger

3 parts licorice root

2 parts green, bitter orange peel

2 parts ligusticum wallichii

2 parts mint leaves

1 part gastrodia

Supplements

- Beta-carotene: 15–30 mg per day
- Vitamin B$_1$: 25 mg, once daily
- Vitamin B$_6$: 2–10 mg per day
- Vitamin C: 100 IU, once daily
- Vitamin E: 100–400 IU per day
- Calcium: 1000 mg per day
- Flaxseed oil: 1–1½ tablespoons per day

Fibroid Tumors of the Uterus

SYMPTOMS

Typically, fibroids are symptomless, especially if they are small. However, a large fibroid can erode the lining of the uterus, resulting in heavy and prolonged menstrual periods. Large fibroids can exert pressure on the bladder, causing discomfort or urinary frequency; or on the bowel, causing constipation and backache. In some cases, a fibroid can cause the uterine wall to become twisted, triggering pain in the lower abdomen, and, in some cases, miscarriage or infertility.

WHAT IS A FIBROID TUMOR OF THE UTERUS?

From Modern Western Medicine

Fibroids may be detected by a routine pelvic examination. Usually, they require no special treatment, though regular examinations may be called for to determine if they are growing. Fibroids that cause serious symptoms or side effects require surgical removal. If the fibroids are numerous, a hysterectomy (removal of the uterus) may be performed. In some cases, a surgery called myomectomy is performed in which the fibroids are shelled out of their capsules. Fibroids tend to shrink after menopause.

From Traditional Medicine

According to Chinese medicine, fibroids are caused by stagnant blood, which itself is the result of insufficient qi in the sex organs to maintain healthy circulation. The stagnant blood coagulates or congeals and forms tumors. Blood stagnates because it is filled with toxins, waste materials, and tiny particles of fat, all of which diminish the life energy, or qi, in the blood and make it difficult to move through the vessels. The blood becomes viscous, sometimes literally like fatty milk. In such a condition, the blood moves slowly and sometimes not at all; it congeals and forms tumors. All remedies from traditional medicine are designed to promote circulation, especially in the area of the sex organs, and increase blood qi.

In addition, it's important to note that fibroids tend to disappear after menopause, when estrogen levels fall dramatically, because fibroids are estrogen-dependent. Estrogen is produced by fat cells. In obese postmenopausal women, fat cells are the leading producers of estrogen in the body. Therefore, to eliminate fibroids, the diet must be exceedingly low in fat so that fat cells shrink and stop producing high levels of estrogen.

REMEDIES

Foods to Eat

The following foods and spices disperse stagnant blood.

- Sweet rice, unless there is deficient digestive fire (see the section on Chinese medicine in Part III); watery stools; pale, swollen tongue; and feelings of coldness
- Adzuki beans
- Eggplant, especially for dissolving uterine tumors
- Kohlrabi
- Turmeric
- Seaweed
- Chives
- Garlic, unless the person has signs of heat (see the section on Chinese medicine in Part III), which include aversion to heat; sensation of feeling too hot; flushed face; bloodshot eyes; deep red tongue with possible yellow coating; and/or great thirst for cold fluids or signs of deficient yin, including tidal fevers, hot palms and soles, fresh red cheeks and tongue, frequent light thirst, and/or night sweats
- Ginger (same precautions as for garlic, above)
- Vinegar (same precautions as for sweet rice, above)
- Basil
- Scallions and leeks
- Chestnuts
- Cayenne (same restrictions as for garlic, above)
- Rosemary
- Nutmeg
- White pepper

Foods to Avoid

- Cold food or drinks
- Sweets
- Meat
- Dairy products
- Eggs
- Ice cream

Herbs to Treat Fibroid Tumors of the Uterus

The following herbal remedy is invaluable in speeding the reabsorption of tumors in the lower abdominal region.

1 part turmeric
1½ parts licorice root

4 parts cinnamon bark

5 parts peach seed (found in Chinese herb outlets or can be collected from inside peach pit and sun-dried)

For those with excessive heat:

- If there is heat or other deficient signs (see the section on Chinese medicine in Part III), substitute black fungus (wood ear) for the cinnamon bark. Use four parts black fungus.
- Turmeric is a good blood purifier. It can be used alone by decocting 1 tbsp. per cup of water or using 3–9 g; drink 3 cups a day; mix 1 tsp. per cup of water, drink 2 cups a day. Avoid during pregnancy, with acute jaundice and hepatitis, ulcers, or irritable stomach.

Flatulence

SYMPTOMS

The passing of abnormal amounts of gas through the anus, with or without discomfort.

WHAT IS FLATULENCE?

From Modern Western Medicine

Intestinal gas is created when air is swallowed and makes its way into the intestine. Fermented foods and bacteria in the intestines may also produce gas, which is released through the anus.

From Traditional Medicine

Flatulence occurs when imbalances exist within the digestive system, most often in the spleen. When the spleen is deficient of qi, it cannot send adequate life force to the small and large intestine, resulting in incomplete digestion. Partially digested foods easily ferment and produce gas, which becomes flatulence.

In addition to a weakened spleen, another cause of flatulence may be foods that the body has trouble digesting, such as beans, dairy products, and glutenous grains. Beans and grains can be made more digestible by soaking them overnight and then cooking them in fresh water. Finally, certain foods and food combinations can produce indigestion and flatulence. Spicy and acidic foods combined with dairy products or sugar weaken the spleen and begin the cycle that results in gas.

Other factors include drinking with meals, overeating, rushed meals, eating when under stress, and failure to chew adequately. Finally, constipation may also contribute to flatulence.

REMEDIES

General Recommendations

- Eat as simply as possible.
- Place highest-protein foods at the beginning of the meal.
- Eat salty foods first, before foods of other flavors.
- Proteins, fats, and starches combine best with green and nonstarchy vegetables.
- Fruit and sweetened foods should be eaten alone or in small amounts at the end of the meal.

Foods to Eat

CHINESE MEDICINE

- Apricot, carrot, fennel, and black pepper congee (see the section on herbology in Part III for how to make congee)
- To remove liver excess, unrefined apple cider vinegar, brown rice vinegar, or other quality vinegar. Mix with honey to improve its effect. If someone has heat signs (see the section on Chinese medicine in Part III), vinegar may worsen the condition, as it is a warming food. In that case, it is better to use lemon or lime.
- Grapefruit peel: Simmer fresh or dried peel for twenty minutes, then drink.
- Lemon and lime are good for flatulence and all indigestion.
- Bitter foods such as rye, romaine, asparagus, amaranth, quinoa, radish leaves (use sparingly if you are a frail, generally deficient person; see the section on Chinese medicine in Part III)
- Coriander, cumin, and ginger: added to bean dishes
- Watercress
- Alfalfa contains eight enzymes that help assimilate protein, fats, and carbohydrates. Use as sprouts, in tablets, capsules, or powder.

Foods to Avoid

- Fried food
- Hydrogenated fat
- Sugar
- Refined carbohydrates
- All junk food
- Ice-cold drinks
- Poor combinations of food

Herbs to Treat Flatulence

- Charcoal tablets: 1 or 2 per hour for acute flatulence (This treats symptoms and is not for long-term use.)
- Goldenseal: 25 drops in water, 3 times per day
- Ginger tea: Grate two inches of fresh gingerroot to yield 1½ ounces grated root and make an infusion with 1 pint of water
- Chai tea: Make a big pot and drink regularly. Traditionally enjoyed in India.

    1 ounce freshly grated ginger
    7 peppercorns
    1 cinnamon stick
    5 cloves
    15 cardamom seeds

1 orange peel
1 pint water

Cover the pot, heat, and simmer for ten minutes. Sweeten with honey.

Homeopathy

- Carbo vegetabilis: for gas and belching a half hour after eating, when even the simplest food causes gas. The person wants his or her clothing loose around the abdomen, and the abdomen is bloated. Dose is 2 tablets, 3 or 4 times per day. When pain is severe, take 2 tablets every thirty minutes to one hour. Decrease frequency of dose with improvement.
- China: for gas that won't come up or go down. Belching gives no relief. The stomach feels full and heavy. Dose is the same as for carbo vegetabilis.
- Chamomilla: for an abdomen distended with gas, a bitter taste, cramping, anger or irritability, and sweat after eating or drinking. Dose is the same as for carbo vegetabilis.
- Lycopodium: for a feeling of fullness even before finishing eating or after a light meal, bloating, rumbling of gas, discharge of flatus, burning belching, heartburn, or a craving for sweets. Dose is the same as for carbo vegetabilis.

FUNGAL INFECTIONS OF THE SKIN

WHAT IS A FUNGAL INFECTION?

From Modern Western Medicine

Fungal infections range widely in their severity and significance. Fungus is a form of plant life, often a single cell, that lacks chlorophyll. It includes yeast, molds, and mushrooms. Fungi are so ubiquitous that they are constantly in contact with the skin, mucous membranes, and tissues of the body. Most of these are harmless; some are mildly irritating; others are quite severe; and still others are lethal. Called mycoses, fungal infections are dealt with through the body's immune system. They are most severe in people who have been taking antibiotics over a long period because antibiotics weaken immune response and kill off bacteria that destroy fungi in the body. Corticosteroid drugs and other immunosuppressive drugs also predispose people to fungal infections.

Common fungal infections include candidiasis, tinea (including ringworm and athlete's foot), sporotrichosi, aspergillosis, histoplasmosis, cryptococcosis, and blastomycosis.

From Traditional Medicine

Fungal infections arise because of an impaired immune system. The immune response has been weakened by accumulated toxins that already exist within the lymph, liver, intestines, and spleen, which require ongoing protection by the immune cells. All natural remedies are designed to cleanse the system and boost immune response.

REMEDIES

See Part IV for foods and lifestyle recommendations that promote immune response.

Foods to Eat

- Raw, saltless sauerkraut
- Chlorophyll-rich foods stop the spread of bacteria, fungi, and other microorganisms. Good sources are: barley grass and wheat grass (probably the most effective of all in treating yeasts), parsley, kale, collards, dandelion greens, chard, watercress, romaine lettuce, cabbage, and microalgae, such as spirulina, chlorella, and wild blue-green algae. Avoid taking these with juice.
- Seaweed contains selenium and many other minerals that rebuild immunity. Seaweed is rich in iodine, which was the preferred treatment for

yeasts before antifungal drugs. Seaweeds are contraindicated when there is emaciation and loose stools because they are extremely cooling and cleansing.

- Raw garlic

Foods to Avoid

- Excess salt. (It is good to eat seaweed and to put a little salt in with grains and beans.)
- Fruit

Herbs to Treat Fungal Infections

- Citrus seed extract, a natural antibiotic, has been found to inhibit members of several classes of microbes and parasites, among them protozoa, amoebas, bacteria, viruses, and at least thirty different types of fungi, including the candida yeastlike fungi. It is available as a major ingredient in liquid extracts, capsules, sprays, ointments, and other forms.
- Pau d'arco excels in controlling candida. Use it with caution when there is weakness.
- Yerba mansa: for external use as tincture or ointment on fungal infections
- Bloodroot: external tincture for fungus
- Chaparral is especially good when candida has arisen because of overuse of antibiotics. Use for three weeks to draw out the residues resulting from antibiotic suppression of disease processes. Tincture, 10–20 drops, 3 times daily; infusion, steep 5–15 minutes, take 6 oz., 3 times daily; powder, 2–10 #0 capsules, 3 times daily.
- Echinacea
- Burdock root
- Dandelion
- Goldenseal

A healing remedy is to combine echinacea, burdock root, and dandelion as a decoction. Boil 3 cups of water, then lower the flame; add 1 tsp. of each herb and simmer for ten minutes; turn off flame and steep for another ten minutes. Drink 1 cup of the tea.

Hydrotherapy

- Ozone-generating machines have been shown to be effective in the treatment of systemic candidiasis. They have not yet been approved by the Food and Drug Administration for medical use in the United States and as a result are being sold by individuals who cannot make claims for their medical benefits.
- Hydrogen peroxide is a remedy that occurs in nature as moisture interacts with ozone in the atmosphere. It is also found in the cells of the body and in foods that are raw and unprocessed, such as vegetables,

grasses, and wild plants and herbs. This remedy is taken internally. The peak dosage is usually twenty-five drops, three times daily, for up to three weeks; then the dosage is tapered at the same rate it was increased, to fifteen drops, three times a day, until symptoms clear. Expert advice is recommended to tailor the dosage to individual needs. Food-grade 35 percent hydrogen peroxide must be used (obtain it in health food stores or order through Vital Health Products, P.O. Box 164, Muskego, WI 53150, or Lighthouse, P.O. Box 4315, Brownsville, TX 78520). The common drugstore variety has 3 percent hydrogen peroxide and may be used externally.

GALLBLADDER DISEASE
(GALLSTONES AND CHOLECYSTITIS)

SYMPTOMS

Headaches, irritability, quick temper, chronic constipation, nervous tension, and pain between shoulder blades, center of chest, or right shoulder. For some, fever and chills manifest, as well.

WHAT IS GALLBLADDER DISEASE?

From Modern Western Medicine

Gallstones are the principle disorder associated with the gallbladder. Gallstones are composed mostly of cholesterol and bile acids. They develop when the gallbladder has too much cholesterol and not enough bile acids and detergents to keep the cholesterol in solution. The consequence is that the cholesterol becomes crystallized. Around that hardened crystal forms a stone.

Although gallstones are common in the Western world, only about 20 percent of people with gallstones have symptoms that require the removal of the gallbladder (an operation called a cholecystectomy). Severe abdominal pain arises when the gallbladder attempts to rid itself of the stones. Bile may become trapped in the gallbladder and in the organ's opening, causing the walls of the organ to become inflamed and infected, a condition called acute cholecystitis. The initial phase of acute cholecystitis is often fever and abdominal tenderness, but as the disorder persists, acute cholecystitis leads to chronic cholecystitis, in which the gallbladder shrinks, the walls of the organ become thick, and the gallbladder ceases to function.

From Traditional Medicine

Gallbladder disease and gallstones are the result of Western dietary practices and lifestyles. Gallstones form when cholesterol within the gallbladder becomes too high to remain in solution, and thus become hardened into stones. The stones would not form if the blood were not carrying so much fat and cholesterol in the first place. In many cases, gallstones can disappear if blood cholesterol declines sharply and bile acids and detergents are allowed to dissolve the stones inside the gallbladder.

WHO GETS GALLSTONES?

Every year, one million people develop gallstones. The disorder is rare in children, but common in middle-aged adults. Women are affected four times as often as men.

REMEDIES

Foods to Eat

Eat smaller and more frequent meals.

- Olive oil cleanses the gallbladder. Include it in your diet five times a week in small amounts in sautéed vegetables, as dressing for vegetables and salads, and in cooking.
- Apple juice
- Beet root tops, beet juice
- Grapefruit juice
- Carrot juice

After the stones have passed, eat:

- Lots of fruit, olive oil, and lemon juice for three days
- Vegetables that stimulate the liver, including cabbage, turnip root, kohlrabi, cauliflower, broccoli, and brussels sprouts
- Figs
- Pears
- Radishes (Eat one or two between meals for three weeks.)
- Prunes
- Dandelion greens
- Chicory
- Beets and tops
- Carrot juice
- Olive oil
- Grated apples
- Flaxseed and flax oil (Pour five teaspoons over food at one meal.)
- Sesame seeds
- Lemons
- Oranges
- Celery
- Garlic
- Onions
- Tomatoes
- Dates
- Melons
- Pineapple

Foods to Avoid

- Meat
- Eggs
- Refined carbohydrates

- Dairy products
- Hydrogenated fats
- Nuts and nut butters
- Sugar
- Alcohol

Herbs to Treat Gallbladder Disease

- Chamomile tea (to dissolve stones)
- Dandelion tea and greens (clears obstruction)
- Use the following formula:

  1 part wood betony
  1 part dandelion root
  1 part wild yam
  1 part parsley root
  1 part licorice root

Simmer one ounce of this formula in one and one-half pints of water for forty-five minutes; strain. Drink one-half cup three times per day. This tea should be taken during a three-day apple juice fast. (Clean the bowels with a warm water enema before and after the fast.) Drink a cup of tea made of one part goldenseal, two parts dandelion, one-half part peppermint every two hours the day before you are going to flush out the gallstones. This will liquify the bile.

Hydrotherapy

Castor oil pack: Place over the liver and gallbladder area for one hour. After using the pack, drink four ounces of cold-pressed olive oil mixed with four ounces of freshly squeezed lemon juice. Take a strong herbal laxative after the tea such as senna. Lie on right side with hips elevated by a pillow. Place a hot castor oil pack or a fomentation of hops and lobelia over the liver while in this position. The stones will pass within two to six hours.

Chinese Medicine

- Treat liver stagnation with the foods and herbs listed above.
- Acupuncture or acupressure, especially treating liver and gallbladder meridians

Supplements

- Beta-carotene: 15–30 mg per day
- Vitamin B complex: 25 mg, once a day
- Vitamin B$_6$: 2 mg per day
- Vitamin C: 100 mg, once a day
- Vitamin E: 100–200 IU, once a day

Glaucoma

SYMPTOMS

Though no symptoms appear in the early stages, glaucoma causes gradual loss of vision, colored halos surrounding lights, eye ache, headache, tunnel vision, and other visual abnormalities in its more advanced stages. People who suffer from the disease usually require frequent changes of eyeglass prescriptions.

WHAT IS GLAUCOMA?

From Modern Western Medicine

Glaucoma is the name given to elevated intraocular pressure, meaning the pressure of the fluid in the eye becomes abnormally high, causing compression and obstruction of the blood vessels and the optic nerve fibers. The result is often nerve damage and partial or complete loss of sight. The higher the pressure, the more severe the damage and the greater the loss of vision. Vision cannot be regained once the damage has been done to the optic nerve. Routine eye pressure examinations are necessary to prevent the disease.

There may be a genetic predisposition to the disorder, but diabetics are especially prone to glaucoma. Other associated disorders include prolonged stress, a history of eyestrain caused by poor lighting, excessive television watching, and habitual use of sunglasses. Some physicians theorize that glandular imbalances, such as adrenal exhaustion and hypothyroidism, may be the cause of glaucoma. Others suggest that general toxicity is the cause.

Treatment consists of eyedrops designed to reduce fluid production and eye pressure. Surgery is also used, including procedures involving laser technology.

From Traditional Medicine

Pioneer health researcher and teacher Nathan Pritikin said the cause of glaucoma was atherosclerotic plaque buildup within the eye, preventing adequate circulation and causing a gradual increase in pressure. Plaque prevents blood from flowing optimally, much as a big rock prevents a river from flowing. Pressure builds up behind the plaque obstruction, causing damage to the vessels and nerves of the eye. In addition, Pritikin showed how the increase in fat consumption changed the hormone composition of the blood, in turn affecting the ability of the eye to drain fluids and waste, which further increased pressure within the eye. He recommended a low-fat, high-carbohydrate diet as the answer to glaucoma. Traditional societies where such a diet and lifestyle are followed appear to be protected from the disorder. Numerous cases were reported at the Pritikin Longevity Center of people with glaucoma-related eye disorders who experienced recovery of vision after adopting the Pritikin diet.

The best-documented alternative therapy for reducing intraocular pressure is megadoses of vitamin C. Another substance also supported by the scientific research as a treatment for glaucoma is marijuana, which doctors will prescribe for those who suffer from the illness. A prescription is available from some ophthalmologists. Other approaches are therapies designed to balance hormones and improve circulation.

Finally, Chinese medicine maintains that the eyes are nourished with qi by the liver. In acupuncture theory, the liver meridian passes through the eyes and thereby directly affects the condition of the eyes. When the liver is abused by a high-fat, high-cholesterol diet and excessive alcohol consumption, it suffers from poor circulation and deficient qi. The Chinese therefore treat eye disorders, including glaucoma, by treating both the liver and the eyes.

Also, in order to take the stress off the liver, one should undereat and occasionally stop eating late in the afternoon or well before bed. This will allow the liver and the gallbladder time to heal.

The liver is remarkably regenerative. It is capable of restoring up to two-thirds to three-fourths of its tissue if supported by the right healing conditions. Here is a description of precisely those healing conditions.

REMEDIES

Foods to Eat

When the liver is implicated in the disorder, an abundance of vegetables—especially leafy greens, carrots, and other roots—are recommended. Lightly steam or boil these vegetables, but include occasional raw vegetables, as well.

- Vegetable juices, especially carrot juice (Occasionally spend one to two days fasting on vegetable juices if your constitution is sufficiently strong to endure a twenty-four- to forty-eight-hour vegetable juice fast.)
- Green vegetables, especially collard greens and kale
- Carrots
- Chlorophyll-rich foods, including cereal grasses and their products (such as wheat or barley grass juice powders), and also microalgae (spirulina, blue-green, and chlorella)
- Parsley
- Watercress
- Alfalfa
- Seafood
- Seaweed

Foods to Avoid

The following interfere with the normal blood circulation to the eyes and upset hormone stability in the system as a whole.

- Alcohol
- Coffee
- Black tea
- Cigarettes
- Coca-Cola and other artificially sweetened soft drinks

Herbs to Treat Glaucoma

Gum plant: Boil the root and drink as a tea for the liver.

Homeopathy

Gum plant: tincture, 5–30 drops, according to age or condition

Physiotherapy

- Ice-cold baths: Fill a large basin with ice-cold water. Immerse both eyes in the container and rapidly blink eyes open and shut five to ten times. Rest and then repeat two to three times, two times each day.
- Alternate hot and cold eye compresses. Apply a hot, moist towel or folded washcloth to both eyes for two to three minutes; then apply an ice-cold cloth for two to three minutes. Repeat three times, ending with a cold cloth.
- Ice-cold eye compress. Apply on ice-cold moist towel or folded washcloth for two to three minutes, rest one minute, and reapply three to four times. Repeat two times a day.
- Bates eye exercise: found in the book *The Art of Seeing* by Aldous Huxley. (See The Eyes under Part IV for exercises to strengthen sight.)

Supplements

- Beta-carotene: 6–30 mg per day
- Vitamin B_1: 1.5 mg per day
- Vitamin B_2: 1.8 mg per day
- Niacin: 20 mg per day
- Vitamin B_6: 2–10 mg per day
- Vitamin C: 100–500 mg per day
- Vitamin E: 100–400 mg per day

GOUT

SYMPTOMS

Acute joint pain, swelling, tenderness, and redness frequently appear suddenly as flare-ups or attacks. Often, the skin is shiny, red, or purple. Attacks usually occur at night with throbbing and excruciating pain. Initially, the attacks are short-lived, but eventually they become prolonged, sometimes lasting for weeks and even months. When allowed to persist, gout can cause the destruction of joints. In addition, soft nodules may form in the earlobes, tendons, and cartilage.

WHAT IS GOUT?

From Modern Western Medicine

Gout is a form of arthritis that usually attacks a single joint, most commonly the big toe. Other joints that are often affected are the knee, ankle, wrist, foot, and those of the hands. It is associated with kidney stones and can lead to kidney failure.

Pain and inflammation can be controlled with large doses of a nonsteroidal anti-inflammatory drug; in some cases, a corticosteroid drug is injected into the affected joint. Medication is reduced and eventually stopped as the inflammation subsides, usually within two to three days.

The illness is brought on by high blood levels of uric acid, which itself is caused by foods rich in purines and protein, such as liver, organ meats, and poultry. Excess alcohol consumption should also be avoided because it may precipitate an acute attack.

From Traditional Medicine

Gout arises from the overconsumption of protein foods. Protein produces high levels of uric acid, which harms the kidneys and spills into the blood. Once in the blood, these uric acid levels accumulate in the joints and cause an immune reaction and pain. Gout is clearly a disease of affluence, affecting people in Western nations, especially those who eat a diet rich in animal protein and fat. In addition to high protein levels, fat and obesity tend to promote the illness. The elimination of a high-protein, high-fat diet is usually enough to eliminate all symptoms of gout.

According to Chinese medicine, gout is a liver disorder brought on by damp heat, explained in Part III under Chinese medicine. To treat gout, include the vegetables listed below, along with adzuki bean congee (described below).

REMEDIES

Foods to Eat

- Adzuki congee (a traditional breakfast food): Cook brown rice and water in a covered pot four to six hours on a very low flame or warm burner. A crockpot is an excellent way of preparing this dish. Use lots of water to make the grain soupy and easy to digest. The dish strengthens the blood and qi, harmonizes digestion, cools, and is highly nourishing. Other vegetables, such as carrots, onions, shiitake mushrooms, or broccoli; or another grain, such as barley, can be added to the broth. This congee is very healing for the liver, joints, spleen, and digestion.
- Vegetable and fruit juices: especially noncitrus juice, vegetable juice, celery and parsley juice, red cherry juice, and carrot juice
- Purified water (dissolves toxins)
- Celery (renews joints, bones, arteries, all connective tissue; clears digestive fermentation, which causes dampness and acidic blood, according to Chinese medicine)
- Tomato: After digestion, it alkalizes the blood and is good for treating acid blood condition of gout.
- Seaweed
- Cherries
- Lots of vegetables, especially kale, cabbage, parsley, and other green, leafy vegetables
- Bananas
- Strawberries

Foods to Avoid

- Excess protein causes the body to become saturated with uric acid.
- Yeast
- Spices
- Mussels
- Mackerel

People with gout are susceptible to bladder infections. Therefore, avoid the following acid-forming foods.

- Refined sugar and other concentrated sweeteners
- Meat
- Greasy, oily foods
- Refined carbohydrates

Herbs to Treat Gout

- Colchicum: tincture, 5–15 drops, three times per day during acute attack
- Celery: tincture of seeds, 10–30 drops, 2 or 3 times per day. (Eat stalks in very large amounts daily.)
- White bryony: For pain made worse by motion, use the tincture.

Exercise

Exercise is essential to improve circulation and help elimination of uric acid.

- Aerobic exercise daily: Especially helpful is walking, bicycling, and jogging.
- Yoga or stretching exercise
- Tai chi chuan
- Dancing

Supplements

- Vitamin B complex
  Thiamine: 1.5 mg per day
  Riboflavin: 1.8 mg per day
  Vitamin B_6: 2–10 mg per day
  Vitamin B_{12}: 2–10 mg per day
  Niacin: 20 mg per day
- Vitamin C: 100–500 mg per day
- Vitamin E: 100–400 mg per day

Hair Loss (Alopecia)

SYMPTOMS

Loss or absence of hair, usually at the top and front of the head.

WHAT IS ALOPECIA?

From Modern Western Medicine

There are different types of baldness, the most common of which is *hereditary alopecia*. Hair falls out at the temples and crown, usually in stages, the initial phase being the loss of normal hair that is replaced by tufts of finer, downy hair. This hair is also lost and not replaced, leaving a bald area. The bald area gradually becomes wider. Such male-pattern baldness is most common among men but, in fewer instances, also affects some women, especially those who have already passed through menopause.

A second type of baldness, which is very rare, is called *generalized alopecia,* and is characterized by loss of hair in large amounts, leaving short, fine hairs covering the entire scalp. Generalized baldness is usually caused by stress, illness, or chemotherapy.

Localized alopecia, in which hair loss is confined to one area of the head, is caused by damage to the skin from burns, radiation, or other forms of trauma. Fungal infections and some skin diseases can cause localized hair loss.

From Traditional Medicine

Americans have the greatest percentage of men with baldness of any country in the world. In Oriental medicine, the condition of the hair is a direct reflection of the blood (especially the amount of protein, acid, and fat in the bloodstream); the blood-cleansing organs (especially the kidneys); the sex organs; and the adrenal glands. The more toxicity in the blood, the poorer the condition of the hair follicles, which nourish the hair and support its growth. Prolonged or chronic stress can tax the adrenal glands significantly and cause hair loss. A traditional form of Oriental diagnosis suggests that hair that is frizzy and has split ends reflects poor condition of the sex organs, as well.

The first step in hair loss is to improve the quality of the blood by taking the burden off the kidneys. The kidneys are most affected by excessive amounts of animal protein, which can damage them and weaken their ability to cleanse the blood. According to the *Yellow Emperor's Classic of Internal Medicine,* excessive amounts of sweet foods make the hair at the top of the head fall out. The reason is that sweets, acidic blood, and oils all cause excessive rising energy (sometimes referred to as excess fire), which escapes the body through the top of the head. This rising and expansive energy causes the hair follicles to expand, thus forcing them to lose their grip on the hair and allowing it to fall out. Treatment includes drawing the energy back into the body, especially to the body's vital center, known throughout the Orient as *hara*. This restores vitality to the hair follicles and allows them to regain their ability to contract tightly around the roots of the hair.

Many foods and certain physiotherapies cause the energy within the body to move downward and become housed within the vital center, or hara. Among the most effective foods are whole grains, root vegetables, and sea vegetables.

REMEDIES

Foods to Eat

Foods to build spleen/pancreas qi:

- Brown rice
- Oats
- Sweet rice and mochi (pounded sweet rice)
- Root vegetables, such as carrots, rutabagas, parsnips, ginger, turnips, and onions
- Winter squash
- Black beans
- Pumpkin
- Black pepper
- Brown rice syrup

To build or strengthen the blood:

- Seaweed (wakame, arame, hiziki), when consumed daily, can prevent hair loss for many.
- Microalgae
- Vegetables
- Beans
- Whole grains
- Nuts and seeds
- Leafy, green vegetables

Foods to Avoid

- Cold foods and drinks
- Sugary foods and drinks
- Fatty foods
- Animal protein
- Excessive raw foods
- Fruit, especially citrus

- Tomatoes
- Tofu
- Millet
- Salt
- Dairy products

Herbs to Treat Hair Loss

- Mulberries: In the West they are viewed as a general tonic for the whole system. The Chinese view them as having tonic action on the kidneys, liver, and blood.
- Parsley: Infuse as a tea to strengthen the kidneys.
- Raspberry and blackberry leaves make a tea that is good for kidney qi.

Physiotherapy

- Dermal hammer (also called seven star needle and plum-blossom needle) is an acupuncture tool with a long handle and a head that contains small individual acupuncture needles. The needles are dull. By lightly tapping the scalp, especially in the areas of baldness, the needles can stimulate the qi in the scalp and follicles, either by gently massaging them or by creating small punctures in the scalp and thus infusing the dermal layer of the scalp with life energy. The dermal hammer is not painful; instead, it provides a gentle massage that can be quite pleasurable (unless one strikes oneself too hard, of course). Dermal hammers can be purchased at an acupuncture supply store or by mail order from East West Herb Course, Box 712, Santa Cruz, CA 95061; or Oriental Medical Supplies, 1950 Washington St., Braintree, MA 02184.
- Harimake: A kind of cummerbund or wide cotton or wool band worn around the waist to protect the vital center, or hara, along with the kidneys, adrenals, bladder, and the root energies deep within the body. You can make your own harimake by wrapping cotton (for summer) or wool (for winter) tightly around the skin of your waist and hips. The harimake must cover the navel and much of the waist and kidney areas. Sew the ends together. A harimake draws the body's vital energy, or qi, into the center of being (see kidney yin, in the section on Chinese medicine) and can help many people slow or prevent hair loss.

Chinese Medicine

- Psoralea seeds: Eat 3 to 9 grams of the seeds daily. A study examining the effects of psoralea extracts and exposure to ultraviolet light in forty-five bald men found that, within six months, hair was completely restored in 36 percent of the cases and there was a significant restoration in another 30 percent.
- Oyster and clam shell, crushed or whole, can be purchased at Chinese herb stores. Crush and decoct into a tea to increase kidney qi.

HALITOSIS

SYMPTOMS

Offensive mouth odor is known as halitosis.

WHAT IS HALITOSIS?

From Modern Western Medicine

Halitosis is the medical word for bad breath, caused most often by smoking, drinking alcohol, eating garlic or onions, or poor oral and dental hygiene. Contrary to popular belief, neither constipation nor indigestion is a cause. Rarely is halitosis a symptom of illness.

If bad breath is persistent and is not due to any of the above causes, it may be a symptom of a mouth infection, sinusitis, or certain lung disorders, such as bronchiectasis.

From Traditional Medicine

Foul breath is a symptom of an internal disorder, the source of which could be the teeth, gums, sinuses, stomach, liver, and small or large intestine. Very often, the imbalance clears up of itself, which is why bad breath is frequently a temporary problem. The most common underlying cause of halitosis is constipation or generally poor elimination.

Essentially, the mouth is the beginning of the digestive tract, the anus the end. It is a unified and interdependent system. Mouth sores, for example, are often the result of stomach or intestinal imbalances; changes in the formation of the lips reflects changes in the small and large intestine. Failure to fully eliminate waste causes food to putrify and toxins to build up within the intestinal tract, ultimately resulting in foul breath.

But there are other factors, as well. The harmony of stomach acids and digestive enzymes, which in turn can affect the odor of the breath, is dependent upon the liver. When the liver becomes imbalanced, the stomach can be adversely affected. An example is a deficiency of hydrochloric acid or other digestive enzymes, which may result from large meals containing meats, heavy sauces, and other fatty foods. Very spicy foods and disharmonious food combinations can throw off the liver balance and result in bad breath, as well.

Finally, the absence of adequate fiber in the diet prevents full elimination from the intestines. Diets that are low in fiber also result in diverticulosis, or pockets forming within the large intestine. Food matter and waste can accumulate in these pockets and cause odors to be released.

REMEDIES

Foods to Eat

All meals should be small and taken dry. Drink soup and other liquids between meals, not less than a half hour before the meal and an hour after. This helps prevent digestive juices from becoming diluted.

- Lemon/lime destroys putrefactive bacteria and purifies the breath.
- Millet retards bacterial growth in the mouth.
- Parsley
- Watercress
- Good-quality water between meals
- Follow the diet for constipation.

The following foods are cooling and reduce heat signs such as halitosis, according to Chinese medicine.

- Apples
- Pears
- Cantaloupes
- Watermelon
- Citrus
- Lettuce
- Radishes
- Cucumbers
- Celery
- Cabbage (green or Napa)
- Bok choy
- Broccoli
- Cauliflower
- Sweet corn
- Tofu and tempeh
- Whole grains such as millet, barley, and wheat
- Seaweed
- Microalgae such as spirulina, blue-green, and chlorella

Foods to Avoid

In Chinese medicine, this is a heat condition and the following should be avoided.

- Red meat
- Chicken
- Alcohol
- Coffee

- Cigarettes
- Dairy products
- Eggs
- Clams
- Crab
- Yogurt

Herbs to Treat Halitosis

Chew any of the following:

- Anise seeds
- Cardamom seeds
- Fennel seeds
- Whole cloves
- Caraway seeds
- Coneflower

Drink the following herbal teas:

- Peppermint tea (for indigestion)
- Goldenseal (for internal causes)

Chinese Medicine

See the sections above on foods to eat and foods to avoid.

Supplements

- Beta-carotene: 15–30 mg/day
- Vitamin B complex
    Thiamine: 1.5 mg per day
    Riboflavin: 1.8 mg per day
    Vitamin B_6: 2–10 mg per day
    Vitamin B_{12}: 2–10 mg per day
    Niacin: 20 mg per day
- Folic acid: 400 micrograms (mcg) per day
- Pantothenic acid: 10 mg per day
- Vitamin C: 100–500 mg/day
- Vitamin E: 100–400 mg/day

Exercise

When halitosis is chronic, physical exercise, especially walking, jogging, or running, can assist in eliminating stored waste by strengthening the muscles in the stomach and lower abdomen, thus assisting bowel elimination. All forms of aerobic exercise, especially exercises that cause you to sweat, can be a good way of eliminating stored toxins within tissues. Aerobic exercise also increases circulation and promotes healthy bowel function.

HEADACHES

SYMPTOMS

Irregular and sometimes prolonged periods of pain occur in various parts of head or in the sinuses.

WHAT IS A HEADACHE?

From Modern Western Medicine

A mild to severe pain localized in the head, most headaches are the body's reaction to various forms of internal and external disturbances, including physical tension, emotional upset, hunger, sleeplessness, hangover, travel, excessive sleep, stress, toxic food substances, weather, noise, air pollution, irritating chemicals, and odors. Many illnesses, such as the common cold and flu, cause headaches, as do toothache, ear infection, head injury, and sinusitis. Tension headaches, the most common form of headache, are caused when muscles in the face, neck, scalp, and back contract, causing pressure on nerves and reducing circulation to cells and tissues. Most headaches clear up in a matter of hours and have no lasting side effects. If headaches are persistent and do not respond to self-help treatment, medical advice should be sought.

From Traditional Medicine

Headaches must be understood as a form of communication by the body alerting us to the fact that there is an imbalance in our lives that is having an adverse effect on the body. Chronic headaches mean that the imbalance is prolonged and is being ignored. In this case, it is likely that more severe symptoms will emerge, since the cause is left unresolved. Therefore, the first step in treating a headache is to recognize it as a symptom rather than the primary problem. The second step is finding the true cause of the pain and then treating that disturbance.

The most common causes of headaches are imbalances in the liver or intestines, poor circulation, stress, muscle tension (especially in the pelvis and low back), menstrual disorders, and hypoglycemia (see the section on hypoglycemia). The key to treating all of these problems is to improve circulation of blood, lymph, and electromagnetic energy, or qi, within the organs themselves and the body in general. That is accomplished by eliminating the extremes that are most often the source of physical tension and stagnation. Excess work must be balanced by exercise and play; physical and muscular tension must be balanced by massage, walking (preferably in nature), relaxing music, soft lighting; hard and contracting foods must be balanced with soft grains, vegetables, and fruits; isolation must be balanced by social activities and intimacy with others and oneself; fear must be balanced by faith.

See also the section on migraines.

REMEDIES

Foods to Eat

- Hot water and lemon (for liver congestion)
- Grapefruit juice (for liver congestion)
- Apple juice, warmed
- Black sesame seeds
- Tomato in small amounts relieves liver heat resulting in headache.
- Lots of leafy greens, such as collard, kale, and mustard greens
- Small amounts of salad, especially in the springtime

Foods to Avoid

- Chocolate
- Caffeine
- Alcohol
- Additives, preservatives, and all chemicalized foods
- Fats
- Meat
- Cheese
- Eggs

Herbal Treatments

Take either of the following herbs for a headache. Both contain salicin, an aspirinlike compound. A common dosage is ½ teaspoon of tincture, three to four times daily:

- White willow bark
- Meadowsweet
- Feverfew (especially effective against migraines)
- Milk thistle (for liver congestion)
- Dandelion (to move energy out of liver to heart)

Milk thistle and dandelion can be combined in tea, infusions, and tinctures. Mix together equal parts of the following:

Skullcap
Rosemary
Peppermint

Make as an infusion and drink warm. Drink one cup whenever needed.

Use any of the following herbs to help reduce the nervous tension that frequently contributes to headaches. A common dosage is ½ to 1 teaspoon of tincture, 1 cup of tea, or 2 capsules three or four times daily.

- Valerian
- Passionflower
- Spearmint
- Rosemary
- Chamomile
- Skullcap

Homeopathy

- Bryonia: for acute frontal headache that may be accompanied by constipation
- Nux vomica: for hangovers
- Belladonna: for throbbing headaches accompanied by fever and dilated pupils

Chinese Medicine

- Acupuncture to restore the balance to the liver and spleen qi
- Acupressure to remove tension from muscles and restore qi to blocked areas of the body

Hydrotherapy

- Ice compress to base of head while lying in darkened room
- Ice to forehead with simultaneous hot footbath is helpful to abort headache
- Make a hot footbath with a tablespoon of mustard in it to draw the blood from the head area. Drink one of the teas in the section on herbal treatments above while taking footbath.

Supplements

- Vitamin B complex
    Thiamine: 1.5 mg per day
    Riboflavin: 1.8 mg per day
    Vitamin B_6: 2–10 mg per day
    Vitamin B_{12}: 2–10 mg per day
    Niacin: 20 mg per day
- Vitamin C: 100–500 mg per day
- Calcium: 500–1000 mg per day (Amount should be less than 1000 mg if leafy greens are eaten daily.)
- Magnesium: 400 mg per day

Essential Oils

Massage or apply compresses of any of the following to the forehead, temples, neck, and shoulders.

- Chamomile
- Lavender
- Peppermint

Exercise

- Daily mild stretching exercises (see the section on exercise in Part III)
- Yoga

Body/Mind

- Part of establishing balance in one's life is to spend time letting go of the daily struggle and to reestablish a conscious link with the true inner self where peace and tranquillity reside. This is accomplished through prayer, meditation, chanting, contemplation, religious ritual, and affirmations.
- Therapeutic massage

HEARING DISORDERS

SYMPTOMS

The failure to sense sound is easier to detect in adults than in children. Parents of infants and young children must be alert to clues of hearing impairment in their children. Typical symptoms in infants and children with hearing disorders include the child's failure to respond to sounds, especially loud noises. Often the child does not make sounds himself, such as the common types of cooing or babbling that precede normal speech. Even though the child may cry normally, he or she does not form rudimentary words or refer to his parents as mommy or daddy. While the condition is often recognized vaguely by a parent, hearing impairment is most often diagnosed by a pediatrician during a routine examination.

In adults, loss of hearing is initially experienced as a distortion of sounds, some of which are too quiet, while others are inaudible, especially the low tones and the sounds of *s, f,* and *z.* Speech is often difficult to discern over background noise, such as in restaurants. Deafness in one ear may be noticed only when the sound clearly comes from the direction at which the impaired ear is pointed.

WHAT ARE HEARING DISORDERS?

From Modern Western Medicine

Deafness is defined as complete or partial loss of hearing. Total deafness is rare and usually present from birth. Partial hearing loss occurs most often from an injury, ear disease (including ear infections), or a more generalized illness (such as rubella) that affects hearing, and degeneration of the inner ear, usually with age. Severe jaundice right after birth can damage the ear and impair hearing. Prolonged exposure to loud noise can cause deafness, as can *Ménière's disease* (increased fluid pressure in the labyrinth). Certain drugs and some viral infections can impair hearing. Organs within the inner ear also degenerate naturally with old age.

Hearing loss can be accompanied by *tinnitus* (ringing and other noises in the ear) and *vertigo* (loss of balance and dizziness). These secondary disorders can result in confusion, psychological imbalances (such as paranoia), and auditory hallucinations, all of which can lead to depression and withdrawal.

Hearing loss can also arise from a hole or perforation of the eardrum, which, like other tissues, can heal itself. Surgery can also be used to heal a perforated eardrum.

Hearing aids increase the volume of sound reaching the inner ear by means of an amplifier and an earphone that fits into the outer ear.

From Traditional Medicine

Hearing disorders are usually the result of poor circulation of blood, lymph, and qi within the inner ear, the instrument within the skull used to detect sound. When blood and lymph cannot circulate freely inside the ear, oxygen, nutrition, and immune cells cannot get to tissues. Without oxygen and nutrition, tissues become deformed. Without immune cells, bacteria and other disease-causing agents proliferate in the warm environment and eventually cause disorders that impair hearing. Whenever lymph is blocked, waste products accumulate in the inner ear. Finally, qi, or life force, is essential for the health of cells and tissues, for the elimination of waste products, and for the support of the immune system.

Chinese medicine maintains that all hearing problems are related to kidney imbalances. This is especially evident in children whose diets include an abundance of refined sugars, fruit juices, and sweets, all of which weaken kidneys and result in ear infections and other ear-related problems. Therefore, in addition to treating the overall circulation and immune system of the body, the Chinese treat the kidneys as well.

Nathan Pritiken, pioneer health researcher and teacher, claimed that diet is the cause of most hearing loss. Researchers compared the hearing capabilities of a random sampling of people living in Wisconsin—the dairy-producing capital of the United States—with the African tribespeople, the Mabaans. The scientists discovered that not a single Mabaan of any age—including seventy-year-olds—could be found with equal hearing loss to the thirty- to thirty-five-year-old Wisconsinites who had been tested. Similar studies were conducted comparing the hearing capabilities of Finnish people with those of Yugoslavians. Finland has the highest per capita rate of coronary heart disease in the world; the average cholesterol level in Finland is 290 mg. The average cholesterol level in Yugoslavia is approximately 180 mg. Researchers found that Finnish children begin to suffer hearing loss at the age of ten, and by nineteen have distinctly impaired capacity to hear the 16,000 to 18,000 cycles per second range of sound. No such hearing loss existed among Yugoslavians.

Other studies have shown that by reducing fat and cholesterol intake, hearing capabilities markedly improve. Pritikin argued that many types of hearing disorders were due to poor circulation to the hearing organs. Plaque development in the blood vessels to the inner ear limits blood and oxygen to the hearing organ and reduces it sensitivity to sound.

WHO SUFFERS FROM HEARING DISORDERS?

Deafness at birth is rare and incurable, occurring in one in a thousand babies. Deafness in young children—usually curable—is common. As many as one-fourth of five-year-olds have some degree of hearing loss as the result of previous middle-ear infections.

The hearing mechanism gradually degenerates with age, and about one-fourth of the population over sixty-five needs a hearing aid.

REMEDIES

General Recommendations

- Strengthen kidneys by eating foods that boost kidney strength and avoiding foods that tax kidneys.
- Avoid foods that contain refined sugars and artificial ingredients; avoid soda pop, excessive amounts of fruit juices, and sweet dairy products, all of which combine to create ear infections that weaken hearing.
- Seek out an acupuncturist to promote qi flow.

Foods to Eat

- Whole grains, especially barley
- Cooked vegetables
- Whole beans, especially black beans (excellent for kidneys)
- Tofu and tempeh
- Cooked carrots and burdock, sautéed in sesame oil and flavored with miso or tamari (excellent dish for kidneys)
- Sea vegetables, especially arame, nori, and wakame (excellent for kidneys)
- Parsley (helps with deafness)
- Mineral-rich foods to boost immunity and strengthen kidneys: sea vegetables, leafy greens (especially collard, kale, and mustard greens), and root vegetables (carrots, beets, rutabagas, and parsnips)

Foods to Avoid

- Meat
- Dairy products
- Poultry
- Eggs
- Sugar
- Refined flour
- Raw fruit and juices
- Nuts and nut butters
- Cold liquids

Physiotherapy

- Roasted sea salt packs over ears to improve circulation: Roast sea salt in dry frying pan until hot. Place salt in cotton packs and hold over ear. Allow ear to drain if fluid or wax begins to loosen and come free.

- Warm or hot ginger compress on kidneys
- Lukewarm ginger compress on mastoid bones, found behind the ear, to promote circulation in ear
- Acupressure massage, especially on kidney and gallbladder meridians

HEART DISEASE

SYMPTOMS

Heart disease is known as the silent killer because it very often presents no external symptoms before a heart attack strikes that could be fatal. When symptoms do appear, they can include angina (gripping pain in the chest around the heart), difficulty breathing, cold hands and feet (from poor circulation), fatigue, dizziness, inability to think clearly, pain in the legs (due to claudication), palpitations, and heart attack. Another major contributing cause of heart disease is stress, which elevates blood cholesterol levels and promotes production of hormones (cortisol or epinephrine) that, over time, weakens the heart.

Among the signs a doctor looks for to detect heart disease are high blood cholesterol, especially a cholesterol level above 200 mg/dL; high blood pressure; enlarged heart; failure of an electrocardiogram or a stress treadmill test.

WHAT IS HEART DISEASE?

From Modern Western Medicine

Coronary heart disease is the condition that arises when the heart is deprived of adequate amounts of blood. The illness is caused by atherosclerosis, or cholesterol plaques that form in the arteries that bring blood to the heart. Atherosclerosis is caused by eating excessive amounts of fat and cholesterol, both of which raise blood cholesterol and create very volatile boils, or plaques, within the arteries. These boils break up and send debris, known as emboli, in the direction of the blood flow. One of these emboli can block blood flow to the heart muscle, thus depriving it of oxygen and bringing on a heart attack. Several tests are used to determine if a person has coronary heart disease, including a blood-cholesterol-level test and a stress treadmill test, which measures the strength and rhythm of the heart.

From Traditional Medicine

The underlying cause of most heart disease is atherosclerosis, brought on by high blood cholesterol levels—which are themselves caused by a diet high in fat and cholesterol and low in antioxidants—and by a lifestyle that is antagonistic to the person's spirit. In fact, an unhealthy diet is a symptom of being out of harmony with one's own inner nature. Therefore, the diet is not the underlying cause so much as a response to a basic lack of understanding of who one really is. In Chinese medicine, the heart is considered the palace of the shen, or the home of the spirit. The spirit is the inner being from which comes

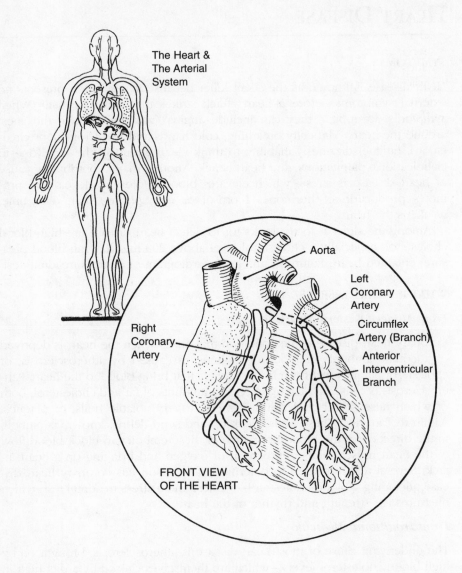

The Heart &
The Arterial
System

Aorta

Left
Coronary
Artery

Circumflex
Artery (Branch)

Anterior
Interventricular
Branch

Right
Coronary
Artery

FRONT VIEW
OF THE HEART

the person's consciousness, or his degree of awareness of himself and his relationship with others and with the universe at large. The spirit has both universal and unique characteristics. The degree to which the person is able to understand and experience his universality—that is, his interdependence with others and the world around him—as well as his unique individual character, including his talents and weaknesses, determines his degree of mental and physical health, including the health of his heart. On the other hand, the more a person conducts his life in opposition to his natural spirit, the more his heart suffers. Chronic stress and poor health habits are symptoms of such an inner conflict.

REMEDIES

General Recommendations

- Reduce blood cholesterol below 150 mg/dL to cause reversal of atherosclerosis and reduce the volatility of the plaques within the arteries.
- Exercise by walking four to six times per week. See your physician before beginning any exercise program, especially if you have already suffered a heart attack.
- Lose weight if you are overweight by following the diet recommended under nutrition (Part III).
- Meditate, pray, or establish some other form of effective stress reduction.
- Do not smoke cigarettes, cigars, or a pipe.

Foods to Eat

- Whole grains
- Plenty of raw vegetables and leafy greens
- Fruit
- Soybeans
- Tofu
- Beans
- Peas
- Cold-water fish: salmon, mackerel, sardines, etc.
- Raw honey and bee pollen
- Onions
- Garlic
- Seeds such as sunflower, flax, pumpkin, and chia
- Seaweeds
- Spirulina

CHINESE MEDICINE

- Wheat germ (improves heart yin)
- Wheat berries (improves heart yin)
- Mung beans (improves heart yin)

Foods to Avoid

- Tobacco
- Red meat
- Eggs
- Dairy products
- Dark meat of chicken or turkey (higher in fat)
- Hydrogenated fats
- Fried foods
- Coffee
- Salt
- Alcohol
- Sugar
- Refined grains

Herbal Treatments

- Ginkgo biloba: 40 mg, 3 times a day of a standardized preparation. Benefits usually show in 4–6 weeks.
- Hawthorn: 100–200 mg a day of standardized extract
- Gugulipid: 500 mg of a standardized preparation, 3 times a day. Also available in more concentrated preparations; take 25 mg, 3 times a day.
- Oat bran: ½–2 cups dry weight per day
- Psyllium (similar to oat bran): 1 teaspoon mixed in 8 oz. of water, 3 times a day
- Angelica, ginger, and prickly ash: Make herb teas to stimulate circulation.
- Motherwort: tincture, 30–60 drops (½–1 tsp.), 3 or 4 times a day

Homeopathy

Arnica is an immediate remedy for heart attack. Homeopaths believe many more lives could be saved if medics carried arnica in ambulances.

Physiotherapy

- Aerobic exercise: Do this only under the supervision of a doctor, as this must be entered into slowly and carefully.
- Alternate hot and cold showers are excellent for stimulating circulation. Do gradually to prevent sudden shock that the heart cannot stand. Take alternate hot then lukewarm showers at first, then alternate between hot/warm every two to three minutes. Slowly, over the next two to six months, increase the difference between the water temperature.
- Daily massage
- Meditation
- Hot compress: In acute angina, apply hot, moist compress to chest or midback, then massage the muscles deeply along the spine.

Supplements

- Vitamin B complex
    Thiamine: 1.5 mg per day
    Riboflavin: 1.8 mg per day
    Vitamin B_6: 2–10 mg per day
    Vitamin B_{12}: 2–10 mg per day
    Niacin: 20 mg per day
- Vitamin C: 100–500 mg/day
- Vitamin E: 100–400 mg per day

Exercise

Do not exercise until after you have changed your diet and lowered your cholesterol level. Exericse can be fatal for someone who eats a high-fat diet. Check with your doctor before you begin an exercise program.

- Walk four to six times per week, for at least thirty minutes per exercise session.
- Do stretching exercises or yoga.
- Tai chi chuan
- Some form of aerobic exercise, such as swimming or jogging

Mind/Body

- Meditation
- Prayer
- Diaphragmatic breathing to reduce stress
- Positive imaging

HEAT STROKE

Loss of consciousness or fainting due to overexposure to high temperatures. If left untreated, the victim could die. The condition is often preceded by heat exhaustion, fatigue, weakness, faintness, and profuse sweating. However, once heat stroke has occurred, sweating diminishes and often stops completely. The skin becomes flushed, hot, and dry; the breathing is shallow; and the pulse is rapid and weak. As the condition progresses, body temperature rises dramatically, and, without treatment, the victim may quickly lose consciousness and die.

WHAT IS HEAT STROKE?

From Modern Western Medicine

A life-threatening condition resulting from overexposure to extreme heat, heat stroke is brought on when the body's heat-regulating mechanisms break down and temperature becomes dangerously high. In some cases, body temperature may reach 107° F or higher, which can cause brain damage and death. Without emergency treatment, the person can lapse into a coma and die.

It is caused by prolonged overexposure to the sun in a climate of unusually high heat. Usually, that climate is also humid, which prevents the body from cooling itself through the production and evaporation of sweat. Very high fever can also bring on the condition, though fever is a rare cause. People who are taking anticholinergic drugs (which reduce sweating), older people in poor health, or those unaccustomed to being in a hot, humid climate (especially if they are dressed in hot clothing) are most at risk.

Emergency medical assistance is essential. Undress the victim and wrap in a cold, wet sheet that is kept continuously wet. Meanwhile, sponge the person with cold water and fan him or her until the temperature is reduced to at least 101° F, or until the body is cool to the touch. If the person is conscious, give him or her salt tablets or a weak salt solution to sip (about one-quarter teaspoon of salt in a pint of water). When heat stroke is treated early, a full recovery can be expected.

REMEDIES

Foods to Eat

CHINESE MEDICINE

These foods protect against summer heat.

- Radish juice
- Bitter melon juice
- Watermelon juice
- Lemons
- Apples
- Cantaloupes
- Papayas
- Pineapple
- Mung beans (in soup)
- Summer squash
- Zucchini
- Cucumbers
- Curries open pores and create perspiration to cool body off.
- Chilies open pores and create perspiration to cool body off.

Foods to Avoid

- Animal foods (meat, dairy, eggs, poultry), as they raise body temperature
- Fried foods

Herbs to Treat Heat Stroke

These herbs will help keep the body temperature down.

- Red clover: 6–15 g in infusion
- Peppermint: ½–6 g
- Chrysanthemum: 3–9 g

Homeopathy

- Veratrum album is useful in most cases of heat exhaustion, when there is prostration with clammy sweat, pallor, nausea, marked weakness, and sometimes rapid pulse.
- Cuprum metallicum: If in addition to the symptoms for which veratrum album is indicated, there are cramps, this will be the appropriate remedy.

HEAVY METAL POISONING

SYMPTOMS

Symptoms vary widely depending on the type of metal and level of toxicity one is exposed to, but common symptoms can include skin rash, headaches, dizziness, immune disorders, joint pain, liver disease, nervous system disorders, loss of memory, and dementia.

If a person experiences extreme confusion, seizures, and disorientation due to heavy metal poisoning, he or she must be treated in the hospital as a medical emergency. Drugs that serve as chelating agents can be used to help the body rid itself of the metal poisoning.

WHAT IS HEAVY METAL POISONING?

Exposure to lead, cadmium, mercury, aluminum, copper, and other less common metals can cause serious disease and can be fatal. Industrial toxicology scientists have established threshold limits that indicate dangerous exposure, depending on the metal in question, but there is widespread controversy over whether any degree of exposure can be considered safe and tolerable. In fact, no one knows if even the smallest exposure to any toxic metal is safe, particularly among people considered sensitive to a particular metal.

Threshold limits are intended to protect the majority of workers from clinical disease. However, many people argue that low-level exposure is triggering subclinical changes in human health that may not manifest as disease until many years after the initial exposure. Concerns have been increasing steadily as people begin to suffer symptoms related to long-term exposure from air, water, and soil pollution. Such pollution arises from cigarettes, auto exhaust, lead cans, aluminum cookware, food additives, pesticides, fertilizers, fungicides, water piping, cosmetics, hair dyes, antacids, and deodorants.

Getting rid of toxins from one's system requires, first, that the toxin be eliminated from one's environment. From there, the toxin should be cleansed from the body gently and gradually, beginning with a diet that is rich in nutrients and low in fat. All fasts should be supervised by a physician or health care professional who is knowledgeable about the effects of fasting and who knows how to respond to the physical side effects of fasts. Toxins are stored in the fat cells within tissues. When a person fasts, he quickly draws on fat reserves as a source of stored calories, which means that the toxins held in fat cells are released into the bloodstream and can overwhelm the liver, kidneys, and spleen and affect the nervous system, thus causing more damage than they did in the stored state. Rather than doing any sort of severe fast, eat a diet that is low in fat and high in nutrition and fiber. Such a diet will cause fat reserves to be burned gradually, allowing toxins to be released into the system at a rate that is more compatible with the blood-cleansing organs. The high-nutrient diet will also boost immune response and protect against the possible side effects of such toxins. The diet also must be high in fiber to maintain healthy bowel elimination, which is the primary method the body rids itself of heavy metals. If constipation develops while attempting to eliminate toxins, use enemas to encourage elimination. Finally, eat sea vegetables daily. Sea vegetables contain sodium alginate, which has been shown at McGill University and other research centers to bind with heavy metals and leach them from the system. Once bound to the sodium alginate, the metal is eliminated from the body by the large intestine.

REMEDIES

Foods to Eat

If poisoning is suspected:

- A diet low in fat and cholesterol
- Whole grains provide nutrition, energy, and fiber.
- Seaweeds (daily)
- Green vegetables, such as collard, Chinese cabbage, kale, mustard greens, watercress, broccoli, brussels sprouts, and others are rich sources of nutrients.
- Root vegetables, including carrots, onions, rutabagas, parsnips, and turnips
- Hot water and lemon juice promotes liver cleansing.
- Grapefruit and other sour citrus fruits promote liver cleansing.
- Apples contain pectin, which removes toxic metals.
- Carrot juice promotes liver function.
- Freshwater fish from unpolluted waters
- Cooked beans
- Bran
- Spirulina
- Raw vegetables
- Spring water
- Garlic

Foods to Avoid

- Meat
- Dairy products
- Sugar
- Eggs
- Poultry
- Canned food

- Frozen food
- Tuna
- Marlin
- Swordfish
- Shellfish (if caught near industrial towns)
- Poor-quality water

Supplements

- Vitamin C: 200–500 mg per day
- Vitamin E: 100–400 mg per day
- Vitamin B complex
    Thiamine: 1.5 mg per day
    Riboflavin: 1.8 mg per day
    Vitamin B_6: 2–10 mg per day
    Vitamin B_{12}: 2–10 mg per day
    Niacin: 20 mg per day
- Zinc: 15 mg per day
- Magnesium orotate: 300 mg per day
- Potassium iodide: 1000 mcg per day for 1–2 months
- Selenium: 70–100 mcg per day

Exercise

Do not overtrain. It is immune-depressing and can promote overelimination of toxins from fat cells, overwhelming blood-cleansing organs, just as fasts do.

- Mild aerobic exercise daily, such as walking, jogging, bicycle riding, or some athletic sport, such as tennis
- Stretching exercises and yoga are ideal for promoting qi throughout the system and supporting blood-cleansing organs, as well as eliminating waste from tissues.

HEMORRHOIDS

SYMPTOMS

Rectal itching, discomfort, pain, and occasional to routine bleeding from the anus, especially on defecation. Internal hemorrhoids, meaning hemorrhoids that exist inside the anus, usually produce a mucous discharge and itching around the anal opening. Complications can arise from hemorrhoids that protrude from the anus (called prolapsed hemorrhoids), including thrombosis, or the formation of a clot in the vein that can reduce the blood supply to the area and cause severe pain. If bleeding is prolonged and significant, iron deficiency anemia can result.

WHAT ARE HEMORRHOIDS?

From Modern Western Medicine

Hemorrhoids are expanded and distended veins that emerge from the interior tissues inside or at the opening of the anus. Hemorrhoids are common, especially during pregnancy and after childbirth. Most often, they occur from straining to overcome constipation or move hard feces. The modern diet, which is made up of animal tissues and refined foods that lack fiber, prevent normal and healthy bowel elimination. Mild cases of hemorrhoids may be treated by increasing fibrous foods, such as whole grains, vegetables, and fruit, and by drinking adequate water. Pain and swelling of hemorrhoids are reduced by taking rectal suppositories and corticosteroid creams.

Hemorrhoids that appear within the anus can be treated with minor surgery on an outpatient basis. Distended hemorrhoids are eliminated by wrapping a tiny rubber band around the vein, which causes it to wither within a few days. A hemorrhoidectomy, or the surgical removal of the vein, is used for prolapsed hemorrhoids.

From Traditional Medicine

According to Chinese medicine, the spleen governs the health of veins and arteries by sending life force, or qi, to the vessels. The spleen also keeps the blood flowing in its natural courses. Internal bleeding, for example, is caused when the spleen cannot supply adequate life force, or qi, to the vascular system, causing fissures to develop within veins or capillaries. Typically, when the spleen is imbalanced, it becomes swollen with blood. During stress and physical exertion, the spleen can contract, sending a rush of blood into the vessels, causing some to swell beyond their normal confines within tissues, and thus creating hemorrhoids.

The five elements system reveals that the spleen also supplies qi to the large intestine, and is considered the mother of the large intestine. When the spleen is weakened, especially by a highly refined diet and excess sugar, the large intestine is deprived of qi and becomes weakened, often resulting in constipation. This causes people to strain during elimination, which further contributes to the creation of hemorrhoids.

REMEDIES

Foods to Eat

Chinese medicine: To correct deficiency of the spleen/pancreas, the following foods are especially helpful.

- Brown rice
- Oats
- Sweet rice and mochi (pounded sweet rice)
- Onions
- Leeks
- Black pepper
- Ginger
- Cinnamon
- Garlic
- Brown rice syrup
- Barley malt

Generally, eat plenty of the following foods:

- Water
- Whole grains
- Beans
- Vegetables
- Nuts
- Seeds
- Agar-agar: Use this seaweed in cooking.
- Bananas
- Figs

Foods to Avoid

- Excessive raw food
- Sprouts
- Citrus
- Coffee
- Hot spices
- Alcohol

Herbs to Treat Hemorrhoids

Take any of the following externally. Place the herbal preparation on a cotton ball and apply it to sore tissue around the rectum after each bowel movement and as needed.

- Calendula has antibacterial properties, stops itching, and speeds healing.
- Aloe gel is soothing and astringent.
- Witch hazel is soothing and astringent. Helps shrink blood vessels. Disposable witch hazel pads are available in pharmacies and natural food stores.
- Goldenseal: Use nightly as suppository or in ointment or salve.
- Stoneroot strengthens the veins; apply externally. Also, take two capsules internally twice a day.

Homeopathy

- Aesculus: for sharp, burning pain in the rectum accompanied by a dull ache in the lower back
- Arnica: for hemorrhoids that come on after childbirth
- Collinsonia: if there is chronic bleeding, itching, and a feeling of sharp sticks in the rectum
- Nux vomica: for overwhelming itching or a constant uneasy feeling in the rectum
- Sulphur: if the rectum feels sore and bruised and there is redness around the anus
- Aesculus or hamamelis: Apply ointment to help relieve pain, itching, and inflammation

Hydrotherapy

Continuous compresses of witch hazel may be applied.

Exercises

- All abdominal strengthening exercises
- Stand with hands at sides at attention. While inhaling, raise the hands over the head and rise on toes. Stretch as far as possible, then breathe normally and lean as far forward as possible without falling. Retain this position for three to five minutes. Repeat two times daily.

Supplements

- Vitamin C (strengthens the capillaries and veins): 100–500 mg/day
- Vitamin E (helps heal blood vessels): 100–400 IU/day

Add the following fiber supplements to the diet to prevent constipation and to create soft, bulky stools.

- Psyllium: 1 teaspoon of powder in a glass of water, followed by another glass of water with meals
- Pectin: 1 tablespoon, 3 times per day

Essential Oils

Apply compresses to the anal area and sit in warm sitz baths using the following oils.

- Cypress: astringent, antiseptic, constricts blood vessels
- Myrrh: anti-inflammatory, antiseptic, astringent

HEPATITIS

SYMPTOMS

Initially, the symptoms of hepatitis appear as weakness, drowsiness, nausea, fever, headache, loss of appetite, aching muscles, joint pain, and malaise. The liver becomes enlarged and tender, causing pain in the upper abdomen and chest area. Jaundice may develop, along with depression. Stools may become gray, urine dark. As the disease progresses, the liver may develop cirrhosis (hardening due to scar tissue) or necrosis (death of tissue). If left untreated, hepatitis can be fatal.

WHAT IS HEPATITIS?

From Modern Western Medicine

Literally, hepatitis is inflammation of the liver. When the illness becomes chronic, there is growing inflammation and destruction of cells causing scar tissue within the organ. Ultimately, cirrhosis sets in. Cirrhosis of the liver is both a cause of hepatitis and a result. Other causes include an autoimmune reaction, viral infection, a reaction to medication or a chemical toxin, and metabolic disorders. The autoimmune-related disorder is treated with corticosteroid drugs to reduce the swelling, while the metabolic cause is addressed by treating the underlying disorder.

Apart from cirrhosis, the most common cause of hepatitis is viral, which is designated as A or B. Hepatitis A is often called infectious hepatitis, and it is contracted by ingesting contaminated food or water. Hepatitis B is communicated via blood transfusion, sexual contact with an infected person, or through the use of a contaminated intravenous needle.

From Traditional Medicine

Hepatitis is often the result of an immune-depressing lifestyle, with alcoholism, intravenous drug use, poor diet, and unhealthy ways of living the primary causes. In these cases, the liver is often congested with fatty acids, which prevent the blood from flowing freely through the organ, thus allowing toxins to stagnate inside the tissues and creating the underlying conditions for disease. If poor health habits are not a cause, then exposure to infectious agents and chemical toxins are important considerations when attempting to create a healing program.

REMEDIES

General Recommendations

- See Part IV for ways to promote liver health.
- Eat at least two servings of leafy green vegetables a day, especially collard, kale, and Chinese cabbage.
- Eat soft grains, especially wheat, bulgur, barley, and brown rice.

Foods to Eat

It is especially important not to overeat, to chew thoroughly, and not to eat up to three hours before bed.

- Whole grains, especially barley, wheat, bulgur, and brown rice
- Leafy green vegetables
- Spirulina
- Lecithin
- Wheat or barley grass juices
- Wheat germ
- Tofu
- Soybeans
- Button mushrooms (to treat contagious hepatitis)
- Garlic (Use every day for several weeks.)
- Grape juice
- Oats
- Kukicha tea

Foods to Avoid

- Alcohol
- Red meat
- Dairy products
- Poultry
- Eggs
- Sugar
- Stimulants
- Refined flour
- Oils (as much as possible)
- Cold drinks
- Spices
- Nuts and nut butters

Herbs to Treat Hepatitis

- Milk thistle: 15–30 drops of tincture in water, twice daily, for two weeks
- Combine equal parts of dandelion, blessed thistle, Oregon grape, and

pipsissewa with fennel seed. Three cups taken daily are an excellent liver tonic.

- Michael Tierra's Planetary Herbs: Formula 12 removes liver stagnation, smooths and regulates qi, and is very useful for hepatitis. (Can be purchased or ordered through your health food store.)
- Goldenseal treats liver diseases. Infusion, 1 teaspoon in 1 cup of boiling water; tincture, 10–30 drops; 3–6 g in formula
- Barberry is one of the mildest and best liver tonics known. Tincture, 10–30 drops; standard decoction or 3–9 g
- Celandine: tincture, 1–10 drops, 3 or 4 times per day
- Culver's root: tincture, 10–60 drops, 3 or 4 times per day

Physiotherapy and Hydrotherapy

- Coffee enemas
- Alternate hot and cold compresses over the liver area
- Rest

Supplements

- Beta-carotene: 10–30 mg per day
- Folic acid: 5 mg per day
- Vitamin B complex, oral: 50 mg per day
- Vitamin C: 500 mg per day
- Vitamin E: 400–600 IU per day

HERPES GENITALIS

SYMPTOMS

The herpes simplex virus may manifest as itching and burning blisters and sores located in the genital area. Eventually, the blisters open, leaving painful ulcers that heal within ten to twenty-one days. Symptoms tend to flare up and then disappear for periods. When the symptoms arise, the person may feel sick and suffer from fever, headaches, and swollen lymph nodes, especially those located in the groin. Cold sores may appear around the mouth.

WHAT IS HERPES?

From Modern Western Medicine

This illness is created by the herpes simplex virus, which is communicated during sexual contact with an infected person and manifests around the genitals. The illness flares up in periodic attacks that often occur after sexual intercourse, sunbathing, or when the immune system is weakened. The affected person should avoid sexual activity when the symptoms assert themselves to protect one's partner from infection.

Once infected, the person cannot be cured, but approximately 40 percent of infected people never have a second attack, while most others experience between four and five attacks annually for several years. Eventually, the flare-ups become wider apart and less severe in nature. Although herpes cannot be cured, early treatment may prevent or reduce the severity of the symptoms. The blisters and sores are treated with antiviral medication, the pain with over-the-counter analgesics. Warm baths with a tablespoon of salt are recommended to soothe and assist in the healing process. Pregnant women may require a cesarean section if a flare-up occurs while giving birth; this prevents the baby from being infected.

From Traditional Medicine

Treatment of herpes requires that the person maintain a strong immune system, which is boosted by the recommendations described below. With vigilance and a balanced, healthy lifestyle, herpes flare-ups can be limited or made to disappear permanently.

REMEDIES

Foods to Eat

For at least six months:

- Whole grains, at least twice a day: especially brown rice, barley, wheat, oats, sweet rice, millet, and whole-grain noodles
- A wide variety of green vegetables, steamed, twice a day
- Root vegetables, such as carrots, rutabagas, onions, turnips, ginger, and parsnips, at least once a day
- Chlorella and wild blue-green algae
- Beans, four to seven times per week
- Seaweeds, especially nori, arame, and wakame, one to two tablespoons, daily
- Miso soup with wakame and vegetables, daily, to alkalize blood and make it more resistant
- Sprouts
- Parsley
- Bee pollen
- Garlic
- Apples

Foods to Avoid

- Meat
- Dairy products
- Eggs
- Fried foods
- Oils
- Sweets
- Spirulina (increases dampness in lower warmer in cases of herpes)
- Refined carbohydrates
- Alcohol
- Fruit
- Tomatoes
- Nuts and nut butters
- Chocolate
- Coffee
- Minimal raw foods

Herbs to Treat Herpes

- Make a decoction of the roots of sarsaparilla, dandelion, and gentian in equal parts. (If the stools become loose, use only sarsaparilla.)
- Make a tincture using two ounces Oregon grape root, one ounce chaparral, one ounce echinacea, and ¼ ounce prickly ash bark. Mix the four ounces of herbs in one pint of vodka. Let it stand in a cool, dark area for fourteen days, shaking twice daily. Strain on the fourteenth day through a fine cheesecloth. Put the tincture in a dark, tightly capped bottle. Take one teaspoon three times a day in warm water, or one tablespoon morning and night.

- Goldenseal: Apply topically.
- Green kukui nut: Apply sap to lesion three to four times per day.
- Oregon grape root: 1 oz. herb to 1 pint water, 1 cup, 2 or 3 times per day.
- Michael Tierra's Formula 14 disperses damp heat from the lower warmer. Take 2–4 tablets, 3 times daily, with warm water. (Purchase or order through your health food store.)

Hydrotherapy

- Bathe in common black tea leaves. Add at least 6 oz. tea leaves to very hot bathwater, allow to cool, and then sit in it for about an hour.
- Ice packs relieve pain and itching.

Physiotherapy

Meditation and chanting help deal with stress, which is important for avoiding outbreaks.

Chinese Medicine

Herpes is characterized as dampness combined with heat in the lower burner, the reproductive and eliminative area of the body. Eat foods recommended for dealing with this condition.

Supplements

- Beta-carotene: 6–30 mg per day
- Vitamin B_1: 1.5 mg per day
- Vitamin B_6: 2 mg per day
- Vitamin C: 100–500 mg per day
- Zinc: 15 mg per day
- Vitamin E: 100–400 IU per day; topical application 1 or 2 times a day during flare-ups

HIATAL HERNIA

SYMPTOMS

Dyspepsia, including heartburn, chronic stomachache and pain, difficulty swallowing, abdominal inflammation, ulcer, gastrointestinal bleeding, reflux (especially when reclining and often with pain), fibrositis, and sometimes stricture of esophagus.

WHAT IS HIATAL HERNIA?

From Modern Western Medicine

Hiatal hernia occurs when the stomach protrudes through the diaphragm and pushes up against the chest wall. In some cases, supportive garments are used to push the stomach back into correct position. However, if there is considerable pain and the stomach cannot be replaced behind the diaphragm, surgery is required.

From Traditional Medicine

Hiatal hernia is uncommon in underdeveloped nations where people subsist on traditional grain-based diets and have active lifestyles. Overweight and overeating are the major causes of hiatal hernia. Large meals slow stomach and intestinal transit time; food tends to sit for prolonged periods in the stomach, causing the organ to become distended and bloated. At the same time, qi is blocked to the stomach and along the stomach meridian, diminishing the life force flowing to the organ. If these conditions persist, the stomach becomes stretched and swollen. Eventually, it can lose its integrity and push its way through the muscular diaphragm. In addition to the size of the meals and their overall weight, hiatal hernia is promoted by diets that are rich in animal protein. Protein is digested primarily in the stomach. The more animal tissue and protein consumed, the harder the stomach must work to break down the sinewy mass of animal flesh and its protein constituents. These foods contribute to the distention, bloating, and swelling that eventually cause the stomach to violate the diaphragm. Finally, highly refined foods, along with high-protein diets, contribute to an increase in stomach acids that reflux into the esophagus, a common symptom of hernia.

REMEDIES

Foods to Eat

- Whole grains
- Beans

- Seaweed
- Vegetables

Foods to Avoid

- Sweets, especially chocolate
- Coffee
- Tea
- Alcohol
- Spicy foods

Herbs to Treat Hiatal Hernia

- Comfrey: decoction (root), simmer 30 minutes and take 3 ounces frequently.
- Goldenseal: tincture, 20–90 drops, 3 times daily; decoction, simmer 15–30 minutes and take 1–2 teaspoons, 3–6 times daily.
- Slippery Elm: tincture, 15–30 drops, 3 or 4 times daily; decoction, simmer whole bark 5–15 minutes and take 3 oz., 3 or 4 times daily.

Chinese Medicine

A good cure for hernia is fennel congee. Cook rice and water in a covered pot four to six hours on warm, or use the lowest flame possible; a crockpot works very well. Add a few grains of salt. Use too much water rather than too little. The longer the congee cooks, the more powerful it becomes. Add fennel to taste. This soup is easily digested and assimilated, tonifies the blood and qi energy, harmonizes the digestion, and is demulcent, cooling, and nourishing. Since rice will strengthen the spleen and pancreas, any food added to it will be more completely assimilated and its properties will be enhanced.

Supplements

- Beta-carotene: 6–30 mg per day
- Thiamine (B$_1$): 1.5 mg per day
- Vitamin C: 100–500 mg per day
- Vitamin E: 100–400 mg per day

HICCUPS

SYMPTOMS

Repeated spasms of the diaphragm followed by sudden closure of the glottis.

WHAT ARE HICCUPS?

From Modern Western Medicine

Hiccups are a very common and usually minor disorder that occurs without obvious causes. In the vast majority of cases, hiccups stop without treatment. In rare cares, hiccups may arise from an irritation of the diaphragm or its nerve supply, conditions that may indicate several disease states, including pleurisy, pneumonia, disorders of the stomach or esophagus, pancreatitis, alcoholism, and hepatitis. Medication or surgery may be needed in those extremely rare cases of prolonged attacks.

From Traditional Medicine

Hiccups are an energetic imbalance of the stomach, spleen, and diaphragm, caused by foods, drinks, and ways of eating that have energetically conflicting effects on these organs. Typically, hiccups are brought on by rapidly eating a meal; by extremely cold or carbonated drinks that have a shocking or irritating effect on the stomach, spleen, and diaphragm; or by eating foods that have an expansive effect on the stomach and spleen (spices or sweets, for example), along with salty or highly alkaline foods (such as those rich in fat) that have a contracting effect. The two extremes cause the stomach, spleen, and diaphragm to go into spasm and bring on a case of the hiccups.

Some healers believe that a high blood carbon dioxide level inhibits hiccups, a theory that has given rise to an endless array of home remedies, including holding one's breath, placing a bag over one's head, and drinking long gulps of water to inhibit breathing. Other common techniques are listed below:

- Take ten sips of water in rapid succession.
- Lie on the left side for ten to fifteen minutes.
- Chew and swallow ice for ten to fifteen minutes.
- Drink a glass of water from the opposite side of the glass.
- Apply pressure with the flat hand just below the breastbone.
- Hold breath while extending the head as far back as possible.
- Eat some sugar.
- Apply ice to neck.

- Take a hot bath.
- Stand on your head.
- Take a roller coaster ride.

REMEDIES

Foods to Eat

- Lemon and lime juice
- Raw onion juice every half hour
- Tangerines

Foods to Avoid

- Cold and/or carbonated water
- Alcohol
- Caffeine
- Tobacco

Herbs to Treat Hiccups

- Chestnut leaves: 10 drops in warm water whenever needed
- Skunk cabbage: Make a tea and take teaspoonfuls every ten minutes; or take the tincture (15 drops in ½ cup of warm water).
- Wild carrot: infusion, 3–9 g (contraindicated in pregnancy)
- Pomegranate: 3–9 g
- Elecampane: 3–9 g; tincture, 10–30 drops

Hydrotherapy

- Soak both feet in hot water for ten to twenty minutes, then massage them with a stimulating massage oil.
- Apply hot water fomentation over the stomach and chest. Make a tea from lobelia and apply.

Body/Mind

Meditate while you wait 'em out.

HIVES (URTICARIA)

SYMPTOMS

Itchy bumps, patches, and rash on the surface of the skin, often white at their caps, surrounded by red, inflamed tissue. Hives most commonly appear on the limbs and trunk, but in severe cases can spread elsewhere on the body. Hives usually last only a few hours.

WHAT ARE HIVES?

From Modern Western Medicine

Though the cause is unknown, the most common stimulus is an allergic reaction to certain foods, such as milk, eggs, shellfish, strawberries, or nuts; certain food additives or artificial colors; and pharmaceutical drugs, such as penicillin or aspirin. The allergic reaction triggers the production of the chemical histamine from cells, which in turn causes capillaries to leak fluid into the tissues of the skin. Less commonly, heat, strenuous exercise, and sweating can bring on a flare-up of hives, as can overexposure to sunlight or cold temperatures. Calamine lotion and antihistamine drugs can relieve the irritation and itching. Severe cases may require corticosteroid drugs.

From Traditional Medicine

Hives are the body's effort to eliminate toxins that have temporarily overloaded the liver and kidneys and thus been shunted to the skin surface in the hope of eliminating such waste products through the skin's pores. Hives usually appear when the bloodstream, lymph system, liver, kidneys, and large intestine are already burdened by toxins. At that point, some toxic food substance or chemical is added to an already overworked immune system, blood-cleansing organs, and digestive tract, and thus becomes the proverbial straw that broke the camel's back.

The first thing to do is to take these burdens off the blood-cleansing organs and systems (such as the lymph) and boost the eliminative organs, especially the large intestine. If constipated, take a laxative and then promote healthy elimination through the bowels.

REMEDIES

Foods to Eat

Omega-3 oils boost immunity.

- Soybeans
- Green, leafy vegetables
- Microalgae such as spirulina, chlorella, and blue-green alga
- Flax, chia, and pumpkin seeds
- Salmon, mackerel, sardines, and other deep/cold-water fish

The following fluids will help to eliminate toxins.

- Carrot and green vegetable juice
- Distilled water

Foods to Avoid

The following foods are common allergens.

- Shellfish
- Milk
- Eggs
- Wheat
- Pork
- Onions
- Some fruits
- Food dyes, additives, and preservatives

Also avoid:

- Saturated fats
- Fried foods
- Sugar
- Refined carbohydrates
- Dairy products
- Spices
- Tobacco
- Coffee
- Alcohol

Herbs to Treat Hives

- Chickweed tea and oil
- Burdock seed tea
- Catnip tea
- Nettle juice: 1 tsp., 3 times per day
- Sassafras tea
- Infusion: 1 part nettle, 1 part yarrow, 2 parts dandelion, ½ part gold-enseal.
- Echinacea: tincture, 30 drops, four to five times daily

- Tea made from equal parts burdock, sassafras, red raspberry, and red clover. Drink in cupful doses two or three times daily to clean the blood.

Hydrotherapy

To draw out toxins from skin, take a hot bath with one pound of baking soda or Epsom salts added to the water.

Hyperactive Children

SYMPTOMS

Restlessness, aggressiveness, impulsive activity, nervous tension and anxiety, low stress tolerance, emotional instability, anger, destructive behavior, short attention span, distractedness, confusion, and, occasionally, awkwardness and poor coordination.

WHAT IS HYPERACTIVITY IN CHILDREN?

From Modern Western Medicine

The cause of hyperactivity is unknown, though many theories abound. Most children have periods in which they appear hyperactive, but the diagnosis is not applied unless the child chronically exhibits hyperactive symptoms past the age of four. The disorder may run in families; hyperactive children often have fathers who were also hyperactive.

Drugs that stimulate the nervous system, paradoxically, have a calming effect on hyperactive children and therefore are used as a treatment. The calming effect of stimulants has given rise to the theory that hyperactivity may be the result of an underarousal of the midbrain, which may fail to control movements and effectively filter sensations in the affected child. This may cause the child to experience too much stimuli. Stimulant drugs may arouse the midbrain sufficiently to suppress the extra activity. Professional counseling and behavioral modification for all family members has been helpful. Restriction of artificial colorings, additives, or foods is very popular, but research so far has been inconclusive.

From Traditional Medicine

Traditional medicine, such as naturopathy, has treated hyperactivity by eliminating all refined foods, artificial ingredients, pesticides, and herbicides from the diets of hyperactive children, meaning the sensitive child must be placed on a 100 percent organically grown diet. Rarely is there one food that triggers the condition. Rather, hyperactive children may be sensitive to a wide array of foods; also, two hyperactive children may have sensitivities to very different sets of foods. In general, traditional medicine recommends that hyperactive children eat organically grown foods that contain no artificial additives, colorings, preservatives, pesticides, herbicides, or any other chemical additive. Adherence to such a diet is important. Also important is physical exercise, which promotes the elimination of toxins through the skin and exhalation; regular hours; adequate sleep; avoidance of hunger by eating many little meals, including vegetable and fruit snacks (such as raw carrots or celery); and daily intake of whole grains, such as brown rice. Whole grains boost production of serotonin, a chemical neurotransmitter in the brain that promotes a sense of well-being, clarity of thought, the ability to concentrate, and enhances sleep.

Hyperactive children may have an overabundance of the neurotransmitter dopamine, which causes heightened states of arousal, alertness, and aggression. It also creates restlessness and greater need for activity. Dopamine is boosted in the brain by eating protein foods, especially those composed of animal tissues. Serotonin balances dopamine and creates greater feelings of calm and relaxation. Serotonin is increased in the brain by eating carbohydrates, especially whole grains, vegetables, and fruits.

REMEDIES

Foods to Eat

All food must be organically grown. Labels must be read carefully.

- Whole grains, especially brown rice, wheat, barley, oats, and corn
- Beans
- Green and root vegetables
- Seaweed
- Spirulina
- Nuts
- Seeds
- Fruit

Foods to Avoid

- Dairy products
- Wheat
- Sugar
- Chocolate
- Coca-Cola
- Salt
- Nonorganic soy sauce
- Yeast
- Commercial baked goods
- Restaurant foods
- Canned food
- Frozen food
- Processed food

Herbs to Treat Hyperactivity

- Chamomile tea: Drink regularly to calm, relax, and promote better sleep.
- Michael Tierra's Formula 5 is especially designed for hyperactivity in

children. It is a soothing, calming, gentle, and nourishing nerve tonic. Purchase or order through a health food store. Take one or two tablets, three times daily. It may be crushed and mixed with maple syrup or honey.

Physiotherapy

- Saunas: one to two times per week.
- Massage: once or twice a week along the spine with cocoa butter

Supplements

For children, a multivitamin and mineral taken daily that includes the following nutrients will help to stabilize the nervous system and boost immunity.

- Beta-carotene
- Vitamin B complex
- Vitamin B_3
- Vitamin B_6
- Pantothenic acid
- Vitamin C
- Essential fatty acids
- Calcium
- Magnesium
- Zinc

Exercise

Any aerobic exercise is beneficial, especially those sports that require individualized effort and skill development, such as tennis, swimming, bicycling, and the martial arts.

HYPOGLYCEMIA

SYMPTOMS

Sweating, weakness, hunger, dizziness, trembling, headache, palpitations, confusion, and sometimes double vision. Behavior is often irrational and aggressive and movements are uncoordinated; this state may be mistaken for drunkenness. The victim may lapse into coma due to extremely low blood sugar. Symptoms are usually episodic, being related to the time and content of the previous meal. Symptoms are usually improved by eating.

WHAT IS HYPOGLYCEMIA?

From Modern Western Medicine

Hypoglycemia is an abnormally low level of glucose (sugar) in the blood. Almost all cases occur in sufferers from insulin-dependent diabetes mellitus. In this disease, the pancreas fails to produce enough insulin (a hormone that regulates the level of glucose in the blood), resulting in an abnormally high level of glucose. To lower it, diabetics take either hypoglycemic drugs by mouth or insulin by injection. Too high a dose of either can reduce the blood sugar to too low a level, thus starving the body cells of energy. Hypoglycemia can also occur if a diabetic person misses a meal, fails to eat enough carbohydrates, or exercises too much.

Rarely, hypoglycemia can result from drinking a large amount of alcohol or from an insulinoma (an insulin-producing tumor of the pancreas); it also occurs for no known reason in some children, but is usually only temporary.

Insulin-dependent diabetics should always carry sugar with them to take at the first sign of an attack. If a person is unconscious and it is suspected he suffered a hypoglycemic attack, a physician should be called immediately.

From Traditional Medicine

Hypoglycemia, or low blood sugar, often develops from the same kind of dietary extremes that cause diabetes, but instead of a diabetic shortage of insulin, an excess is produced. In time, if insulin overproduction continues, the pancreas becomes overworked and loses its ability to produce sufficient and/or effective insulin, the result being diabetes. Therefore, hypoglycemia is often a precursor to the onset of diabetes.

The hypoglycemic person usually has a long history of sugar abuse and is often drawn to sugar in an attempt to placate some underlying emotional disharmony. Often, too much meat in the diet causes excessive sugar cravings. This is an attempt at establishing a protein/carbohydrate balance. Excessive meat-eating also generates prostaglandins that may cause pain, inflammation, and depression, and sugar and alcohol can temporarily reduce these burdens.

To resolve a hypoglycemic condition, one must avoid denatured and refined foods, because these foods lack the minerals and other nutrients that control all metabolic activities, including insulin production. Refined flour or sugar, for example, is composed primarily of carbohydrates that deliver energy and warmth. The minerals that are refined away would have been incorporated into the blood, hormones, and various body fluids to cool, moisten, and subdue the burning of sugars into energy. The hypoglycemic body robs its own tissues of these needed minerals, thereby losing the deep, controlling reserves that stabilize it during dietary extremes and stress in general. Thus, those with low blood sugar may notice major fluctuations in blood sugar levels according to what they ate at the last meal.

High-protein diets have been considered a cure for hypoglycemia, because protein digests slowly, supplies energy gradually, and does not trigger excess insulin production. But a high-protein diet causes other serious problems. The best dietary remedy seems to be to eat complex carbohydrates (as shown below) along with the general advice to chew thoroughly, eat small and frequent meals, and do simple food combining.

REMEDIES

Foods to Eat

- Whole grains, such as rice, millet, and oats
- Beans, especially mung and garbanzo
- Tofu and soy products
- Chlorophyll-rich foods such as wheat grass or barley grass, spirulina, and chlorella
- Seaweeds (Soak before using.)
- Vegetables, especially string beans, carrots, Jerusalem artichokes, asparagus, yams, spinach, and avocados
- Fruits, especially blueberries and huckleberries in small doses
- Nuts and seeds, in small quantities
- Flax oil
- Sweeteners, such as rice syrup and barley malt, in small quantities

Foods to Avoid

- Salt (Eat only in small amounts because salt reduces blood sugar.)
- Fruit juices
- Sugar
- Alcohol
- Tobacco
- High-protein foods such as meat, poultry, and dairy products
- Flour products

- Spices
- Honey
- Coffee
- Dried fruit
- Refined carbohydrates
- Vegetable juices

Herbs to Treat Hypoglycemia

- Michael Tierra's Formula 25: Purchase or order through your health food store. One of the best formulas to use for hypoglycemia.
- The following is a specific formula for hypoglycemia:

  1 part goldenseal
  1 part juniper berries
  1 part uva ursi
  1 part cedar berries
  1 part dandelion root
  1 part bistort
  1 part licorice root powder
  1 part huckleberry leaves

Powder the herbs and put them into #00 capsules. Take two capsules, three times a day, between meals. This can also be taken as a decoction in doses of two ounces twice daily on an empty stomach.

- Dandelion tea: A cup one-half hour before meals acts as a tonic to the liver and stomach and helps to regulate blood sugar levels. Combine the following herbs to build up the digestive system:

  1 part dandelion root
  1 part calamus root
  1 part gentian
  ¼ part ginger
  ¼ part cinnamon

Hydrotherapy

Alternate hot and cold packs morning and night for ten minutes over the kidney area, pancreas, and adrenals.

Supplements

- Vitamin B complex
    Thiamine: 1.5 mg per day
    Riboflavin: 1.8 mg per day
    Vitamin B_6: 2–10 mg per day

Vitamin B_{12}: 2–10 mg per day
Niacin: 20 mg per day
- Vitamin C: 100–500 mg per day
- Vitamin E: 100–400 IU per day
- Zinc: 15 mg per day
- Lecithin: 1 tsp., three times daily
- Bran: 1 tsp., two or three times daily

IMMUNE DISORDERS

SYMPTOMS

Recurrent infection; slow or incomplete recovery from illness or injury; slow or poor response to proven treatments; fatigue, lethargy, extended sleep requirements; susceptibility to colds, flu, or cancer. All of these illnesses stem from weakness of the immune system. Diseases that stem from an overreactive immune system include allergies (see the section on allergies for symptoms) and immune disorders in which the immune system attacks the tissues of the body, such as multiple sclerosis (see the section on multiple sclerosis). Symptoms that occur when the immune system attacks healthy tissues include fatigue, lethargy, weakness, tingling in the fingertips, numbness, heavy extremities, spastic muscle activity, stiffness, and incontinence.

WHAT ARE IMMUNE DISORDERS?

From Modern Western Medicine

There are two types of immune disorders, which have very different sets of symptoms. One set stems from immune deficiency in which the body's defenses fail to respond adequately to a pathogen, toxic agent, or cancer, and therefore allows the disease-causing agent to proliferate. Human immunodeficiency virus (HIV) weakens immune response by destroying macrophages and CD4 cells (the immune system's governing cells). As the number of macrophages and CD4 cells decline, the number of CD8 cells—the cells that turn off the immune response—increase, thus causing the system to shut down. Meanwhile, opportunistic diseases, such as pneumonia, *Candida albicans,* or certain types of cancer gain a foothold within the body, either causing further illness or death.

The second group of immune disorders arise from an overreaction of the immune system, in which the immune system is hypersensitive to antigens, as in the case of allergies, or when the immune system attacks the body's own tissues, as in the case of multiple sclerosis. Science doesn't know why the immune system attacks the body's tissues.

From Traditional Medicine

In general, immune deficiency arises out of exhaustion, which itself occurs from excessive amounts of work, irregular hours, inadequate sleep, the intake of drugs, promiscuity, and a nutrient-deprived diet.

An overreactive immune response occurs when the toxins build up within the tissue fluid, cells, and the blood-cleansing organs, especially the liver and spleen. When toxins build up, the immune system reacts to ordinarily harmless antigens, such as pollen, dust, and a multitude of other substances. As for cases in which the immune system attacks tissues, one theory posed suggests that the cells of those tissues themselves may well have degenerated and now appear to immune cells as foreign substances and are therefore attacked by the body's defenses. (See the sections on allergies and multiple sclerosis for an explanation of causes of specific immune disorders.)

REMEDIES

General Recommendations

- Eat a diet rich in whole grains; green, leafy vegetables; roots; sea vegetables; and low-fat white fish.
- Follow instructions in Part IV for healing the liver, spleen, large intestine, and immune system.
- Adhere to a balanced lifestyle, including ample time to work, play, meditate, and enjoy social activity.

Foods to Eat

- Whole grains
- Vegetables, especially green, orange, and yellow vegetables and roots, all of which boost immunity
- Beans, especially soybeans and soybean products, such as tempeh, tofu, tamari, and miso
- Seaweeds: small amounts daily to increase trace mineral consumption
- Nuts and seeds in very small amounts
- Shiitake and reishi mushrooms are powerful immune boosters.
- Chlorophyll-rich foods, such as microalgae and cereal grasses, are anti-inflammatory and immune-enhancing.

Foods to Avoid

In addition to avoiding the following foods, do not eat too much food, do not eat late at night, and eat simpler food combinations.

- Meat
- Dairy products
- Alcohol
- Refined food
- Chemicalized food
- Processed food
- Oils and fats (minimize)
- Recreational drugs

Herbs to Treat Immune Disorders

- Shiitake mushrooms
- Garlic
- Cumin
- Turmeric
- Green tea
- Cinnamon
- Mint
- Chamomile
- For the more robust individual, decoct equal parts of:
  Chaparral leaf
  Pau d'arco (inner bark)
  Suma root
  Dried ling zhi (reishi) or shiitake mushrooms
  Peach seed
- For someone who is more deficient or debilitated, combine equal parts of:
  Suma root
  Dried ling zhi (reishi) or shiitake mushroom
  Job's tears seeds
  American ginseng root
  Astragalus root

Supplements

- Beta carotene: 15–50 mg/day
- Vitamin B complex
    Thiamine: 1.5 mg per day
    Riboflavin: 1.8 mg per day
    Vitamin B_6: 2–10 mg per day
    Vitamin B_{12}: 2–10 mg per day
    Niacin: 20 mg per day
- Vitamin C: 100–500 mg/day
- Vitamin E: 100–400 IU/day
- Magnesium: 400 mg/day
- Selenium: 20 mcg/day
- Zinc: 15 mg per day

Exercise

- Light aerobic exercise four to five times per week: walking, jogging, bicycling
- Yoga and stretching

Mind/Body

- Meditation, prayer, chanting: daily
- Social support (See recommendations for the immune system in Part IV.)
- Journal writing: Studies have shown that confessing painful memories, shame, and guilt to a journal can be immune-enhancing.
- Confessing to a friend or counselor painful memories, shame, or guilt can boost immune function and help to resolve long-standing conflicts that impair immunity.
- Seek professional counseling

IMPOTENCE

SYMPTOMS

Impotence is the inability to achieve or maintain an erection.

WHAT IS IMPOTENCE?

From Modern Western Medicine

Psychological factors are the cause of impotence in the majority of men. Among the most common are fatigue and stress (which cause temporary impotence) or guilt, anxiety, and long-standing psychological disorders involving sexual abuse, relationships with parents, or depression.

A minority of cases of impotence are caused by physical impairment (such as neurological disorders), disease (such as diabetes), or alcohol or drug abuse. Certain prescription drugs (such as those for high blood pressure) may also cause impotence. Finally, circulatory disorders can be a cause of impotence by preventing adequate blood flow to the penis. Poor circulation may also result in lower levels of testosterone, the male hormone.

From Traditional Medicine

According to Chinese medicine, the kidneys are the source of sexual energy. Specifically, kidney yang, or the outward flow of energy from the kidneys, warms and energizes the sex organs and ignites sexual desire. The spleen and spleen meridian support kidney yang. Therefore, treatment of both the kidneys and spleen are essential to the restoration of sex drive and function. Another set of organs that must be treated is the heart and circulatory system (regarded in Chinese medicine as the fire element).

Often, the tiny vessels within the penis can become blocked by atherosclerosis, causing the inability to experience or maintain an erection.

REMEDIES

General Recommendations

- See Part IV for strengthening kidneys, spleen, and circulation to overcome impotence.
- Avoid high-fat and cold foods, which decrease circulation.
- Exercise regularly.
- Maintain body warmth.

Foods to Eat

- Whole grains (Brown rice, congees, oats, and sweet rice are especially good.)
- Carbohydrate-rich vegetables, such as winter squash, carrots, rutabagas, turnips, parsnips, sweet potatoes, yams, and pumpkins
- Onions, leeks, black pepper, ginger, fennel, garlic, and other pungent tastes

To strengthen kidney yang:

- Cloves
- Fenugreek seeds
- Anise seeds
- Black peppercorns
- Ginger (preferably dried)
- Cinnamon
- Walnuts (one of the best remedies)
- Black beans
- Onion family
- Quinoa
- Salmon
- Trout

Also good for impotence:

- Green vegetables
- Seeds, especially sunflower and pumpkin
- Free-range, fertilized eggs
- Cold-pressed oils
- Sprouted seeds and beans
- Wheat germ
- Fish
- Seaweeds, especially kelp (moderately)
- Walnuts

Foods to Avoid

- Excessive raw vegetables cool and weaken kidney yang.
- Fruit, especially citrus, cools and weakens kidneys.
- Sprouts
- Tomatoes
- Spinach
- Chard
- Tofu
- Vinegar

Foods that weaken kidney yang:

- Cold foods and drinks
- Salty food

Foods to avoid for anyone who suffers from impotence; these foods will especially weaken circulation and kidney health.

- Meat
- Poultry
- Dairy products
- Sugar
- Alcohol
- Cigarettes
- Drugs

Herbs to Treat Impotence

- Ginkgo biloba
- Yellow dock (also known as curly dock)
- Raspberry
- Cinnamon (warming)
- Ginseng (warming)
- Blackberry

Physiotherapy

- Alternate hot and cold sitz baths. This is the most effective measure in rejuvenating the sexual organs. Repeat one or two times per day, if possible.
- Ice-cold plunges are an excellent tonic for the body generally, and especially for the pelvic region if the plunge is confined to below the waist. Precede ice plunge with sauna wherever possible.

Supplements

- Beta-carotene: 15–30 mg/day
- Vitamin B complex
    Thiamine: 1.5 mg per day
    Riboflavin: 1.8 mg per day
    Vitamin B_6: 2–10 mg per day
    Vitamin B_{12}: 2–10 mg per day
    Niacin: 20 mg per day
- Vitamin C: 100–500 mg/day
- Vitamin E: 100–400 mg/day
- Zinc: 15 mg/day

INCONTINENCE

SYMPTOMS

Several types of incontinence exist, each exhibiting its own symptoms. Stress incontinence is the involuntary release of small amounts of urine when coughing, laughing, picking up a heavy object, or engaging in excessive activity. It is very common in women, especially after childbirth when the urethral sphincter muscles are stretched.

Urge incontinence is the strong desire to urinate, accompanied by an inability to control the bladder. Urge incontinence may occur when walking or sitting, but is frequently triggered by a sudden change in position.

Total incontinence is the inability to control the bladder, resulting from the loss of sphincter function.

Overflow incontinence occurs when a person is unable to empty the bladder fully due to the presence of an obstruction. The bladder remains full, but is constantly dribbling small amounts from the overflow. Elimination of the obstruction restores continence.

WHAT IS INCONTINENCE?

From Modern Western Medicine

Incontinence is a localized disorder of the urinary tract caused by infection, bladder stones, tumors, or a prolapse of the uterus or the vagina. Other causes of incontinence include a nervous system disorder that causes the loss of bladder control and weak pelvic muscles that are unable to control the urethra sphincter. Exercises that strengthen these muscles can restore bladder control.

Special padded underwear can be purchased to reduce discomfort. A minority of people are able to pass a catheter into the bladder four or five times a day to urinate. If these measures are unsuccessful, surgery may be needed.

From Traditional Medicine

Urinary tract infections, constipation, muscle and sphincter weakness, hormonal imbalance, neurological disorders, and overweight can all cause bladder problems. In general, however, these problems all cause or arise from weak qi to the kidneys and bladder. Treatment is designed to promote the increase in qi to the kidneys and bladder. These include foods, herbs, and exercises that promote bladder qi.

REMEDIES

Foods to Eat

- Sweet brown rice
- Wheat berries (in sourdough bread, plain cooked berries, or herb tea)
- Parsley

Foods to Avoid

- Caffeine
- Alcohol
- Sugar
- Acidic juices and foods
- Spicy foods
- Milk products
- Tobacco
- Cocoa
- Sodas high in caffeine

Herbs to Treat Incontinence

- Parsley tea
- Celery seed: 5–30 drops of the fluid extract; can be combined in herbal tea
- Yarrow: infusion, 1 teaspoon to 1 cup of boiling water is given in wine-glass to cup amounts, 3 or 4 times a day.

Homeopathy

- Couch grass (especially helpful when there is a burning sensation and constant desire to urinate): 10–20 drops in water, two or more times per day
- Damiana: 15–30 drops, once a day
- Mullein: 15–40 drops in warm water, every 2–4 hours

Exercises

Do the bladder drill. This technique requires that you urinate only at scheduled times during the day, usually one to two hours apart. Then, over a few weeks, gradually extend the periods between urinations, with a goal of reaching two and a half hours, then three hours. You should empty your bladder as completely as you can at your scheduled time, regardless of whether you feel an urge to go. If you feel an urgency to go again before your next scheduled trip to the toilet, try to distract yourself with work or some pleasant activity. If the urge becomes too great to be suppressed, of course you should go after you have made a significant effort to resist. It may take up to six months to regain the desired amount of control, but this method of bladder training has been shown to be highly effective against incontinence.

Kegel exercises should be done daily. Pelvic muscle exercise has been used as an effective treatment for more than a century. It calls for stopping and starting the flow of urine several times every time the bladder is being voided. Like any muscle-training regimen, these exercises must be done correctly and daily to have sustained benefits. To do this:

1. Locate the proper muscles by placing your hands on your thighs and buttocks as you stop and start the urine flow. If these are tensed, you're doing the Kegels wrong. Focus instead on closing and opening the muscles that control the urethra and anus, which are the ones you want to strengthen.
2. Tighten the muscles slowly to the maximum extent you can; hold the contraction for ten seconds; slowly release.
3. Repeat the exercise at least ten times throughout the day.

Do yoga and stretching exercises daily, especially those designed to cleanse and eliminate blockages from bladder meridian.

Chinese Medicine

- To strengthen the kidney and bladder qi, obtain crushed or whole oyster and clam shells in a Chinese herb store. If they are whole, crush them before decocting into a tea. Oyster shell calcium supplements can also be taken.
- Acupressure, especially to restore the strength of and eliminate blockages from the bladder and kidney meridians
- Acupuncture for bladder and kidneys

INFERTILITY

SYMPTOMS

Infertility is the inability to conceive. Either the man or the woman or both can be the source of the infertility. Infertility is suspected when pregnancy has not occurred within a year of unprotected sexual intercourse.

WHAT IS INFERTILITY?

From Modern Western Medicine

Infertility can occur at any step during conception or maturation of the developing fetus. In order for conception to occur, a healthy sperm and egg must join as a result of sexual intercourse, and the resulting zygote must implant in the uterus where its cells can multiply and the fetus can grow. Once this has occurred, the developing embryo needs a healthy environment that supports the growth of the baby through the nine months of pregnancy.

The majority of cases of male infertility occur because the man has failed to produce enough healthy sperm. Several factors can damage sperm, including a blockage in the spermatic tubes caused by a sexually transmitted disease; varicose veins in the scrotum; damaged testes; abnormal development of the testes; or toxins in the blood that lower sperm count, such as from cigarettes, alcohol, and drugs. Chromosomal damage, though rare, can also cause infertility. In addition, the man's ejaculation can fail to project the sperm far enough into the fallopian tube in order for the sperm and egg to meet.

The most common cause of female infertility is the failure to ovulate, or produce eggs, which can be caused by hormonal imbalance, stress, or a disorder of the ovary (such as the presence of a cyst or tumor). A blocked fallopian tube can prevent the sperm and egg from meeting. Other causes include disorders of the uterus and the production of antibodies in the cervical mucus that kill sperm. In rare instances, an allergy to a partner's sperm can occur or some form of chromosomal damage may be present.

Tests on both partners can determine the cause of the infertility. Changes in diet and relaxation exercises are sometimes recommended. Drugs intended to treat male infertility have limited success; for women, medication may be helpful to promote ovulation. Fallopian tubes can be repaired by surgery. More technologically advanced procedures, such as in vitro fertilization or the insemination of a man's semen into the woman's cervix (used when a woman's mucus contains antibodies that are hostile to a man's sperm) may be tried.

Forty percent of infertility cases stem from disorders affecting both members of the couple. Thirty percent are caused exclusively by men, and another 30 percent by women.

From Traditional Medicine

Before consulting a holistic healer, the couple should have had a complete physical examination by a medical doctor to determine the cause of the infertility. Once this is done, the health of the man and woman can be promoted by natural healing methods. Very often, fallopian tubes are inflamed or blocked because of pelvic infection, which can be treated by diet, supplementation, and hydrotherapy. In Chinese medicine, the sexual vitality of both men and women depends on the health of the kidneys and adrenal glands, which are located on top of the kidneys. Infertility is seen as a kidney yang deficiency, meaning the absence of warmth and outgoing energy (sometimes referred to as fire energy). The remedies listed below are designed to increase kidney and adrenal strength by restoring kidney yang.

REMEDIES

Foods to Eat

Add all the foods under incontinence to this list as both are Chinese medicine remedies for insufficient kidney yang.

- Whole grains, especially barley, a tonic for the kidneys
- Cooked vegetables
- Seaweed in small amounts (two-tablespoon serving) daily strengthens kidneys, bladder, and adrenals.
- Beans, especially black beans, are especially strengthening to kidneys and adrenals and restore kidney yang.
- Nuts, especially walnuts
- Fish, especially low-fat white fish and salmon, which strengthen kidneys

Foods to Avoid

- Coffee (especially weakening to kidneys, adrenals, and sex organs)
- Alcohol
- Drugs
- Cigarettes
- High-fat foods block circulation and can cause obstructions in the sex organs.
- Excessively cold foods shock the stomach, digestion, and kidneys and weaken circulation in the kidneys (kidney fire).
- Raw foods: Especially avoid these in fall and winter when kidneys, bladder, and adrenals are being strengthened. (See the description of the five element theory in the section on Chinese medicine in Part III.)
- Excess fruit and sugar weaken the kidneys.
- Soft drinks tax the kidneys.

Herbs to Treat Infertility

- False unicorn: decoction, simmer 5–15 minutes, take 6 oz., 3 times daily; tincture, 15–30 drops, 3 times daily; fluid extract, ½–1 tsp., 3 times daily; powder, 2–5 capsules (15–30 grains), 3 times daily
- Add dong quai and ginger to chicken soup for an excellent female hormone tonic.
- Saffron: 100–500 mg (not to be used during pregnancy)

Hydrotherapy

- Hot and cold sitz baths are very effective in removing internal congestion and inflammation.
- Avoid excessively long showers. They drain minerals from the body and weaken kidneys.
- Loofah brush the body vigorously when showering to promote qi flow.

Chinese Medicine

- Acupuncture to strengthen kidneys and adrenals
- Wear a cotton cummerbund around the kidneys, adrenals, and bladder beneath your shirt to keep kidneys warm.

Exercise

- Pelvic exercises (see the section on incontinence)
- Daily swimming
- Daily aerobic exercise, including walking, jogging, or any athletic sport that is enjoyed

Supplements

For men and women:
- Vitamin B complex
    Thiamine: 1.5 mg per day
    Riboflavin: 1.8 mg per day
    Vitamin B_6: 2–10 mg per day
    Vitamin B_{12}: 2–10 mg per day
    Niacin: 20 mg per day
- Folic acid: 200 mcg/day
- Vitamin E: 100–400 IU

For men, also include:

- Selenium: 20–50 mcg/day
- Zinc: 15 mg/day
- L-carnitine: 300 mg per day
- L-lysine: 500 mg per day
- Vitamin C: 100–500 mg/day (increases sperm motility)
- Vitamin E: 100–400 mg/day

INFLUENZA OR FLU

SYMPTOMS

Physicians classify influenza, or flu, into three types, each with a slightly different set of symptoms. Types A and B symptoms include chills, fever, headache, muscular aches, loss of appetite, and fatigue. Type A is more debilitating than type B. Type C is a mild illness that is indistinguishable from the common cold. The symptoms include cough, sore throat, runny nose, fever, joint ache, and fatigue. After two days, the symptoms tend to subside, and after five days they have disappeared. However, the lungs may still be affected and the person may feel weak and depressed after the main symptoms subside. The illness is usually gone in seven to ten days.

WHAT IS INFLUENZA?

From Modern Western Medicine

Influenza is a viral infection of the respiratory tract that is spread through water droplets that contain the virus and are coughed or sneezed into the air. Outbreaks of flu tend to occur in the winter. Flu viruses alter themselves just enough so that even when you contract a type of flu and become immunized to it, you may still be vulnerable to that same type in the future, if it is altered sufficiently to overcome your body's immune protection. This is the case with the type A flu, which is highly unstable and constantly creating new strains. Such mutant strains have created pandemics during the course of the twentieth century, such as the Spanish flu in 1918, the Asian flu in 1957, and the Hong Kong flu in 1968.

Flu vaccines for the A and B types are 60 to 70 percent effective, though the resulting immunity is short-lived. The vaccine, therefore, must be readministered each year before the flu attacks.

Once you get the flu, bed rest, painkillers, and medication to reduce fever, sore throat, and respiratory congestion are recommended.

From Traditional Medicine

Flu is not distinguished from the common cold and is looked at as a way for the body to eliminate stored-up waste and poisons that have accumulated over months of poor eating, stress, lack of exercise, and inadequate rest. Eating smaller meals and getting plenty of rest will help to alleviate the symptoms and speed recovery. Overeating will prolong the condition or send the underlying toxins deeper into the body. Elimination of mucus and waste through the nose, bladder, and intestines should not be suppressed, since this is doing considerable good work to cleanse the system.

REMEDIES

Foods to Eat

- Fast on apple, citrus, or lemon juice.
- Cabbage with hearts is high in bioflavonoids.
- Peppers with their insides are high in bioflavonoids.
- Parsley
- Carrots
- Broccoli
- Turnips
- Kuzu
- Parsnips
- Garlic
- Scallions
- Grapefruit
- Cooked fruit

Foods to Avoid

- Meat
- Dairy products
- Poultry
- Flour products
- Eggs
- Sweets
- Salty foods
- Fried foods or excess oil
- Coffee
- Tea
- Alcohol
- Tobacco

Herbs to Treat Influenza

Garlic can often halt a cold or flu if taken soon enough. Take it every three hours during the day that symptoms first appear. Hold, without chewing, half a peeled garlic clove between the cheek and teeth for twenty to thirty minutes. Move it around occasionally to avoid burning delicate mouth tissue. If the juice is still too strong, use an uncut clove for a longer period. Use garlic when there is a need for warming herbs, as in the case of chills, lack of sweating, and body aches. These are diaphoretics to increase circulation.

When the person feels weak:

- Hyssop: standard infusion or 3–9 g; tincture, 10–30 drops
- Freshly grated ginger tea: Steep 2–6 slices of the fresh root in a cup of

boiling water. Ginger teabags can also be purchased at your health food store. For sweating to help dispel toxins.

- Cinnamon branch: standard infusion or 3–9 g
- Peppermint: standard infusion or ½–6 g
- Lemon balm: standard infusion or ½–6 g
- Burdock seed: standard infusion or 3–9 g
- Feverfew: standard infusion or 3–9 g

Cooling, diaphoretic herbs are used to dispel toxins through sweat, and are appropriate when there is high fever. They are contraindicated for individuals with low metabolism who are complaining of cold when there is no fever present.

Supplements

- Beta-carotene: 15 mg per day
- Vitamin C: 100–500 mg per day

INSECT BITES

SYMPTOMS

The irritation you experience after an insect bite is an allergic reaction to the insect's saliva and/or feces, often left on or near the bite by the insect and then rubbed into the skin when scratching. Reactions to bites and stings vary widely from a harmless red pimple that itches to more severe and painful swelling and rash. About one person in two hundred suffers a dangerous immune reaction that can cause *anaphylactic shock* unless the toxin is eliminated from the body by an injection of epinephrine. These people must carry an epinephrine kit with them at all times.

For the vast majority of people, the irritation is gone after forty-eight hours. Hundreds of bites or stings are necessary to be life-threatening to the average adult.

REMEDIES

From Modern Western Medicine

If stung by a bee, remove the stinger or sac from the wound by scratching the skin or digging it out with a knife. Do not squeeze the sac with your fingers and risk injecting more venom into the wound. Wash thoroughly with soap and water and apply an ointment, such as calamine lotion. Call a physician immediately if there is a severe reaction.

Itching of the scalp or pubic hair could indicate the presence of lice or fleas, which can be removed by an insecticide. In this case, your entire home and everyone living there must be treated to remove the insects.

From Traditional Medicine

Anyone who suffers an allergic reaction to an insect bite or sting must be treated medically. For those who develop the normal irritation, however, the following recommendations will reduce the discomfort.

General Recommendations

- Remove the stinger, if present, then immediately apply ice to the area.
- Ice water and baking soda made into a wet paste will draw out the toxins of bee stings and reduce the pain.
- Clay packs: Mix green clay with a little water and apply to the affected area to draw out toxins.
- Vinegar plus lemon juice applications reduce the toxic effect and pain of insect bites. Apply regularly.
- Onion (grated; apply topically) draws out swelling and reduces pain.

Herbs to Treat Insect Bites

- Echinacea (excellent blood purifier, used for snake and spider bites): tincture, 30–60 drops, 3–6 times daily; fluid extract, ½–1 teaspoon, 3–6 times daily, taken internally
- Witch hazel: tincture, 15–60 drops as needed; fluid extract, ½ teaspoon as needed, taken internally
- Agrimony: Apply a fomentation externally.
- Aloe vera: Apply gel externally.
- Yerba santa: Apply fomentation externally.
- Lobelia: Apply poultice externally.

Foods to Eat

- Citrus fruits for vitamin C
- Soft grains with chopped-up carrots, onion, and ginger to encourage digestion and elimination
- Green, orange, and yellow vegetables to boost immunity

Homeopathy

For bee, hornet, and wasp stings:

- Apis mellifica is one of the most widely used homeopathic remedies for bee stings. It is made from the whole honey bee. Use it when there is burning and stinging pain and puffiness. Rush to the nearest hospital if the person is allergic to bee stings, and give apis mellifica in the highest potency you have.
- Ledum: Apply a drop or two with a cotton swab or cotton ball. Used for puncture wounds and stings, numbness or great sensitivity to touch, pain that moves upward, or when the sting and surrounding area may be cold.
- Other choices: arnica, calendula, urtica urens or Hypericum tincture.

For poisonous spiders or scorpions, rush the person to the nearest hospital, but apply the following remedies along with ice as a first aid measure.

- Carbolicum acidum: Use when the patient has a red face, is pale around the mouth and nose, and is languid but is highly sensitive to smells.
- Crotalus horridus: Use when there is a lot of swelling and discoloration around the bite.
- Oxalicum acidum: Use when the affected area is cold and numb, with violent pains and trembling.

Supplements

- Vitamin C: 100–500 mg per day
- Vitamin E: 100–400 mg per day

INSOMNIA

SYMPTOMS

A person with insomnia has difficulty falling asleep or staying asleep. Once awakened in the middle of the night, the person has trouble returning to sleep. The result of any sleep disturbance is often irritability, depression, emotional disturbances, or poor memory. Conversely, insomnia can be a sign of depression, as well.

WHAT IS INSOMNIA?

From Modern Western Medicine

One in three American adults has trouble sleeping. Drugs that induce sleep are among the most widely used medications today. Most insomnia is caused by worry, but other causes include sleep apnea (a breathing problem), restless legs, noise or light, excess caffeine before bed, lack of exercise, and drug use, including the overuse of sleep-inducing drugs. Other factors include chronic anxiety and/or depression, mania, and schizophrenia.

People with insomnia should try to be very active during the day and go to bed when tired.

From Traditional Medicine

Traditionally, insomnia is most often the result of a liver and gallbladder imbalance. This is especially the case when the person has trouble sleeping between 11 P.M. and 3 A.M, when the body is channeling its energy to the gallbladder and liver, which means these organs are receiving their peak amounts of qi or life energy. Just as Western science has established a circadian rhythm, so, too, did Chinese healers, who maintained that each of the major organs receives optimal amounts of energy during a two-hour period through the course of the day. (See Part III for a discussion of the Chinese clock.) A weak liver and gallbladder cannot remain stable and relaxed during the hours of 11 P.M. to 3 A.M. when they are receiving an abundance of energy. This is especially the case for those who have eaten before bed or have consumed alcohol or heavy or spicy foods.

Any food that taxes the liver and gallbladder and is consumed before bed can cause insomnia. Overeating, food additives, preservatives, artificial colors, or foods that do not combine well can all disturb the liver and gallbladder before bed, and therefore can keep you awake.

Insomnia can also be caused by an excess of other foods and drinks consumed during the day, including too much coffee, tea, chocolate, and soda.

Other dietary factors include a deficiency of B vitamins and calcium, and too much salt or excessive amounts of liquids.

Finally, eating whole grains and getting physical exercise are essential to a good night's sleep. Whole grains promote the production of serotonin, a brain neurotransmitter that promotes better concentration, feelings of well-being, and deep sleep. Exercise works off physical tension that can keep you awake during the night.

REMEDIES

Foods to Eat

- Chlorophyll-rich foods, such as leafy, green vegetables, steamed or boiled
- Microalgae, such as chlorella and spirulina
- Oyster shell can be purchased in health food stores and taken as a nutritional supplement.
- Whole grains: Whole wheat, brown rice, and oats have a calming and soothing effect on the nervous system and the mind. Carbohydrates also boost serotonin, which promotes better sleep.
- Mushrooms (all types)
- Fruit, especially mulberries and lemons, which calm the mind
- Seeds: Jujube seeds are used to calm the spirit and support the heart. Chia seeds also have a sedative effect.
- Dill
- Basil

Foods to Avoid

In addition to the foods listed below, also avoid too many ingredients in a meal and too much food late at night.

- Coffee
- Tea
- Spicy foods
- Cola
- Chocolate
- Stimulant drugs
- Cigarettes (Nicotine is a stimulant that causes the adrenals to secrete adrenaline. This leads to increased heart rate, elevated blood pressure, and hyperactivity.)
- Alcohol (For many people, this is a stimulant.)
- Refined carbohydrates (They drain the B vitamins.)
- Sugar
- Additives
- Preservatives

- Non-organic foods containing pesticides
- Canned foods or any source of toxicity or heavy metals

Herbs to Treat Insomnia

- Rose hips: Take with any of the other herbs in this list. The vitamin C is calming to the nerves.
- Chamomile tea is a mild sedative. It can be mixed with hops in equal parts.
- Hops are a mild sedative. It can be mixed with chamomile in equal parts.
- Passionflower is a sedative. Take 30–60 drops of tincture forty-five minutes before bed.
- Mix together equal parts:

  Skullcap
  Valerian
  Lemon balm
  Lady's slipper

Drink as an infusion when needed, using one ounce to a pint of boiling water. Steep for twenty minutes.

Homeopathy

- Nux vomica, known as the student's remedy, is helpful when you're sleepless after mental strain and can't turn off your mind.
- Arsenicum: when you're sleepless from worry or anxiety
- Cocculus is known as the nurse's remedy, because it treats those who can't get to sleep after their late-night duty is done.
- Coffea: for sleeplessness from excitement or joy; less effective for the big coffee drinker
- Pulsatilla: for sleeplessness from recurring thoughts

Physiotherapy

- Hot footbaths draw blood away from the head, making sleep easier.
- Warm baths are relaxing, but if they are too hot, they become stimulating.
- Alternate hot and cold showers
- General exercise plus fresh air

Exercise

- Vigorous aerobic exercise daily, for at least twenty to thirty minutes per exercise session can combat insomnia. Among the best choices are walking, jogging, bicycling, playing a sport, or swimming.
- Yoga or some form of stretching exercise
- Sleep-inducing exercises, such as progressive contraction/relaxation ex-

ercises: Lie on a bed and relax as much as possible. Breathe deeply. Feel your body sink into the mattress while concentrating on your breath. Ignore any thoughts or feelings that pass through your mind. Contract your face, making a grimace, and then your neck, and then let both go, allowing the relaxation to sink into the muscles of the face and neck. Do the same for your arms: contract the upper arms and chest, then release. Continue the same contraction and releasing of the muscles of your lower arms, hands, abdomen, buttocks, thighs, lower legs, and finally the feet. Finish with one final contraction of your entire body and then release all at once. Repeat the cycle two or three times. Resume relaxation while breathing deeply. Continue to focus on your breath until you fall asleep.

Supplements

- Vitamin B complex
  Thiamine: 1.5 mg per day
  Riboflavin: 1.8 mg per day
  Vitamin B_6: 2–10 mg per day
  Vitamin B_{12}: 2–10 mg per day
  Niacin: 20 mg per day
- Vitamin C: 100–500 mg per day
- Pantothenic acid: 250 mg per day
- Calcium: 800–1000 mg per day
- Magnesium: 100 mg per day
- Zinc: 15 mg per day
- Manganese: 1 mg per day

ITCHING

SYMPTOMS

Intense, distracting irritation or tickling sensation in the skin may be generalized (felt all over the skin's surface) or local (confined to one area).

WHAT IS ITCHING?

From Modern Western Medicine

The cause of itching is not understood. Though it is the most prominent symptom in skin disease, it does not itself necessarily indicate an underlying skin disorder. People differ widely in their tolerance, with thresholds altering according to stress levels and emotions. Warm conditions and few distractions—such as occur at nighttime—make itching worse.

Itching can occur all over the body or at a specific site. Generalized itching can occur from excessive bathing or the use of harsh soaps, both of which remove the skin's natural oils and may leave the skin excessively dry and scaly. This is a very common cause of itching. Pharmaceutical drugs, including antibiotics, can cause itching. Certain illnesses, such as chicken pox, produce generalized itching; the elderly sometimes suffer from itching for no apparent reason. Itching can also be caused by diabetes, disorders of the thyroid, and those of the blood.

Local itching can occur for many reasons (see the section on anal itching). The most common cause is, of course, insect bites. Other common causes include worm infestation, lice, scabies, candidiasis, hormonal changes, and the use of spermicides, ointments, and deodorants.

Scratching an itch provides only temporary relief and makes it worse in the long run. Treatment includes cooling lotions such as calamine to relieve irritation and emollients to reduce dryness. Apply a soothing lotion, salve, or wet compress to the affected areas.

From Traditional Medicine

Itching occurs because the body is attempting to discharge waste products that the kidneys and liver have not been able to remove from the blood. The skin is an eliminative organ and will attempt to rid the body of toxins when the liver and kidneys are either overworked or sluggish.

Liver stagnation, a major cause of skin irritations and itching, is referred to in Chinese medicine as liver wind, which refers to the presence of excessive heat and turbulence within the liver, both caused by the stagnation. Traditional Chinese healers characterize the imbalance as "heat gives rise to wind."

Sufficient yin fluids would help to stabilize the liver and inhibit the generation of yang influences such as wind and heat. (See the list of foods to eat, below.)

REMEDIES

Foods to Eat

The following foods counteract dryness in the body.

- Soybean products, including tofu, tempeh, and soy milk
- Spinach
- Barley
- Millet
- Pears
- Apples
- Persimmons
- Loquats
- Seaweeds
- Black and white fungus
- Almonds
- Pine nuts
- Peanuts
- Sesame seeds
- Honey (cooked)
- Barley malt
- Rice syrup
- Eggs
- Clams
- Oysters
- Mussels
- Herring
- Dairy products (Good-quality dairy may be appropriate for those with signs of deficiency.)

The following foods nurture yin fluids:

- String beans
- Black beans
- Mung beans and sprouts
- Kidney beans
- Kuzu root
- Watermelon and other melons
- Blackberries
- Mulberries
- Blueberries

- Water chestnuts
- Spirulina
- Chlorella
- Black sesame seeds

Foods to Avoid

- Spices (Especially hot spices will warm the body and dry the person.)
- Herbs (Many herbs are warming.)
- Animal foods (Warming foods will dry the person.)
- Bitter foods can be depleting if the condition is deficient.

Herbs to Treat Itching

INTERNAL

- Cocklebur: decoction, 3–12 g
- Caltrop: 6–12 g
- Burdock root: tincture, 30–60 drops, 3 or 4 times daily; infusion (leaves), 1 cup, 3 or 4 times daily; decoction (root and seeds), 1 oz. root to 1½ pints water, boiled down to 1 pint, take 3 oz., 3 or 4 times daily

EXTERNAL

- Goldenseal as fomentation
- Buckthorn as fomentation for itchy skin
- Alum as fomentation

KIDNEY DISEASE

SYMPTOMS

Chills, fever, low back pain, bladder irritation, pain on urination (dysuria), frequency, and possibly edema. Each acute episode causes some permanent kidney damage.

WHAT IS KIDNEY DISEASE?

From Modern Western Medicine

There are many disorders that affect the kidneys. High blood pressure damages the nephrons, or the functional unit of the kidneys, but nephrotic damage can also result from some other cause. Nephrotic syndrome occurs when fluid collects in the body and large quantities of protein are lost in the urine. Acute or chronic renal failure is another serious and even life-threatening disorder of the kidneys.

Many people suffer from congenital kidney abnormalities. A person might be born with only one functional kidney, or with both kidneys on one side, or with a kidney that has two ureters and partially duplicates itself (duplex kidney). Such conditions are rarely life-threatening, however.

A wide variety of illnesses can give rise to kidney disease, including diabetes mellitus and hemolytic-uremic syndrome; an autoimmune disorder known as glomerulonephritis, or the inflammation of the filtering units of the kidneys; kidney stones (see the section on kidney stones); and infection (known as pyelonephritis), most often caused by a blockage of the urine flow.

Renal cell carcinoma is the most common form of kidney cancer in adults over forty, while nephroblastoma (Wilm's tumor) is the kidney cancer that affects children, most of them under four years of age.

Allergies to pharmaceutical drugs can also cause kidney disease.

The techniques used to diagnose kidney disease include blood tests, urinalysis, renal biopsy, ultrasound scanning, intravenous or retrograde phylography, angiography, and CT scanning.

From Traditional Medicine

Among the most common causes of kidney disease related to lifestyle in the West is excess protein in the diet. Protein converts to uric acid, which the kidneys excrete from the blood. Excess uric acid damages kidneys. Anyone with a kidney disorder should minimize protein by avoiding animal foods, except for small amounts of fish. Temporarily adopting a vegetarian diet can be helpful to those with kidney problems.

In Chinese medicine, the kidneys are regarded as part of the water element, which is responsible for the health of the kidneys, bladder, and sex organs. The kidneys are said to be the seat of the will, meaning that willpower emanates from these organs. The kidneys also provide qi, or life force, to the entire body. Any damage to the kidneys will weaken the body and the will.

Most kidney disorders are the result of deficiencies, either inadequate yang (expansive energy) or yin (contractive energy). Deficiencies of kidney yin—a common cause of premature ejaculation in men and frequent urination—is caused by inadequate amounts of yin fluids. Without sufficient yin fluids, all other parts of the body are affected, including the heart, liver, and lungs. Common symptoms of deficient kidney yin include low backache, weak legs, rapid pulse, dry mouth and throat, ear problems (including tinnitus), anxiety, and fear. (See the lists of foods to eat and foods to avoid in order to nurture kidney yin).

Kidney yang, regarded as the fire within the kidneys, is needed to warm the body, energize it, and provide the outgoing energy that supports willpower, courage, self-expression, and social interaction. When the kidneys are deficient in yang, the person is said to lack spirit and will suffer from fatigue. He may become introverted, lack physical and mental vitality, and suffer from poor sex drive. Women experience irregular periods and vaginal discharge. People often experience the inability to urinate (not enough outgoing energy), weak legs, and low backache (from tightness). Asthma may also result. (See the lists of foods to eat and avoid for warming kidney yang and providing kidney yang.)

REMEDIES

Foods to Eat

In acute cases, fast on the following liquids:

- Cranberry juice
- Mullein tea
- Watermelon seed tea
- Parsley water
- Barley water
- Watermelon juice

Incorporate the following foods into the dietary regimen, as they are excellent for healing kidney disease.

- Garlic
- Green vegetables, such as asparagus, kale, parsley, watercress, dandelion greens, and turnip greens
- Watermelon
- Celery

- Potato skins
- Horseradish
- Apples
- Pears
- Cucumbers
- Parsnips
- Carrot, celery, and parsley juice
- Kidney beans

CHINESE MEDICINE

To nurture kidney yin:

- Millet
- Barley
- Tofu
- String beans
- Black beans and all other beans
- Mung beans and sprouts
- Seaweeds
- Spirulina and chlorella
- Black sesame seeds

To nurture kidney yang:

- Onion family, such as garlic, onions, leeks, and scallions
- Salmon
- Quinoa
- Herbs, such as cloves, fenugreek seeds, fennel seeds, anise seeds, and dried ginger
- Walnuts

To nurture kidney qi:

- Parsley
- Wheat berries
- Sweet rice

Foods to Avoid

For kidney yin deficiency:

- Animal foods, especially eggs, pork, and cheese
- Coffee
- Alcohol
- Tobacco

- Cinnamon
- Cloves
- Ginger
- Hot spices

For kidney yang deficiency:

- Cooling foods and fruit
- Raw foods
- Excessive salt
- Use seaweed cautiously

Herbs to Treat Kidney Disease

- Crushed or whole oyster or clam shell (good for deficient kidney qi): Crush if whole (find them on the beach) and decoct into a tea or else purchase at Chinese herb store.
- Prepared rehmannia root is the main herb in the Chinese Rehmannia-Siz formula found in all Chinese pharmacies as well as many other herb shops. (Builds kidney yin; most widely used tonic.)
- Stinging nettle (diuretic): tincture, 10–40 drops, 3 or 4 times/day
- Buchu (diuretic, antispasmodic): tincture, 10–15 drops, 3 or 4 times/day

Massage

Massage the following mixture across the kidney area and abdomen:

1 oz. dissolved mutton tallow
20 drops spirits of gum turpentine
40 drops camphor
20 drops benzoin
3 drops sassafras

Supplements

- Beta-carotene: 15–30 mg per day
- Vitamin B complex: 25 mg per day
- Vitamin C: 100–500 mg per day
- Vitamin E: 100–400 IU per day
- Magnesium: 100 mg per day

KIDNEY STONES (CALCULUS OR CALCULI)

SYMPTOMS

Kidney stones are usually felt as a dull, intermittent low backache, or as pain in the testicles, groin, or legs. The pain often gets worse with activity. When the stones move into the ureter, there can be hemorrhaging, severe pain, pallor, nausea, and vomiting.

WHAT ARE KIDNEY AND URETHRAL STONES?

From Modern Western Medicine

Men are three times more likely to suffer from kidney stones than women. Once a person develops a kidney stone, he has about a 60 percent chance of developing another within seven years. The summer months see the highest incidence of kidney stone attacks, perhaps because of the body's loss of water from sweat. This causes the urine to become more concentrated, and thus increases the likelihood of stones.

There is no known cause of kidney stones, though mild dehydration may be a factor.

Most kidney stones are composed of calcium oxalate and/or phosphate, both of which are end products of metabolism and must be excreted from the urine. They are not easily soluble, which is why they can easily form stones. High levels of oxalate in the blood from diets rich in foods or drinks containing oxalic acid, increase the likelihood of kidney stones.

Calcium stones are often the first sign of metabolic disorders, including hyperparathyroidism. People with disorders related to protein may have stones that consist mostly of uric acid. Such stones may indicate the presence of gout, some cancers, or chronic dehydration.

Bed rest, painkillers, and increased fluid intake to encourage the passage of the stone are the primary means of treatment. Most stones are smaller than 0.2 inch in diameter; these are passed at home with few, if any, problems. Larger stones may require surgery to prevent kidney damage. Probes, such as ultrasonic lithotripsy, and shock waves (produced by extracorporeal shock-wave lithotriptor) that disintegrate the stones from outside the body are also used today.

From Traditional Medicine

The standard American diet, rich in oxalic acid, calcium, phosphorus, and protein, is the perfect formula for kidney stones. In addition, there is very little pure water drunk with this diet. Instead of water, coffee and soft drinks are the primary liquids consumed, both of which weaken kidneys and increase the likelihood of stones. In addition, excess salt and sugar may also play a role in the creation of stones.

Citric acid, vitamin E, and magnesium promote elimination of waste products that cause stone formation. Adequate intake of clean water also decreases the chance of a kidney stone forming.

Recent research suggests that deficiencies of vitamin B_6 and magnesium may lead to kidney stones. B_6 helps to regulate the body's production of oxalic acid. It also increases oxalate elimination. Magnesium helps to break down oxalate and make it more soluble in the urine. When combined with a healthy diet, B_6 and magnesium therapy is effective in preventing future stone formation, especially when urine oxalate levels are high. A urine test is needed to determine if oxalate levels are high.

REMEDIES

Foods to Eat

Stage one is the acute phase until all pain has ceased for at least twenty-four to forty hours.

- Mullein tea, watermelon seed tea, unsweetened fruit juice. Drink tea first thing in the morning. Watermelon seed tea should be taken two times a day. To make watermelon seed tea, grind a handful of watermelon seeds; steep in hot water for ten to fifteen minutes and strain; add a little honey; and drink the tea.
- Fresh juices such as watercress, parsley, carrot, and celery
- Liquids

Stage two:

- All the drinks listed above
- Fresh noncitrus fruit juice, especially cranberry
- Watermelons, papayas, and bananas
- Raw, grated salad composed of leafy greens such as lettuce, celery, watercress, parsley, cucumber, cabbage; alfalfa sprouts; and dressing of olive oil with lots of lemon and garlic and/or herbs
- Steamed vegetables
- Tofu
- Brown rice
- Miso
- Seaweed
- Fish
- Baked potato

CHINESE MEDICINE

- Black bean juice: Simmer one cup of beans in five cups of water for an hour. Drink ½ cup juice ½ hour before meals.
- Corn silk tea
- Parsley promotes urination and is good for stones (not for severe kidney inflammation or nursing mothers).
- Radish: one tablespoon of grated radish taken every day for several weeks (People who are deficient and cold should avoid radishes.)

Herbs to Treat Kidney Stones

- Mix together the following herbs:

    1 part gravel root
    1 part parsley root
    1 part marshmallow root
    ¼ part lobelia
    ¼ part ginger

Take one ounce of herbs and simmer for twenty minutes in one and one-half pints of distilled water. Drink one-half cup three times a day.

- Gravel root: decoction, 1 cup, 2–6 times per day to clear kidneys and dissolve stones
- Birch tea dissolves stones and removes uric acid.
- Cleavers (helps prevent reoccurrence): 10–15 drops, 2 or 3 times per day.
- Marshmallow: infusion, steep flowers/leaves for 5–15 minutes, drink one cup at a time, frequently; tincture, 30–60 drops, 3 times daily; fluid extract, 1–2 tsp., 3 times daily.

Physiotherapy

- Mullein poultice: Obtain a large amount of mullein herb. Moisten ¼ inch of herb with very hot water, lay on a large piece of gauze, and cover with gauze or cloth. This poultice should be large enough to cover the area from the navel to the pubic region in front, or over the kidney area in back. Apply the poultice and cover with hot, wet towels. Keep these as warm as possible, either by replacing the towels with a second set of heated, wet towels, or by using a hot water bottle or other source of heat. Keep this poultice on for thirty minutes.
- Spirits of gum turpentine pack: Alternate the mullein poultice with this pack. Mix 2 oz. spirits of turpentine with 1½ qt. hot water. Saturate a folded towel and apply to the prescribed area (bladder to pubic area in front or kidney area in back). Apply hot, wet towels as above. Apply this pack for thirty minutes every one, two, or four hours.

- Hops and lobelia poultice (for severe pain): Mix 1–2 oz. of the herbs and apply as per directions for mullein poultice.
- Hot sitz baths help urine flow.

Supplements

- Beta-carotene: 15 mg per day
- Vitamin B complex: 25 mg per day
- Vitamin B$_6$: 50 mg per day
- Vitamin C: 100 mg per day
- Vitamin E: 100–400 IU per day
- Magnesium helps keep calcium in solution and mobilizes calcium from the stone. Take 100 mg two times per day.

KNEE PROBLEMS

WHAT ARE COMMON KNEE PROBLEMS?

From Modern Western Medicine

Sprains of the ligament within the knee or the tearing of the meniscus, the small piece of cartilege within the knee joint, are usually the result of a sudden twist. Fragments of the meniscus can be torn free from the cartilage and cause the knee to become temporarily locked in one position.

Severe injuries, such as from sports activities or car accidents, can cause bleeding within the knee (hemarthrosis); minor injuries usually cause only inflammation of the lining of the joint (synovitis); running and other repetitive motion activities can cause inflammation of the tendon. Children sometimes experience temporary swelling of the prominent bone just below the knee (tibial tubercule) after repeated injury, such as from falling.

Excessive pressure on the front of the knee can cause bursitis (inflammation of the bursa, which are fluid-filled sacs within the joint). When fluid appears to be leaking from the knee or from one of the bursae, there may be a cyst within the joint, called a Baker's cyst.

Osteoarthritis, rheumatoid arthritis, and retropatellar arthritis (inflammation of the under surface of the patella) all affect the knee. Dislocation of the kneecap (patella) can occur after a sharp blow to the knee. Fractures of the bones of the knee are also common.

Children commonly suffer from knock-knees and bowlegs, but the vast majority of them outgrow these temporary abnormalities.

From Traditional Medicine

Knee problems are the result of a deficiency of kidney yang (see the section on kidney disease) and kidney jing, or the energy that is considered the deep essence within the kidneys that determines vitality, resistance to disease, and longevity. Chinese medicine teaches that each person has only a certain amount of jing. When it's used up, we cease to live. Certain foods provide jing, and protect existing jing. To strengthen jing, you should begin by eliminating those factors that weaken it, among which are stress, fear, insecurity, and overwork; excess ejaculation in men; too many births for women; toxins in food and water, intoxicants, heavy metals; excessive sweet-flavored food; and too much protein.

To nourish the jing, see the foods to eat listed below.

REMEDIES

Foods to Eat

See foods to eat to enhance kidney yang in the section on kidney disease. Foods to enhance the kidneys in general, according to Chinese medicine:

- Millet
- Wheat
- Black sesame seeds
- Black beans and black soybeans
- Chestnuts
- Mulberries
- Raspberries
- Strawberries
- Walnuts

Foods to nourish jing:

- Microalgae, such as chlorella, spirulina, and wild blue-green algae
- Bone-marrow soup (chop up the bones of an organic chicken) is especially good when there is deficiency characterized by frailty, pale or sallow complexion, weak radial pulse, introverted personality, and/or little or no tongue coating. Use cautiously when there are signs of heat. People who have an aversion to heat, great thirst, red tongue, yellow tongue coating, flushed face, and/or bloodshot eyes should use this warming remedy cautiously.
- Fish (Those with heat signs should use cautiously.)
- Cereal grasses repair damaged nucleic acid in the cells and are a rich source of provitamin A and omega-3 oils. (Those with cold signs, characterized by frequent feelings of coldness, aversion to the cold, pale complexion, and/or attraction to warm food and drink should avoid cereal grasses.)
- Almonds, high-quality milk, and clarified butter are especially good for those with cold signs.
- Nettles: Eat as a cooked green. Avoid when there are cold signs.
- Royal jelly contains the most complete range of human nutrients of any food. It is an energy tonic used for general deficiency. Royal jelly promotes phenomenal physical growth, reproductive ability, and longevity in the queen bee. In humans, it strongly stimulates sexuality and may help extend human life as well.

Foods to Avoid

- Cold food and liquid
- Fruit
- Sugar
- Processed food
- Stimulants
- Intoxicants
- Excessive amounts of protein

Herbs to Treat Knee Problems

- Pyrola relieves knee pain. Take 9–30 g.
- Michael Tierra's Formula 33 tonifies the kidney yang. Purchase or order through a health food store. Take two tablets, two or three times per day with warm water and a little miso, tamari, or sea salt.
- Lycium berries tonify liver and kidneys. To treat sore knees, take 6–15 g daily.

LEG CRAMPS

SYMPTOMS

Shooting pain or dull ache in legs, especially in thighs and back of calves.

WHAT ARE LEG CRAMPS?

From Modern Western Medicine

Leg cramps are extremely common. They may affect anyone and occur while walking or in bed. The cause is often a simple mineral imbalance. Athletes often get leg cramps due to excessive exercise and sweating, which leads to mineral depletion. The best remedy for this is a proper diet and replacement of fluids. (See the list of foods to eat below.)

Other forms of leg cramps are more complicated. Older people may suffer leg cramps associated with arteriosclerotic changes in the circulatory system and should be evaluated by a doctor well-trained in cardiovascular disease. (See the section on heart disease.)

From Traditional Medicine

Leg cramps are typically from weak and tired kidneys, along with a depletion of minerals and antioxidants, especially magnesium and vitamin E.

REMEDIES

Foods to Eat

- Beans (to strengthen kidneys)
- White fish (to strengthen kidneys)
- Green and leafy vegetables, especially collard greens, kale, and mustard greens (all rich in calcium, other minerals, and antioxidants)
- Sea vegetables, such as arame, nori, wakame, and kelp (to strengthen kidneys and increase mineral content of blood)
- Fresh fruit juice
- Fresh vegetable juice
- Fruits
- Vegetables (If denture wearers find eating vegetables difficult, the only recourse is vegetable soups, potassium broth, and raw vegetable juices daily.)
- Whole grains, especially barley, which strengthens kidneys (All grains contain vitamin E.)

Foods to Avoid

- Meat
- Soft drinks
- Dairy products

Supplements

- Vitamin B_6: 2–10 mg per day
- Vitamin C: 100–500 mg per day
- Vitamin E: 100–400 IU per day
- Calcium: 1000 mg per day
- Magnesium: 100 mg per day
- EPA: 1–2 capsules, 2 or 3 times per day

LOW BACK PAIN

SYMPTOMS

Pain or ache in the back; pain, ache, or altered sensation in the buttocks, thigh, calf, and foot. Muscle wasting may occur late in life, along with reduced reflexes and muscle weakness.

WHAT IS LOW BACK PAIN?

From Modern Western Medicine

Back pain can arise from a number of causes affecting the spine. The disorders can cause back pain with or without sciatica (pain in the buttock and down the back of the leg). Most people suffer from back pain at some time in their lives. In many cases, it is labeled nonspecific and no exact diagnosis is made. Some kinds of back pain can be linked to a specific disorder. For example:

- Osteoarthritis: pain and stiffness in the back due to degeneration of the joints between the vertebrae in one (or more) of the cervical, thoracic, or lumbosacral regions
- Fibrositis: pain and tenderness in the larger back muscles
- Pyelonephritis: pain in the loin due to infection of the kidney
- Sciatica: pain in the buttock and down the back of the leg into the foot due to pressure on a nerve
- Coccygodynia: pain and tenderness at the base of the spine, sometimes after a fall
- Nonspecific back pain: pain that commonly affects the lower back but may occur in other parts due to ligament, muscle, joint, or disk damage

Treatment includes painkillers, anti-inflammatory drugs, muscle-relaxant drugs, acupuncture, spinal injection, exercise, spinal manipulation, wearing an elastic brace, or spinal surgery.

From Traditional Medicine

Even when someone's spine is in good condition, pain may result from a fall, an auto accident, any sudden, unusual, or extreme movement, or from another traumatic cause. The cause of pain may be a result of muscle or ligament strain, in which case rest and physiotherapy are all that is needed.

Low backache is primarily from weak kidneys, deficient kidney yin, or excess weight in the stomach area, causing pulling on vertebrae, which in turn

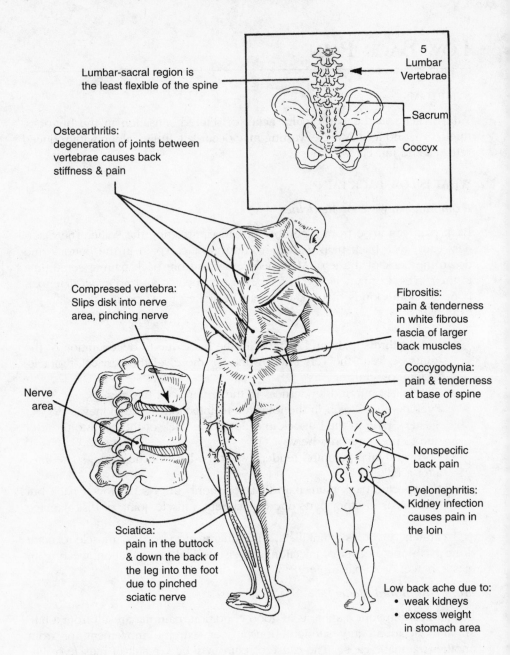

5 Lumbar Vertebrae

Sacrum

Coccyx

Lumbar-sacral region is the least flexible of the spine

Osteoarthritis: degeneration of joints between vertebrae causes back stiffness & pain

Compressed vertebra: Slips disk into nerve area, pinching nerve

Nerve area

Fibrositis: pain & tenderness in white fibrous fascia of larger back muscles

Coccygodynia: pain & tenderness at base of spine

Nonspecific back pain

Pyelonephritis: Kidney infection causes pain in the loin

Sciatica: pain in the buttock & down the back of the leg into the foot due to pinched sciatic nerve

Low back ache due to:
• weak kidneys
• excess weight in stomach area

pinches disks and nerves and causes pain. The pain is usually severe, but it often becomes less severe after a week or two if left untreated. Unfortunately, the lessening of pain is interpreted as a sign of recovery by the patient. What's really happening is that the acute hot problem is now cooling and becoming chronic. If proper spinal manipulation does not occur (such as acupressure massage) then this area can create secondary changes in other spinal levels as the body attempts to reestablish a semblance of spinal balance. In general, the longer you wait to begin treatment, the longer it will take for the treatment to work.

Another common cause is taut muscles caused by emotional stress. In his book, *The Back Pain Book: A Self-Help Guide for Daily Relief of Neck and Back Pain,* Mike Hage writes, "When you feel angry, anxious, tired, ill, or depressed, your brain automatically increases your sensitivity to pain. Feelings of fear, anger, or anxiety tend to increase muscle tension around the face and head and along the spine. This crams joints together and overworks your muscles, aggravating your pain."

As vertebrae compress, the disks in between can bulge or slip, a condition called a herniated disk. Once a disk goes out of alignment, it can press against the sciatic nerve that runs along the spinal column and down the leg.

Releasing the tension and strengthening the muscles that support the back are the best ways to deal with back pain.

WHO GETS BACK PAIN?

According to Leonard Faye, D.C., a chiropractor and author of *Good-bye Back Pain!* 85 million Americans suffer from back pain.

REMEDIES

Foods to Eat

The following foods will nurture kidney yin:

- Millet
- Barley (to strengthen kidneys)
- Tofu
- String beans
- Black beans
- Black soybeans
- Mung beans and sprouts
- Beans, especially kidney
- Kuzu root
- Watermelon and other melons
- Blackberries, blueberries, and mulberries
- Water chestnuts

- Seaweeds
- Spirulina
- Chlorella
- Black sesame seeds

Foods to Avoid

According to Chinese medicine:

- Animal products stimulate the liver into a heat condition, which will drain kidney yin.
- Coffee
- Alcohol
- Tobacco
- Cinnamon
- Cloves
- Ginger
- Hot spices

Herbs to Treat Back Pain

According to Humbart Santillo, author of *Natural Healing with Herbs,* drink an infusion of:

2 parts uva ursi
1 part dandelion root
1 part marshmallow
1 part ginger
1 part plantain

Simmer two ounces of herbs in one quart of distilled water for ten minutes with the top on tightly. Steep for ten minutes; strain. Drink one cup, three times daily.

Physiotherapy

- Complete bed rest for twenty-four to forty-eight hours: Use supportive mattress or lay mattress on the floor.
- Ice packs for the first twenty-four hours. Apply for ten to thirty minutes with a ten- to thirty-minute break between applications.
- Heat will loosen tight spinal muscles and give pain relief. Apply local moist heat. Hot, moist, folded towels are good for home use. Apply steaming hot and cover with dry towels to retain heat. Follow heat applications with gentle stretching.
- Epsom salt baths are relaxing and antispasmodic.

Exercise

The following exercises are outlined in Dr. Faye's book. He says you should see improvement in your range of motion and diminishing pain within a month. Try to warm up your muscles by taking a ten-minute walk before you begin. Start stretching gently and slowly, and stop any exercise that causes sharp pain or pain that lingers. A dull ache or pain can be relaxed into. Attempt to hold each of the following stretches for twenty-five to thirty seconds, and do the exercises daily for twenty minutes. Breathe regularly and easily, exhaling for the last five seconds of each exercise.

- Lean into it: Sit on a chair and lean forward. At the point where you begin to feel pain, breathe out and try to relax into the pain slightly. This will stretch the spine, back muscles, and ligaments.
- Pull your knee: Sit upright in a straight-backed chair. Lift your right knee and take hold of it with both hands, pulling it toward your chest until it's up as high as possible. Repeat with the left leg.
- Stretch your pelvis: Take the same position as in the previous exercise. Lift your right leg toward your chest by grasping your knee, and move the knee gently toward your left shoulder. This stretches the pelvis and lumbar muscles even farther than the previous exercise. Repeat the stretch, this time moving your left knee toward your right shoulder.
- Push your thigh: Sit in a chair and place your right foot on your left thigh, near the knee. Gently push your inner right knee and thigh down toward the floor, stretching your groin and lower back muscles. Repeat, using the left leg.
- Pull your ankle: Stand behind a straight-backed chair, and hold on to it for support. Take hold of your right ankle with your right hand and pull your leg back until your heel touches your right buttock. Repeat, using the left ankle. If you are able, add more stretch by moving your knee backward.
- Stretch lying down: Lie on your back on the floor or a firm mat. With both hands, take hold of your right knee and pull it toward your chest. Repeat with the other leg.
- Do both at once: Lying down, take hold of your knees. Bring both legs up to your chest.
- Rotate those knees: Lie on your back, bending your knees while keeping your feet on the floor. Gently lift your buttocks as high as you can and hold for a count of eight. Repeat the exercise as many times as you can without overdoing it. Gradually work your way up to ten repetitions without pain.
- Touch your forehead: Get down on your hands and knees and lift your right knee off the floor and bring it to your forehead. Do not force it if you cannot touch your forehead. Now push your right leg backward

until you can stretch the leg straight out, parallel to the floor. Bring your knee back to the floor, and repeat the exercise with the left leg.

- Improving abdominal strength will help back pain: Do crunch sit-ups. Start on your back with your knees bent, feet flat on the floor, your lower back pressed into the floor. Either cross your arms over your chest or place your fingers lightly behind your ears. Slowly lift your upper body, bringing your shoulder blades off the floor four or five inches, without swinging your elbows forward. Now lower your shoulder blades to the floor without letting your head touch the floor. Start out with about three to five, four times a week.

MEMORY DISTURBANCES

WHAT ARE DISTURBANCES IN MEMORY?

From Modern Western Medicine

Memory can be broken down into three stages: registration, long-term memory, and recall. Registration is the process of perceiving and understanding. Once it is understood, the information goes into a short-term memory system that has limited storage space. Unless the material is repeated over and over again, it will be forgotten and replaced with new information.

In the long-term memory stage, a person associates the new material with words, meanings, visual imagery, or other experiences such as smell or sound. Finally, in the recall stage, stored information is brought from the unconscious mind into the conscious mind. The strength of the recall stage depends on how well the new material was associated with other experiences and put into long-term memory.

Poor memory can happen at any of the three stages. Usually, the problem involves an inability to recall past events. In some cases, the problem occurs at the registration stage, perhaps because the person is distracted or preoccupied.

In the case of amnesia, the storage of information in long-term memory and/or the recall of such information is impaired. Amnesia is caused by damage to or disease of brain regions.

From Traditional Medicine

Traditional Chinese medicine sees memory as a function of both a balanced liver and heart. It's not as if the memory is actually located in these organs but that the function of specific parts of the brain are dependent upon a balanced liver and heart, both of which provide their own unique types of qi, or life, to the memory center of the brain. The liver is associated with all mental activities, especially with study and retention of ideas and events. The heart is associated with identifying with emotional and psychological events, especially those that leave a lasting imprint. Memory loss is usually the result of either a weak liver, weak heart, or both. In general, mental function is dependent upon a strong and well-balanced liver. The more blocked the liver becomes, the poorer the memory. Fatty foods and alcohol, both of which can be destructive to the liver, weaken memory, especially the capacity to remember facts, names, places, dates, and intellectual concepts. The heart, which is referred to in Chinese medicine as the palace of the shen, or the seat of the spirit, is responsible for supporting the memory of important life events.

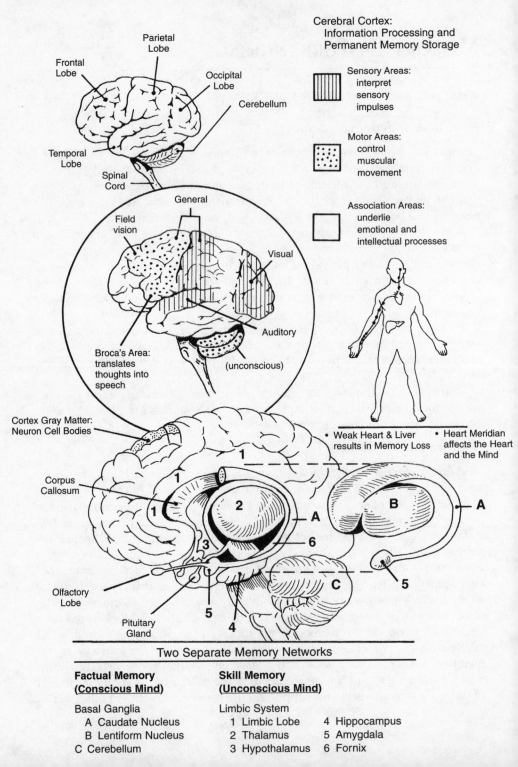

Cerebral Cortex:
Information Processing and
Permanent Memory Storage

Sensory Areas:
interpret
sensory
impulses

Motor Areas:
control
muscular
movement

Association Areas:
underlie
emotional and
intellectual processes

Parietal
Lobe

Frontal
Lobe

Occipital
Lobe

Cerebellum

Temporal
Lobe

Spinal
Cord

General

Field
vision

Visual

Auditory

Broca's Area:
translates
thoughts into
speech

(unconscious)

Cortex Gray Matter:
Neuron Cell Bodies

Corpus
Callosum

Olfactory
Lobe

Pituitary
Gland

• Weak Heart & Liver
results in Memory Loss

• Heart Meridian
affects the Heart
and the Mind

Two Separate Memory Networks

**Factual Memory
(Conscious Mind)**

**Skill Memory
(Unconscious Mind)**

Basal Ganglia
  A Caudate Nucleus
  B Lentiform Nucleus
C Cerebellum

Limbic System
  1 Limbic Lobe   4 Hippocampus
  2 Thalamus   5 Amygdala
  3 Hypothalamus 6 Fornix

The heart is considered the center of mental and emotional consciousness. It is also related to the nervous system and the brain. Acupuncture theory treats the heart meridian as affecting both the physical heart and the mind.

Memory is also a function of optimal blood flow to the brain. The better the circulation to the brain, the better the memory, and vice versa. Therefore, to improve memory, foods rich in fat and cholesterol should be reduced to improve circulation to the brain.

Finally, the brain neurotransmitter called acetylcholine, which plays a role in the coordination of smooth muscle function, has been shown to boost memory when acetylcholine levels are boosted in the brain. Brain levels of acetylcholine are increased by eating foods rich in choline, an amino acid that is found in abundance in soybean products and eggs. In addition to poor memory, low brain levels of acetylcholine are also associated with Alzheimer's disease.

REMEDIES

Foods to Eat

- Whole grain products (good source of zinc, which is found to improve memory function)
- Soybeans and soybean products, such as tofu, tempeh, natto, and soy milk
- Lots of green, orange, and yellow vegetables, which increase circulation to the brain

According to Chinese medicine, the following will reduce excesses of the liver, which drain the yin of the heart:

- Vinegar (apple cider, brown rice, or other quality vinegars): Best results occur when mixed with honey. Take one teaspoon each in a cup of water. This is a strong, quick-acting remedy, which should not be taken over a long period of time.
- Lemon, lime, or grapefruit act more gradually and can be taken for a longer period of time.
- Romaine lettuce
- Asparagus
- Amaranth
- Quinoa
- Seaweed, especially kelp
- Mung beans and sprouts
- Celery
- Tofu

The following tonify kidney yin and heart yin:

- Wheat germ
- Wheat berries
- Mung beans

Foods to Avoid

- Coffee
- Alcohol
- Tobacco
- Cinnamon
- Cloves
- Ginger
- Hot spices
- Animal foods that are rich in fat

Herbs to Treat Disturbances in Memory

- Calamus increases memory and concentration: 3–9 g; tincture, 10–30 drops. In Ayurvedic medicine, this is regarded as an herb that promotes wisdom by improving mental focus.
- Blessed thistle: infusion, steep 5–15 min., take 3 oz. as needed; tincture, 5–20 drops, as needed; fluid extract, ½–1 tsp., as needed; powder, 5–10 #0 capsules (30 to 60 grains), as needed (This is a brain food and stimulates memory. Do not take undiluted or in large amounts during pregnancy.)

Exercise

Aerobic workouts will increase oxygen efficiency to the brain and spark an increase in glucose metabolism. Studies have shown significant improvement on verbal memory tests in those who exercised.

MENOPAUSE

SYMPTOMS

Menopause means the last period, or the cessation of menstruation. About 70 percent of women experience hot flashes and night sweats during a two- to five-year period when menses become infrequent and eventually end. About 25 percent of women seek medical help for the hot flashes, night sweats, and other symptoms of menopause.

Menopause also is associated with physical changes in the vagina, including shrinking of the vaginal wall, loss of elasticity, and dryness. These changes may also increase minor infections. Psychological changes occur, as well. Among them are poor memory, poor concentration, tearfulness, and anxiety. Some women report a loss of sex drive; others say that menopause was accompanied by an increase in their sex drive. Not all women experience discomforts or negative emotional states during menopause, however. Many experience a kind of relief after losing their periods; they also report feeling a new freedom and a rebirth into a new and exciting stage of life.

Menopause marks a significant reduction in estrogen production. With the reduction in estrogen also comes an increase in bone loss, a lowering of HDL (the good cholesterol), and an increase in cholesterol. These changes result in an increase in atherosclerosis, coronary heart disease, and stroke.

WHAT IS MENOPAUSE?

From Modern Western Medicine

Menopause usually occurs between the ages of forty-five and fifty-five, when the ovaries stop producing eggs (ova). The woman also undergoes a number of hormonal changes, including a reduction in estrogen production, an increase in pituitary hormone (gonadotropin), and higher amounts of male hormones (androgens).

Hormone replacement therapy (HRT), or taking oral estrogens, often with progesterone, is recommended for some women to treat the physical and psychological symptoms of menopause and to prevent such diseases as osteoporosis and heart disease.

From Traditional Medicine

The ancient Greeks referred to menopause as the climacteric or change of life, and regarded it as a step in the ladder of life. In other words, it was an important step in the maturation of a woman. In traditional cultures, even those of today, there is little or no evidence of the negative symptoms modern people associate with menopause, in large measure because the traditional human diet is low in fat and animal proteins. In health, the body adjusts for the ovarian reduction in estrogen by signaling other glands (especially the adrenal glands) to produce more estrogen, which prevents the complete loss of the female hormone. However, if the adrenal glands are weakened after a lifetime of poor diet and health habits, they may be unable to meet the needs of the body when menopause begins.

HRT is associated with a dramatic increase in uterine cancer, along with a smaller but still significant increase in the risk of breast cancer. Progesterone is given to reduce the risk of uterine cancer, but progesterone also reduces HDL cholesterol, which means the woman will be more susceptible to heart disease and stroke.

Traditional healers prescribe foods that are rich in phytoestrogens, which are plant-produced estrogens that promote bone health and prevent cancer. (See the list of foods to eat below.)

REMEDIES

Foods to Eat

A low-fat, high-fiber diet will help the body to adjust more easily to changing hormonal levels.

- Whole grains
- Fresh vegetables
- Beans
- Seaweed
- Miso
- Tofu and tempeh
- Seeds and nuts, especially sunflower seeds

According to Chinese medicine, the following foods will build the yin:

- Wheat germ and wheat germ oil
- Mung beans and sprouts
- Tofu
- String beans
- Black beans
- Kidney beans
- Barley
- Black sesame seeds
- Royal jelly tonifies the female hormonal system. A normal dose is just 100–400 milligrams daily.

Foods that contain phytoestrogens help prevent hot flashes and other symptoms of estrogen depletion:

- Tofu and other soy products
- Yams
- Carrots
- Apples
- Potatoes

Foods rich in calcium help prevent osteoporosis:

- Sesame seeds
- Almonds
- Low-fat yogurt
- Dark, leafy greens, such as kale, collards, and broccoli
- Sardines

Foods to Avoid

- Animal foods
- Fat found in fried foods, dairy products, nut butters, etc.
- Sugar and refined carbohydrates contribute to mood swings.
- Caffeine can cause hot flashes.
- Alcohol can cause hot flashes.
- Tobacco

Herbs to Treat Menopause

- Chaste berry: ½ teaspoon of tincture, 3–4 times a day, stimulates the production of progesterone and helps balance the hormones.
- Dong quai, alfalfa, or black cohosh: ½ teaspoon of tincture or 2 capsules, 3 times a day, stimulates estrogen production.
- Motherwort: ½ teaspoon of tincture or two capsules, 3 times a day, relieves heart palpitations; combine with sage to relieve hot flashes.
- Siberian ginseng: ½ teaspoon of tincture or 2 capsules, two times a day, helps strengthen adrenal glands.

For tension and anxiety:

- Wild oats or skullcap: tincture, ½ teaspoon, 3 or 4 times a day
- Valerian (for extreme anxiety or difficulty sleeping): tincture, ½–1 teaspoon, 3 times a day.

Apply salves of the following herbs to vaginal tissue to help relieve dryness and thinning:

- Calendula
- Comfrey

Homeopathy

- Lachesis: for mental irritation and hot flashes that are worse in the morning
- Pulsatilla: for frequent mood changes and hot flashes at night
- Sepia: for emotional exhaustion accompanied by tiredness, irritability, and chills

Physiotherapy

- Daily exercise helps build bone mass: walking, dancing, jogging, aerobic dance, or tennis. Resistance training would be excellent.
- Walking on wet grass

Chinese Medicine

In Chinese medicine, the symptoms of menopause imply a deficiency of yin fluids, particularly those yin fluids that calm and relax the liver. A helpful dietary approach, then, is to add foods that especially build the yin. See the list of foods to eat above.

Supplements

- Beta-carotene: 15 mg per day
- Vitamin B complex
    Thiamine: 1.5 mg per day
    Riboflavin: 1.8 mg per day
    Vitamin B_6: 2–10 mg per day
    Vitamin B_{12}: 2–10 mg per day
    Niacin: 20 mg per day
- Vitamin C: 100–500 mg per day
- Vitamin E: 100–400 IU per day
- Calcium: 1200 mg per day
- Magnesium: 400 mg per day
- Zinc: 15 mg per day

MENSTRUAL PROBLEMS

WHAT ARE MENSTRUAL PROBLEMS?

According to Modern Western Medicine

Menstruation is the shedding of the blood that saturates the endometrium, or the lining of the uterus. The cyclical production of female hormones, estrogen and progesterone, bring on menstruation and regulate it according to the lunar cycle. Any change in a woman's hormonal balance can cause disruptions in the menstrual cycle or the characteristics of the period. Changes in menstruation can indicate hormonal imbalances, the presence of fibroid tumors, endometriosis, pelvic inflammatory disease, or more serious disorders.

Painful periods (known as dysmenorrhea) is the most common form of menstrual problem. The cause is unknown.

Pregnancy, stress, malnutrition, starvation, and anorexia can all cause the loss of the period (known as amenorrhea). On the other hand, two periods within a twenty-two-day cycle (called polymenorrhea), scanty periods (oligomenorrhea), and excessive bleeding (menorrhagia) may all be caused by hormonal imbalances, the presence of an IUD, fibroids, or polyps.

PMS, or premenstrual syndrome, which occurs either prior to the period or during it, is associated with a variety of physical and psychological discomforts, including depression, irritability, edema, sore breasts, abdominal distension, and nausea.

From Traditional Medicine

Irregularities in the menstrual cycle must first be checked out by a medical doctor. After serious illness has been ruled out, the underlying causes can be dealt with.

Invariably, those women with PMS, including those with breast tenderness and imbalanced periods, especially heavy bleeding, have high estrogen levels. Typically, these women had an early menarche—usually at twelve years of age or younger—and are on a high-fat, high-cholesterol diet. To correct the menstrual imbalance, the diet must be changed to lower fat and cholesterol and increase fiber.

Fat cells produce estrogen, which disrupts the estrogen/progesterone balance within the body. A significant reduction in fat and cholesterol will reduce estrogen levels quickly, usually within a month. When estrogen levels are reduced, the menstrual cycle usually normalizes, breast tenderness disappears, and symptoms of PMS are significantly reduced or eliminated.

The second step is to improve digestion and elimination. Estrogens are eliminated through the feces. The more efficient the bowel elimination, the greater the estrogen reduction from the body. In addition to improving elimination, the bacterial environment of the intestines must also be improved. Anaerobic bacteria, which characteristically populate the intestines of women on a high-fat, high-protein diet, cause existing estrogens in the body to be circulated through the system several times. In fact, the body attempts to prevent this by binding estrogens with an enzyme that makes reabsorption impossible, but anaerobic bacteria remove this binder and allow estrogens to keep circulating, causing a variety of health problems, including menstrual problems.

The third step is to increase fiber, which binds with estrogen and takes it out of the body through the bowels.

Other factors that disrupt the menstrual cycle include taking birth control pills and stress, both of which disrupt adrenal glands. The adrenals produce about 20 percent of a woman's estrogen. Diets that cause extreme weight loss can disrupt periods, as can hypoglycemia, nutritional anemia, iodine deficiency, and hypothyroidism.

REMEDIES

Foods to Eat

- Whole grains
- Beans
- Fruits
- Vegetables
- Nuts
- Seeds

Foods to Avoid

- Red meat and poultry
- Dairy foods
- Sugar
- Cold foods
- Hydrogenated fats and polyunsaturated cooking oil
- Too much raw fruit or juice
- Salt
- Fat
- Caffeine

Herbs to Treat Menstrual Disorders

- Dong quai (also known as dang gui): ½ teaspoon of tincture or 2 capsules, 3 times a day, taken during the first two weeks of the menstrual cycle, helps regulate hormonal production, particularly estrogen. Do not take during menstruation or pregnancy because it can stimulate bleeding.
- Vitex: ½ teaspoon of tincture or 2 capsules, 3 times a day, especially during the last two weeks of the cycle (after ovulation occurs), helps stim-

ulate the production of progesterone, normalizing the estrogen/ progesterone balance.

- Red raspberry leaf: 1 cup of tea, ½ teaspoon of tincture, or 2 capsules, 3
  or 4 times a day. Gentle but effective nutritive tonic for the reproductive
  system.

For dysmenorrhea: The following have an antispasmodic effect on the uterine muscle and may help alleviate or prevent menstrual cramps. An average
dose is ½–1 teaspoon of tincture or 2 capsules, 3 or 4 times a day.

- Ginger: Use as tea to relieve cramps.
- Valerian calms the nervous system and alleviates cramps.
- Cramp bark helps relax and sedate the entire reproductive system.

For amenorrhea:

- Blazing star (for low ovarian function): tincture, 10–30 drops, 3 times a
  day
- Life root (increases local circulation; uterine tonic): tincture, 10–30 drops,
  2–4 times daily
- Pulsatilla (especially when amenorrhea is due to stress or emotional suppression): tincture, 10 drops, 3 times a day

For oligomenorrhea:

- Blazing star: tincture, 10–30 drops, 3 times per day

For menorrhagia/metrorrhagia:

- Amaranth: tincture, 15–25 drops, 3 or 4 times per day
- Life root: tincture, 15–30 drops, 3 or 4 times per day

For PMS:

- Valerian: tincture, ½–1 teaspoon, 3 times a day
- Chamomile: 1 cup of tea or ½ teaspoon of tincture, 3 or 4 times per day
- Dandelion leaf (when there is water retention): 1 cup of tea

Homeopathy

Take one of the single remedies below.

- Belladonna: for pain centered around the uterus
- Pulsatilla: for delayed menses
- Sepia: for PMS tension, tiredness, and irritability

Physiotherapy

- Alternate hot and cold sitz baths. This will remove pelvic congestion and restore uterine and ovarian health. Take a bath two times a day, if possible.
- For excessive bleeding or pain, apply ice pack to uterus and pubic or sacral region. If one wants to increase the flow of blood, hot compresses applied to the legs and feet will enhance the action of removing blood from the pelvic region.
- Abdominal exercises
- Outdoor exercises; swimming
- Place a hot water bottle over uterus during the period to increase flow and assist in elimination.

Chinese Medicine

At the time of menstruation, the deeper hormonal/emotional qualities surface, while their physical corollary—the heat-bearing blood that results from a natural purification—is discharged. This is a fragile state. Surfacing aspects from the interior, yin, hormonal parts of the being are delicate and sensitive, and need protection from cold and dampness and physical and emotional extremes. During menstruation, one should avoid heavy physical work, emotional stress, and overexposure to cold and damp conditions.

Supplements

- Beta-carotene: 15 mg per day
- Vitamin B complex
    Thiamine: 1.5 mg per day
    Riboflavin: 1.8 mg per day
    Vitamin B_6: 2–10 mg per day
    Vitamin B_{12}: 2–10 mg per day
    Niacin: 20 mg per day
- Vitamin C: 100–500 mg per day
- Vitamin E: 100–500 IU per day
- Calcium: 800–1000 mg per day
- Magnesium: 100 mg per day
- Zinc: 15 mg per day

Essential Oils

- Chamomile: Massage into lower abdomen; place in bath or in vaporizer.
- Lavender: for headaches and anxiety; massage, bath, or vaporizer

Migraines

SYMPTOMS

Recurrent headaches, accompanied by visual disturbances, nausea, vomiting, diarrhea or constipation, and sensitivity to light. Usually, the pain is localized or especially intense on one side of the head or over one eye. The person may also suffer from irritability. He or she usually wants to be left alone and out of any direct light. Attacks are usually preceded by flashes of light, which are caused by constriction of cerebral blood vessels.

WHAT IS A MIGRAINE?

From Modern Western Medicine

Lasting anywhere from two hours to two days, migraines are intense and severe headaches that affect many other areas of the body. For unknown reasons, migraines are three times more common in women than in men. Migraines usually run in families, and most migraine sufferers (about 60 percent) experience their first attack before the age of twenty. Migraines are caused by a variety of reasons, depending on the person's unique sensitivities. Among the most common causes are stress, food sensitivities, excessive stimulation of the senses, menstrual disorders, and the taking of birth control pills.

Migraines are classified as common and classical. The common migraine is associated with a slowly increasing pain, eventually developing into a throbbing headache that is made more intense by even the slightest movements or noise. The pain usually occurs on one side of the head and is accompanied by nausea or vomiting. Many sufferers feel relief after vomiting; this is usually the case with children.

In the case of classical migraines, which are far less common, the person begins by experiencing some degree of blindness or visual impairment that slowly occupies a larger field of vision. The blinded area is often surrounded by a sparkling edge. Up to one-half of the field of vision can be blinded or reduced. The blindness usually lasts about twenty minutes and is followed by a severe one-sided headache with nausea, vomiting, and sensitivity to light.

Migraines are so severe that a person knows very well that he or she is suffering a migraine; consequently, special tests are usually unnecessary. When testing is needed, a complete neurological examination is performed.

Doctors treat migraines by having people keep a record of the events leading up to a migraine. Once those trigger factors are recognized, the person attempts to avoid such situations as a way of preventing the headaches. Aspirin or acetaminophen plus an antiemetic drug are the most common form of treatment. A doctor may prescribe ergotamine, a stronger analgesic. Sleeping in a very quiet, darkened room causes most people to recover more quickly than if they remain in the light or in highly stimulating environments.

From Traditional Medicine

Any headache involving the eyes or sensitivity to light is seen as involving the liver and gallbladder, which provide qi, or life force, to the eyes. According to Chinese medicine, anger and irritability are associated with an imbalanced liver. In the Chinese system, an imbalanced liver destabilizes or injures the spleen (the liver is said to invade the spleen). The spleen is responsible for governing digestion; an imbalanced spleen is the most common cause of nausea, another symptom of migraines. Migraines, therefore, involve the liver, gallbladder, and spleen, primarily, though other organs, especially the intestines, may be involved secondarily.

Specifically, the liver and gallbladder can become congested, filled with bile, and excessive in energy. Once the liver becomes excessive, it usually invades and weakens the spleen, causing nausea. These conditions are often brought on by a variety of foods (especially foods that are rich in fat, spices, and sugar), emotions that are repressed or denied (especially anger and sadness), and a tendency to think excessively, especially about problems.

Finally, food sensitivities may also play a role in the onset of migraines. Among the most common are cheese, wine, citrus, and, to a lesser extent, avocados, plums, bananas, raspberries, and alcoholic beverages. Some naturopaths believe that the amino acid tyramine causes the release of norepinephrine, which in turn creates constriction of the blood vessels in the scalp and brain. The result is reduced blood and oxygen flow to the brain, causing the first stage of the migraine, which is visual impairment. As norepinephrine levels drop, blood vessels expand dramatically, which may bring on the headache.

The liver, gallbladder, and spleen must be treated. Regular exercise is needed, as well as an avoidance of foods that may serve as triggers. Finally, strong emotions and beliefs that are there below the surface but are not being dealt with must be expressed directly, especially to people who may be sources of conflict or emotional conflict.

REMEDIES

General Recommendations

- See Part IV for methods of strengthening liver, gallbladder, and spleen.
- When migraines occur, eat soupy grains, soft foods, and soups. Avoid foods that are difficult to digest or those rich in fat.
- Avoid constipation and if necessary take an herbal laxative.

Foods to Eat

- Brown rice soup with carrots, onions, and about ½ teaspoon of miso per bowl
- Carrot juice (especially good for liver and gallbladder)
- Miso soup with vegetables (especially good for spleen)
- Rye broth or congee
- Black sesame seeds
- Flaxseeds
- Chia seeds
- Soybeans and their products, such as tofu and tempeh
- Dark green vegetables

Foods to Avoid

- Animal products
- Fried and oily foods
- Spicy foods
- Coffee
- Caffeinated tea
- Alcohol
- Tobacco

Herbs to Treat Migraines

- Michael Tierra's Planetary Herbs Formula 9 relieves head wind and blood stagnation. Can be purchased or ordered through your health food store. Contraindicated for pregnant women.
- Feverfew: standard infusion or 3–9 g (Do not use when the migraine results from a weak, deficient condition.)
- Fenugreek: infusion, steep 5–15 minutes, take 1 cup during the day, hot or cold
- Peppermint: oil, 5–10 drops, 3 times daily; fluid extraction, ½–2 tsp., 3 times daily; infusion, steep 5–15 minutes, take 6 oz., 3 times daily
- Rosemary: infusion, steep 5–15 minutes, take 2 oz., 3 times daily; oil, ½–3 drops, 3 times daily; external: Rub diluted oil (1 part rosemary with 10 parts vegetable oil) on forehead and temples. Also use as a nasal vapor bath.

Homeopathy

- Aconitum nappellus: for migraines characterized by a sudden, violent headache all around the head like a band, or in the forehead like a bursting pain. The patient is restless, fearful, and thirsty. Symptoms get worse in evening or night, in a warm room, and on getting up from bed, and improve in the open air. Such a condition often follows exposure to cold wind.

- Arnica montana relieves the headache brought on by a blow or a fall and that is characterized by a sore, bruised feeling anywhere in the head.
- Belladonna: a natural for the headache that comes on suddenly and violently, characterized by throbbing, pounding pain, restlessness, a hot head, and a red, flushed face.
- Bryonia: one of the most commonly indicated remedies for acute headache, when the pain is stitching or tearing and is most apt to be right-sided, and the person feels worse from motion, even moving the eyes or raising the head. There may be a bursting sensation on stooping or on coughing. Constipation often accompanies the headache.
- Gelsemium may be needed by the person who has a vague but distressing headache beginning in the neck and extending up over the head, settling in a band around the head. It may develop into a bursting sensation in the eyes and forehead, and the scalp feels tender. It sometimes comes on after exposure to too much sun or from stress, bad news, or apprehension. It gets worse from lying down. The person feels languid, chilly, and without thirst and wishes to be left alone.
- Iris versicolor: often needed when a migrainelike headache begins with blurring of vision. The scalp may feel tight and there is profuse flow of saliva with burning of the tongue, throat, and stomach. The person may lose his or her appetite and there may be nausea and vomiting. Headaches are usually worse in the evening and at night, and are somewhat relieved by continued motion.
- Kali bichromicum: for a headache that matches the symptoms often referred to as sinus headache: Pain is in the "mask" area, either over, under, or behind the eyes, or at the root of the nose in a small spot that can be pointed to with one finger. Motion aggravates the pain, as does stooping or bending forward. The person feels worse when warm, better in the open air.
- Nux vomica is for the hangover headache, a splitting headache all over the head, with nausea and an out-of-sorts feeling. The person is irritable and oversensitive to everything.
- Sanguinaria canadensis is for the typical "sick headache," which begins in the morning, increases during the day, and lasts until evening. Pain is bursting, beginning in the back of the head, spreading upward, and settling over the right eye; it is accompanied by nausea and often by vomiting and dizziness.

Hydrotherapy

- Ice compress to base of head while lying in darkened room
- Ice to forehead with simultaneous hot footbath to abort an attack

Exercise

- Vigorous daily exercise seems to help as a preventive measure, not during an attack.
- Walk daily
- Play a game that you enjoy, such as tennis, basketball, volleyball, softball, or soccer.
- Ride a bicycle five times per week.

Mind/Body

- Meditation daily: Especially focus on what you are feeling each day.
- Progressive relaxation techniques (see Part III)
- Seek counseling or safe environments that allow you to release emotions regularly. Cry, express anger, sadness, and grief.
- Write in a journal what you are feeling each day.

Multiple Sclerosis

SYMPTOMS

Symptoms vary, depending on the part of the brain and nervous system involved. Common symptoms include tingling, numbness, and heaviness in the extremities. Sometimes the arms and legs feel weak and stiff. Incontinence may also manifest if the nerve fibers of the bladder become involved. If the white cells in the brain are affected, the person may suffer from staggering and erratic gait, vertigo, slurred speech, blurred and double vision, and pain in the face. Chronic constipation, muscle spasms, skin ulceration, and significant swings between euphoria and depression are also common. For some, paralysis may occur.

All of these symptoms may vary in intensity from one person to another. Some people experience only mild symptoms, some of which disappear for a time. Others suffer steady deterioration of the nervous system and a wide variety of related problems, until they become bedridden and incontinent.

WHAT IS MULTIPLE SCLEROSIS?

From Modern Western Medicine

Multiple sclerosis occurs when the myelin sheath or protective covering of the nervous system is attacked by the immune system, causing progressive damage and scarring of the nervous system, including the brain. No one knows why the immune system attacks the body's nerves.

People are eight times more likely to suffer from multiple sclerosis if a member of their family has contracted the disease. Environment also seems to play a role. People living in temperate zones, including the United States and Europe, are far more likely to suffer the illness than those living in the tropics. Some physicians theorize that a virus communicated early in life may be responsible for the onset of the disease later on.

No single diagnostic test is used to reveal the presence of MS. Rather, the illness is diagnosed through a process of elimination. The most common forms of treatment include corticosteroid drugs, which sometimes relieve symptoms, and other pharmaceutical agents used to control incontinence and depression. Physical therapy may also be helpful in strengthening muscles and increasing mobility.

From Traditional Medicine

Macrobiotic educator Michio Kushi has suggested that multiple sclerosis occurs after nerve cells have degenerated to the point that they are no longer recognized as part of the body by the immune system, but rather as an alien substance, which precipitates an immune attack. This degeneration occurs because of a general deterioration of the body, primarily from a deficiency of good-quality minerals, especially from vegetables, and an excess of fat and sugar. Once the nerve cells degenerate beyond recognition of the immune system, they are systematically destroyed by the body's defenses. Although the immune system triggers the illness, MS is not an autoimmune disorder, as medical doctors believe, but a degeneration of the nerve cells to the point that they are recognized by the body's defenses as foreign and therefore a threat to the system. In order to restore health, Kushi recommends a diet centered around grains, vegetables, sea vegetables, beans, and small amounts of fruit.

Pioneer MS researcher Dr. Roy Swank of the University of Oregon Medical School used exercise and a low-fat, high-carbohydrate diet to treat MS. Later, Nathan Pritikin, pioneer health researcher and teacher, used the same methods after studying Dr. Swank's work. Pritikin and Swank reported numerous case histories in which symptoms of patients with MS were significantly reduced after the patients adopted a diet very low in fat and cholesterol and rich in whole grains, fresh vegetables, beans, and fruit. Pritikin recommended that people with MS exercise daily. He recommended that the person walk daily as far as he or she could—say, down to the corner of the street, stop and rest when they became fatigued, and then walk home. Exercise, Pritikin and Swank believed, strengthened muscles and nerve function.

Chinese medicine treats MS by strengthening the liver and heart, both of which are related to the nervous system. The foods recommended below correspond with Kushi's recommendations and those of Swank, Pritikin, and Chinese medicine.

WHO GETS MS?

MS is the most common acquired disease of the nervous system in young adults. In relatively high-risk temperate areas, the incidence is about one in every thousand people. The ratio of women to men sufferers is three to two.

REMEDIES

Foods to Eat

The following foods will strengthen and soothe the nerves:

- Raw oats, soaked
- Sprouted wheat (if there is no gluten sensitivity)
- Rice
- Goat's milk, raw
- Wheat germ
- Wheat-germ oil (When using with flaxseed oil, alternate the days, taking

one tablespoon a day with meals. Double the dose when there is a chronic condition.)

- Flaxseed oil (very anti-inflammatory) (When taking with wheat-germ oil, alternate the days, taking one tablespoon a day with meals. Double the dose when there is a chronic condition.)

Eat foods high in lecithin, which is often deficient in diets of those with MS:

- Tofu
- Tempeh
- Soy sprouts
- Soy milk
- Cabbage
- Cauliflower
- Eggs

The following foods are liver-building, according to Chinese medicine:

- Leafy, green vegetables
- Mung beans
- Mung sprouts
- Millet
- Seaweeds
- Cereal grass concentrates
- Microalgae

The following foods reduce liver-wind, which is what causes the spasms and paralysis of MS, according to Chinese medicine:

- Celery
- Basil
- Sage
- Oats
- Black soybeans
- Black sesame seeds
- Fresh, cold-pressed flax oil

Foods to Avoid

- Dairy and all saturated fat
- Coffee
- Alcohol
- Sugar

Omit the following gluten foods at the beginning to see if the condition improves:

- Wheat
- Rye
- Barley
- Sweet rice

The following foods worsen liver-wind conditions, according to Chinese medicine:

- Eggs
- Crabmeat
- Buckwheat

Herbs for MS

- Saint-John's-wort (pain-relieving, antiviral, good for all diseases affecting the spine; full effect may not be realized for a few months, but benefits can be felt within a few weeks): infusion, 1–2 tsp/cup water, drink 1–2 cups regularly, morning and night; 2 "00" capsules, 3 times/day; tincture, 5–10 drops, 3–9 g in formula.
- The following is a broad, immune-enhancing formula. Prepare as a decoction of equal parts:
  Chaparral leaf
  Pau d'arco (inner bark)
  Suma root
  Dried ling zhi (reishi) or shiitake mushroom
  Peach seed

Hydrotherapy

- Alternate hot and cold showers daily
- Alternate hot and cold compresses or sprays to spine
- Outdoor exercise
- Sunshine
- Ocean swimming
- Outdoor living

Supplements

- Beta-carotene: 15–30 mg per day
- Thiamine: 1.5 mg per day
- Riboflavin: 1.8 mg per day
- Vitamin B_6: 2–10 mg per day
- Vitamin C: 100–500 mg per day
- Vitamin E: 100–400 IU per day

Nail Problems

WHAT ARE NAIL ABNORMALITIES?

From Modern Western Medicine

Nails often become injured from accidents (such as a crushing weight). They can become thick or curved (a condition called onychogryphosis that often appears in the elderly); damaged by bacterial or fungal infections, especially tinea and candidiasis; pitted, called alopecia areata; and separated from the nail bed, which is called onycholysis.

Many disorders that affect the body in general can also affect the nails. The relative strength or weakness of the nails may suggest overall health or a nutritional deficiency. Brittle, ridged, and concave nails can be a sign of iron-deficiency anemia. Fibrous growths on the nails can indicate the presence of tuberous sclerosis; separation of the nail from the nail bed can be a symptom of thyrotoxicosis. Bacterial infection can appear on the nails as a greenish discoloration. Respiratory disease can turn the nails blue, while bronchiectasis and lymphedema can turn the nails yellow.

There are few effective treatments for disorders affecting the nails. Medication usually isn't able to penetrate the nail's hard surface, and oral medication is usually too slow or ineffective to make a difference.

From Traditional Medicine

Traditional medicine has developed its own diagnostic techniques, one of which is based on the condition of the fingernails and toenails. The following are some of the more common associations between health of nails and nutritional status:

- White half moons: excess sugar consumption and calcium deficiency
- Nail ridges: protein deficiency, vitamin A deficiency, excess salt consumption
- Pale nail beds: anemia
- Peeling nails: vitamin A deficiency
- Poor nail growth: zinc deficiency
- Splitting nails: excess sweets and refined foods, acidic blood and mineral deficiency
- Spoon-shaped nails: excess consumption of refined foods, fruit, fruit juice, and deficiency of minerals
- Thin, brittle nails: deficiency of vegetable-quality oils, coupled with mineral deficiency—especially iron and calcium—and vitamin deficiency, especially vitamin D

- Washboard ridges: deficiencies of iron, calcium, and zinc, coupled with consumption of extremes in diet, such as excesses of meat and salt along with excesses of sugar, refined foods, and fruit
- White nails: liver disease, copper excess

REMEDIES

Foods to Eat

To enrich the blood:

- Miso soup
- Grains
- Beans
- Vegetables
- Seaweed
- Microalgae
- Dark green, leafy vegetables
- Sprouts
- Mochi, especially with mugwort (Powdered mugwort leaf could be added to mochi.)

Foods to Avoid

- Sugar
- Coffee
- Tobacco
- Alcohol

Supplements

If supplements are desired, take the vitamins and minerals that are deficient, as suggested by the condition of your nails. Otherwise, get your nutrients from food.

OSTEOPOROSIS

SYMPTOMS

Osteoporosis, or porous bones, often shows no symptoms until the person afflicted with the disorder breaks a bone. Osteoporosis usually affects the bones of the wrist, arm, hip, legs, or spinal vertebrae. When the bones become sufficiently porous, they break, especially after a fall. A common symptom of osteoporosis, especially among the elderly, are minor fractures of the spinal vertebrae, leading to progressive loss of height. In some elderly, the spinal fractures can cause compression on the spinal nerves and considerable back pain.

WHAT IS OSTEOPOROSIS?

From Modern Western Medicine

Osteoporosis is the result of calcium loss from the protein matrix tissue of the bone. In time, the bones become increasingly brittle and vulnerable to fracture. This disorder is a natural part of aging. Osteoporosis is much more common in women than in men, primarily because women lose estrogen after menopause. Estrogen helps to maintain bone density in women, just as testosterone, the male hormone, maintains bone strength in men. Menopause is accompanied by a dramatic diminution of estrogen production by a woman's body, which often is accompanied by bone loss. Since men do not undergo the same type of menopausal decrease in testosterone production, their bone density remains much more stable. Osteoporosis is also much more common in Caucasians than in African Americans, who tend to have denser bones. Overall, more than 25 million Americans suffer from osteoporosis.

Since bone health is dependent upon hormonal health, all drugs, surgery, and illnesses that weaken hormonal balance can contribute to osteoporosis. Among the most common contributing factors are hysterectomy, or the removal of the ovaries; prolonged treatment with corticosteroid drugs, such as prednisone; alcoholism (interferes with estrogen and testosterone production); and hormonal disorders, such as Cushing's syndrome. Other factors include a diet low in calcium, cigarette smoking, and lack of exercise.

Exercise is essential to maintain bone health. Exercise causes tiny fractures in the bone, which must be rebuilt by the bone. This process of breaking down old bone and building up new, a process exercise speeds up and increases, results in stronger and denser bones, overall. People who remain sedentary or immobilized for long periods are at increased risk of contracting osteoporosis.

For reasons not well understood, osteoporosis is also associated with chronic disorders of the lungs. Bone loss can be minimized by taking extra calcium, regular exercise, and by taking estrogens after menopause.

From Traditional Medicine

Although orthodox medicine stresses calcium consumption, more holistic medicine points to a diet rich in protein, salt, and substances that block calcium absorption, such as oxalic acid, insoluble fiber, and phosphates (or phosphorus salts).

Protein, especially from meat and other animal sources, creates high quantities of uric acid in the blood. The high acid levels cause the body to secrete calcium from the bone in order to alkalize the blood. This, of course, causes calcium loss and results in porous bones. Even though Americans eat much more calcium than any other people on earth, they nevertheless suffer from more osteoporosis than any other nation. The Bantus of New Guinea get only 350 mg of calcium each day, but they do not suffer from osteoporosis, even though Bantu women bear and nurse an average of nine children. Studies have shown that most people around the world get only 300 to 500 mg of calcium per day.

Salt and oxalic acid, found in certain vegetables (see the list of foods to avoid, below), interfere with calcium absorption. Increasingly, researchers are finding that the ratio between calcium and phosphorus is a delicate balance that must be maintained if bones are to remain healthy. In the Western diet, phosphorus salts, or phosphates, are particularly high. These high levels of phosphates interfere with calcium absorption. Foods that are rich in phosphates include red meat, soft drinks (especially colas), and coffee. Red meat is especially unhealthy for bones because it is loaded with protein and contains twenty to fifty times more phosphorus than calcium.

Other factors that promote osteoporosis are cigarette smoking, lack of vitamin D, and a diet low in minerals, especially calcium and magnesium, which are essential for calcium absorption.

It is the general lack of raw vegetables in the diet that predisposes many people to osteoporosis. Vegetarians have much less incidence of it. The calcium-to-phosphorus ratio is much more favorable in vegetables than in dairy or meat products.

In order to prevent osteoporosis, the diet must be low to moderate in high-protein foods (especially red meat and dairy products) and rich in whole grains, fresh vegetables, and other mineral-rich foods, such as sea vegetables (see page 314). It must have sufficient calcium, anywhere from 500 mg per day to 1200 mg, and it must be low in foods that contain salt, phosphorus, and oxalic acid.

Scientific research has shown that the average adult needs 20 grams of protein a day (about two-thirds of an ounce of protein). The body uses that protein to replace and repair cells, produce hormones, and grow hair. The average American consumes 90 grams or more of protein each day. Nutritionists have demonstrated that no one can create a diet that is deficient in protein if that diet is composed chiefly of whole foods, such as whole grains, fresh vegetables, beans, and fruit.

Contrary to the American standard, the World Health Organization recommends that people eat only 400 to 500 mg of protein per day. The WHO scientists recommend, however, that protein levels be kept moderate.

REMEDIES

Foods to Eat

- Vegetables especially leafy greens, such as collard, kale, mustard greens, broccoli, cabbage, and dark lettuce.
- Whole grains
- Vegetables
- Legumes
- Nuts
- Sprouted seeds and beans
- Salad (with lemon juice or cider vinegar to aid calcium absorption)
- Microalgae
- Seaweed

To nourish kidney yin:

- Millet
- Barley
- Tofu
- String beans
- Black beans
- Mung beans and sprouts
- Kidney beans and most other beans
- Kuzu root
- Watermelon and other melons
- Blackberries, mulberries, blueberries, and huckleberries
- Water chestnuts
- Potatoes
- Black sesame seeds
- Seaweed
- Spirulina

Foods to Avoid

Avoid foods that contain calcium oxalate, which binds with calcium, making it nutritionally unavailable.

- Spinach
- Chard
- Beet greens
- Chocolate
- Cranberries
- Plums

Avoid the following foods that will drain the kidney yin:

- Meat
- Coffee
- Alcohol
- Cigarettes
- Hot spices

Herbs for Treating Osteoporosis

Combine the following ingredients:

    1 part horsetail
    1 part oat straw
    1 part kombu seaweed or kelp powder
    ⅓ part lobelia

Simmer one ounce of formula in 1 pint water for 25 minutes and drink ½ cup two or three times a day. At the end of every three weeks, stop using the formula for one week. Take during an entire season of the year, ideally in the winter (as recommended by Paul Pitchford, author of *Healing with Whole Foods*).

Physiotherapy

- Sunbathing
- Sea bathing

Exercise

- Aerobic exercise, such as brisk walking: Focus on areas of the body most susceptible to fracture such as legs, hips, wrists, and arms.
- Work out forty-five minutes, three to four times a week. Do three sets of resistance exercises, with eight to ten repetitions per set.
- Chest pull: Using a resistance band or exercise tube, stand with your feet shoulder width apart, and extend your arms in front. Pull your arms apart, stretching the band. Bring your arms back slowly.
- Outer thigh lift: Using an elastic band wrapped around your ankles, lie on your side with your legs straight. Lift your upper leg until the band

is taut. Lower your leg slowly. Roll over on your other side and repeat with your other leg.

- Outer thigh press: Lie on your back, with an elastic band around your ankles and your hands under your buttocks. Lift both legs into the air, and press them apart until the band is taut. Slowly bring your legs together.
- Standing arm row: Stand with an elastic band looped beneath one or both feet, while holding the ends in your hands. Pull your fists up toward your underarms. Lower your fists slowly, then slowly pull the band up toward your shoulders, in a rowing action. Slowly allow the band to recoil. Repeat.
- Lateral raises: Stand, and lift a hand-held weight from your side until it is parallel with the floor, so that your arm forms a ninety-degree angle with your body. Slowly let the weight return to your side. Repeat, alternating arms.
- Triceps press: Lift a hand-held weight straight up above your head, and slowly bring it back down behind your head. Repeat.
- Biceps curl: Hold a hand-held weight in front of your body and curl it to your chest, keeping your elbow at your hip. Repeat.
- Chair push-up: Place a chair with its back against a wall. Kneel in front of the chair, grip the chair seat, and do a push-up against the chair. Repeat.

Supplements

- Thiamine: 1.5 mg per day
- Riboflavin: 1.8 mg per day
- Vitamin B_6: 2–10 mg per day
- Vitamin B_{12}: 2–10 mg per day
- Vitamin C: 100–500 mg per day
- Calcium: 1200 mg per day
- Vitamin D: 10 mcg per day
- Vitamin E: 100–400 IU per day

OVERWEIGHT (OBESITY)

WHAT IS OBESITY?

From Modern Western Medicine

Overweight is a condition of excess body fat that causes body weight to be above the ideal for a person's height. Obesity is classified as being 20 percent above the ideal body weight for a person's height.

Overweight occurs when the number of calories consumed each day exceed the number burned as energy. There are many reasons why a person may become obese, but as of yet, the underlying causes of obesity are not well understood. For example, many obese people do not eat any more food that thin people. Obese people commonly have slow metabolic rates, which means that they expend many fewer calories in a given hour than thin people do. This causes energy to be stored as fat much more easily. The rate at which energy is burned depends a great deal on the level of activity engaged in each day. Obese people tend to be more sedentary than thin people.

Genetic factors may play a role. Children of obese parents are twenty times more likely to be obese themselves than children of thin parents. In a minority of cases, hormonal factors may be involved in creating additional body weight.

Obesity significantly increases a person's risk of contracting other illnesses, particularly heart disease, adult-onset diabetes (type II), high blood pressure, and cancers of the breast, uterus, cervix, colon, and prostate. Other conditions, such as arthritis, can be exacerbated by obesity.

Treatment for overweight and obesity consists of taking in fewer calories than are expended each day. Medical doctors recommend that overweight people eat a diet that provides 500 to 1000 calories less than their daily energy requirements. That will result in an average weight loss of one to two pounds per week. By exercising at least four times a week, more calories are burned and muscle mass is increased. Muscle has a much faster rate of metabolism than fat cells, which means that the more muscle you have, the more weight you burn. Exercise also increases metabolism. (See the section on exercise in Part III.)

From Traditional Medicine

While overweight and obesity have reached epidemic proportions in the United States, people throughout the rest of the world, even in Europe, do not suffer nearly the same rates of the disorder as Americans do. The reason, simply, is that Americans eat more animal foods and foods rich in fat than any other people on earth. Most of the world subsists on a diet that is low in fat and made up primarily of grains, potatoes, vegetables, beans, fruit, and fish. This reduces the amount of fat consumed. Fat is the most calorically dense food available to humans. A gram of fat contains nine to eleven calories, while a gram of carbohydrates (found in grains, vegetables, and fruits) contains only four calories.

Research has demonstrated that diets that require calorie counting fail repeatedly to affect lasting weight loss. On the other hand, studies have also shown that people who change the composition of their diets to regimens similar to those of our ancestors—diets made up largely of grains, vegetables, beans, and fruit—lose weight effortlessly. Moreover, a diet dominated by vegetables and low-fat animal foods does not require any calorie counting. Nor does anyone on such a diet ever have to go hungry. The reason is that grains and vegetables are calorically light, while animal foods and fats are calorically dense.

WHO IS OBESE?

Approximately 25 percent of the U.S. population is overweight. Fifty percent of American children are overweight or obese. Americans on average gained eight pounds during the 1980s.

REMEDIES

General Recommendations

- See the exercise section in Part III.
- Significantly reduce fat by reducing or eliminating red meat, whole milk, dairy products, and fried foods.
- Increase vegetable foods, especially whole grains, fresh vegetables, beans, and fruit. Vegetables are nutritionally rich but calorically light.
- See your medical doctor before starting an exercise program, especially if you are obese or have not been given a routine check-up in the previous year.

Foods to Eat

- Whole grains, especially brown rice, oats, barley, corn (a good diuretic), millet, amaranth, quinoa, and basmati rice (unrefined)
- Beans, especially adzuki beans, black beans, chickpeas, lentils, and others
- Vegetables, especially leafy greens, such as collard, kale, mustard greens, broccoli, squash, carrots, and other roots (Steam, boil, or—in the case of squash—bake them.)
- Sea vegetables are rich in minerals and amino acids. They regulate metabolism and help to control weight.
- Cold-pressed flax oil provides hormonal balance for those who have eaten excess animal products. Two teaspoons of flax oil can be poured over food each day; or eat three tablespoons of soaked or crushed flaxseed. Eat soaked seeds alone to make digestion easier.
- Spirulina
- White fish

- Fruit, such as apples, plums, peaches, berries, oranges, and pears (According to Chinese medicine, a person who has symptoms of dampness such as water retention, yeast overgrowth, fatigue, sluggishness, and/or emotional heaviness should avoid these fruits.)
- Goat's milk normalizes the weight of the body. Take it raw.
- Bee pollen: one-half ounce daily

Foods to Avoid

- Animal fats
- Vegetable fats: nuts, seeds, and oils (Use sparingly, if at all, except for unrefined, cold-pressed flaxseed oil.)
- Salt, except for a small quantity of unrefined whole salt in cooking
- Alcohol

The following will stimulate false appetite:

- Hot spices
- Coffee
- Tea
- Sugar
- Tobacco

Herbs for Obesity

- Evening primrose, borage, black currant: Take 125 mg of any of these.
- Burdock purifies the blood while reducing fat and regulating blood sugar. Decoct the dried herb or eat the fresh root (raw or cooked).
- Alfalfa: Take as tea infusion or in tablet form.
- Chickweed: decoct the dried herb.
- Michael Tierra's Planetary Herbal Formula 11: This formula can be used to open the channels of elimination and assist in a balanced detoxification. It aids assimilation and satisfies hunger. Take two to four tablets, three times daily. Can be purchased or ordered through your natural food store. Take with warm soy milk.

The following herbs are helpful for those with signs of coldness:

- Cumin
- Ginger
- Cloves
- Spearmint
- Fennel
- Cayenne

The following herbs are helpful for those with signs of heat:

- Peppermint
- Chamomile
- Kohlrabi
- Turnip
- White pepper

Hydrotherapy

- Add two cups of Epsom salts to warm, full-body baths with the addition of steam baths three times a week to promote sweating, which reduces water held in the tissue, and to promote circulation. Dry yourself with brisk towel rubbing.
- Saunas
- Alternate hot and cold showers to stimulate the circulation and the endocrine system

Chinese Medicine

According to Oriental tradition, the flavors that will stimulate weight loss are bitter and pungent (see the list of foods to eat above). A limit should be placed on sweet, salty, and sour foods.

Exercise

- Aerobic exercise: continuous for 12 to 20 minutes minimum at 80 percent maximum heart rate, six times per week
- The best exercise is walking. Another good routine is bicycle riding.
- Avoid competitive sports, especially if you are obese.
- See your medical doctor before starting an exercise program.

Supplements

- Beta-carotene: 15–30 mg per day
- Thiamine: 1.5 mg per day
- Riboflavin: 1.8 mg per day
- Niacin: 20 mg per day
- Vitamin B_6: 2–10 mg per day
- Vitamin B_{12}: 2–10 mcg per day
- Vitamin C: 100–500 mg per day
- Vitamin E: 100–400 IU per day
- Iron: 15 mg per day
- Magnesium: 400 mg per day
- Zinc: 15 mg per day
- Folate: 400–800 mcg per day
- Selenium: 70–200 mcg per day
- Chromium: 100–200 mcg per day

PARKINSON'S DISEASE

SYMPTOMS

Muscle tremor, trembling, weakness, stiffness, slow movements, rigid posture, and shuffling and unbalanced walk. As balance is thrown off and movement becomes more restricted, the person is forced to take only the tiniest of steps. His or her head shakes; the body stoops somewhat; and an unblinking, fixed expression takes over the person's face. Routine matters, such as washing, dressing, and eating become difficult to manage without assistance.

WHAT IS PARKINSON'S DISEASE?

From Modern Western Medicine

Parkinson's disease is a degeneration of the neurons or nerve cells in the basal ganglia of the brain causing tremors in one or both hands, arms, or legs. The illness arises from the inability of neurons to produce dopamine, a neurotransmitter in the brain that is essential for coordinated muscle activity. Among the treatments for Parkinson's disease is the use of a drug called L-dopa, which is designed to increase brain levels of dopamine.

In its early phases, the hands, arms, or legs tremble more when they are at rest but come under much greater control when the limb is used. As the illness progresses, the symptoms worsen, with increasing stiffness and weakness of muscles, trembling of the hands, and imbalance that is often worse at rest than in movement.

Although speech and handwriting may be impaired, mental function is usually not affected until very late in the disease. This creates many difficult internal issues for the person, and depression is common.

Treatment is available for those who suffer from Parkinson's disease, but there is no cure. Medication, exercise, special assistance at home, and encouragement all serve to diminish symptoms, increase mobility and self-reliance, and improve morale.

From Traditional Medicine

Parkinson's disease results from the brain's inability to produce adequate levels of dopamine, a neurotransmitter whose production is increased when high-protein foods are consumed. Some researchers have speculated that a lifetime of high-protein, high-fat foods have resulted in the overproduction of dopamine. Production of dopamine becomes weaker with time, until the neurons are unable to produce adequate quantities of the neurotransmitter.

Recent research has shown that people with Parkinson's disease respond better to treatment when placed on a high-carbohydrate, low-protein diet.

Such a diet is composed chiefly of whole grains, fresh vegetables, beans, and fruit, along with occasional low-fat animal foods, such as fish. (See the section on foods below.) Such a diet provides an abundance of vitamins, minerals, trace elements, essential fatty acids, and protein.

It's essential to eat a diet that maximizes oxygen and glucose to the brain, which means the diet must be extremely low in fat and rich in complex carbohydrates, vitamins, and minerals. Brain function declines when oxygen levels fall due to a high-fat diet. The same is true when glucose levels fall. Blood sugar is increased on a diet rich in complex carbohydrates (found in whole grains, vegetables, and fruit), which are the basis for optimal blood sugar levels. Brain levels of both oxygen and blood sugar are also enhanced when a person gets regular exercise, even a daily walk. Other excellent exercises include yoga and gentle stretching.

WHO GETS PARKINSON'S DISEASE?

There are about 50,000 new cases of Parkinson's disease diagnosed each year in the United States, with approximately 1 in 200 adults contracting the disease, usually in their senior years. For unknown reasons, men are at higher risk of contracting the disease than women.

REMEDIES

Foods to Eat

- Spelt (made as congee): At the Hildegard Practice, a clinic in Konstanz, Germany, spelt has been used as an adjunct in the treatment of many disorders, including Parkinson's.
- Fruit
- Vegetables, especially leafy greens
- Vegetable juice, especially carrot
- Seaweeds
- Sprouted grains
- Raw seeds, such as sunflower and pumpkin

Foods to Avoid

- Chemicalized and processed food
- Coffee
- Caffeinated tea
- Sugar
- Tobacco

Herbs to Treat Parkinson's Disease

- Larkspur: 20 grams in 4 cups of boiling water; do not drink more than 3 cups a day, a mouthful at a time.

- Lady's slipper is good for tremors, especially in debilitated conditions; it clears depression. Use a standard decoction or 3–9 g; tincture, 10–30 drops. Take 3 or 4 times a day for maximum effectiveness.
- Skullcap: Combine with lady's slipper for broader action. Strengthens the brain. Standard infusion or 3–9 g; tincture, 10–30 drops (Most of what is sold as skullcap in this country is germander. Ask for the genuine herb.)

Exercise

- Daily walking
- Yoga or gentle stretching

Physiotherapy

- Ozone-producing machines: Ozone may help improve nervous system and brain function in Parkinson's patients. The FDA has not yet approved the machines for medical use; however, they are available through medical doctors and from people who work to make homes and offices more environmentally healthful. (Ozone machines can be purchased through International Ozone Assn., 83 Oakwood Terrace, Norwalk CT 06850.)
- Alternate hot and cold showers
- Alternate hot and cold head douches
- Saunas followed by massage
- Outdoor exercise
- Sun and ocean baths

Supplements

- Vitamin A: 5000 IU per day
- Thiamine (B_1): 1.5 mg per day
- Riboflavin (B_2): 1.8 mg per day
- Vitamin B_6: 2–10 mg per day
- Vitamin B_{12} 2–10 mcg per day
- Vitamin C: 100–500 mg per day
- Vitamin D: 10 mcg (400 IU) per day
- Vitamin E: 100–400 IU per day
- Zinc: 15 mg per day
- Magnesium: 400 mg per day
- Selenium: 70–200 mcg per day

POISON IVY AND POISON OAK

SYMPTOMS

Red welts and blisters that itch and burn appear on the skin after coming in contact with a poison ivy plant and related plants.

WHAT IS POISON IVY?

Poison ivy is a green plant with three leaves that grow from a single shoot. It typically grows close to the ground. Poison ivy contains an allergen on its leaves that can cause skin reactions, which for some people may be extremely severe.

When you come in contact with poison ivy, wash the exposed area of the skin thoroughly, wipe with alcohol, and apply calamine lotion. Also, wash the clothing that may have touched the plant. When the reaction is severe, call a physician.

REMEDIES

Foods to Eat

- Miso soup, once a day, to alkalize the system
- Whole brown rice, boiled together with carrots and onions and a pinch of sea salt; or pressure-cooked with a pinch of sea salt
- Vegetables: Leafy greens, such as collard, kale, and mustard greens, carrots, and burdock root (pressure-cooked with chopped carrots)
- Sea vegetables, such as sushi nori, which does not require cooking; filled with immune-boosting minerals
- Fruit

Foods to Avoid

- Sugar
- Fried foods
- Fats, both vegetable and animal

Herbs for Poison Ivy

- Lycium root: 9–15 g, used both internally and externally for poison ivy

Try any of the following herbs, singly or in combination to assist in detoxifying the system. Dose is 1 cup of tea, ½ teaspoon of tincture, or 2 capsules, 3 or 4 times a day.

- Nettles
- Red clover
- Yellow dock
- Burdock

Apply externally:

- Calendula: antibacterial, anti-inflammatory, and antiviral
- Aloe vera gel: cools and soothes
- Goldenseal: 1 tablespoon of powdered herb to ¼ cup of clay, or mix with an equal part of water and apply. Has antibiotic and astringent properties.
- Comfrey, chickweed, or witch hazel help relieve itching.

Homeopathy to Treat Poison Ivy

- Rhus toxicodendrun treats blisters and rashes
- Sulfur: for burning itch made worse by warm bathing

Hydrotherapy

- Cooling compresses with cold water and vinegar every one to two hours
- Oatmeal baths will help relieve itching.
- Baking soda plaster moistened with water will help relieve itching.
- Swimming in salt water

Essential Oils

Apply as compresses or in baths.

- Lavender: antimicrobial, antiseptic, speeds skin healing
- Patchouli: antibiotic, astringent, anti-inflammatory

Supplements

- Vitamin C plus bioflavonoids: 2–5 g or to bowel tolerance; to boost immune response
- Zinc: 50 mg per day
- Beta-carotene: 10–20 mg per day

POLYPS OF THE COLON

SYMPTOMS

Bleeding from the rectum or blood in the stools are symptoms of colon polyps.

WHAT ARE POLYPS?

From Modern Western Medicine

Polyps are small, stalklike growths that project from the lining of a mucous membrane. They often appear in the large intestine. Polyps are usually benign, but some may become cancerous. They may be removed surgically, especially if there is evidence that they may become malignant.

From Traditional Medicine

Polyps occur much more frequently in the intestines of people who eat a diet rich in red meat and fat. Such a diet slows intestinal transit time and exposes sensitive mucous tissues to toxins and carcinogens for lengthy periods of time. By increasing fiber from grains and vegetables, intestinal transit time is decreased, and bowel elimination is enhanced. Some studies have shown that when the diet is changed dramatically, the polyps recede.

REMEDIES

Foods to Eat

Lots of high-fiber foods:

- Whole grains
- Organic vegetables
- Fruit

According to Chinese medicine, white, pungent foods affect the metal element. Have them very lightly cooked.

- Onion family vegetables, especially garlic
- Turnips
- Ginger
- Horseradish
- Cabbage
- Radishes

- Daikon radishes
- White peppercorns

Mucilaginous foods remove old, thick mucoid deposits and replace them with a clean, moist coating.

- Seaweed
- Flaxseed

Dark green and golden orange vegetables:

- Carrot
- Winter squash
- Pumpkin
- Broccoli
- Parsley
- Kale
- Turnip and mustard greens
- Watercress
- Wheat or barley grass
- Microalgae

Foods to Avoid

- Red meat
- Eggs
- Dairy products
- Fried foods
- Spicy foods
- Coffee
- Tea
- Tobacco

PROSTATE PROBLEMS

SYMPTOMS

A man's prostate gland, located just below the bladder, is vulnerable to a host of afflictions, including benign swelling (known as *benign prostatic hyperplasia,* or BPH), bacterial infection, and cancer. All three may prevent urine from flowing optimally, which can affect the bladder and kidneys.

Symptoms of benign swelling, or BPH, include obstructed urine flow, difficulty urinating, and weak stream. At first, the bladder muscles compensate for the obstruction by becoming stronger in order to force urine through the obstructed urethra, the tube that runs from the bladder, through the center of the prostate, and down through the penis, allowing urine to be evacuated. If the prostate swelling is not reduced, the bladder can become enlarged and cause abdominal swelling.

Symptoms of prostatitis and swelling of the prostate gland are often caused by bacterial infection and can include pain or discomfort while urinating, increased frequency of urination, and, in some cases, fever may develop and a discharge may occur. Pain may also arise in the lower abdomen, rectum, groin, and lower back. Blood may also appear in the urine.

Approximately 122,000 American men get prostate cancer each year, and 32,000 men die from the disease. Symptoms include difficulty starting urination, obstructed urinary flow, and increased frequency of urination. In time, urine flow may stop completely. In more advanced cases, pain may also accompany the disease.

WHAT ARE PROSTATE PROBLEMS?

From Modern Western Medicine

The prostate gland produces the seminal fluid that carries sperm out of the body. The gland is about the size of a chestnut. When the prostate swells, it pinches the urethra, a tube that runs through the center of the prostate, and prevents urine from flowing optimally from the bladder.

Virtually every man over the age of fifty has some prostate swelling. For most men, the condition is mild and harmless, except that it causes symptoms. Symptoms will pass without treatment in about 30 percent of men, according to urologists. For those who need treatment, antibiotics are usually the first line of treatment. The most common antibiotics used are quinolones, which are broad-spectrum antibacterial agents. For most men, the symptoms improve in twenty-four to forty-eight hours. The disorder is diagnosed with a rectal examination. If the prostate remains enlarged and obstruction of urine

Prostate
Male Pelvic Region with Sex Organs

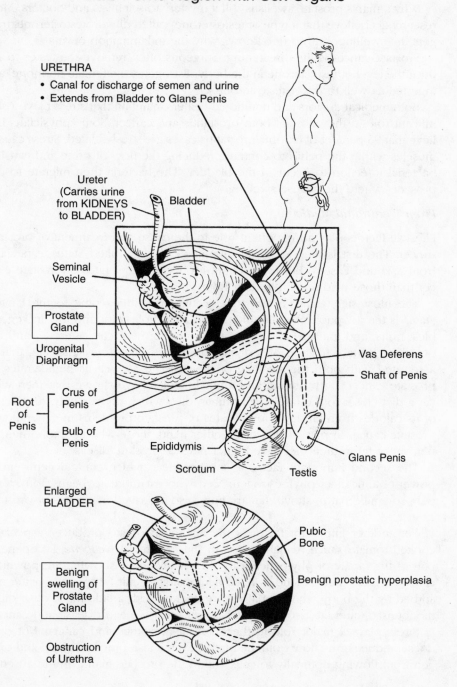

URETHRA
- Canal for discharge of semen and urine
- Extends from Bladder to Glans Penis

Ureter
(Carries urine
from KIDNEYS
to BLADDER)

Bladder

Seminal
Vesicle

Prostate
Gland

Urogenital
Diaphragm

Vas Deferens

Shaft of Penis

Crus of
Penis

Root
of
Penis

Bulb of
Penis

Glans Penis

Epididymis

Scrotum

Testis

Enlarged
BLADDER

Pubic
Bone

Benign
swelling of
Prostate
Gland

Benign prostatic hyperplasia

Obstruction
of Urethra

continues, surgery may be needed to open the urethra passageway or remove the prostate.

Why a man's prostate swells is still a mystery to scientists and doctors. Most researchers believe that a type of testosterone, called dihydrotestosterone, triggers the swelling, but no one knows why the inflammation occurs.

Prostate cancer is life-threatening. Surgeons often remove the testes to reduce the level of testosterone in the body. Estrogens, the female hormone, are ingested as well to lower testosterone.

Both medical doctors and traditional healers maintain that stress plays a significant role in the onset of both prostatitis and cancer. Some physicians believe that 95 percent of chronic prostatitis cases are stress-related. Stress causes muscles within the pelvis to contract, reducing the flow of urine and causing bacterial infection to occur in the bladder. The bacteria then migrate to the prostate, where they cause swelling.

From Traditional Medicine

Lifestyle factors play an important role in the cause and treatment of prostate cancer. The first is diet. Men who immigrate to the United States, especially from Asia and Eastern European countries, have higher rates of prostate cancer than those who remain in their homelands.

The most significant change that occurs once men come to the United States is the adoption of a diet high in fat and cholesterol and low in vegetables, fruits, and grains. Fat elevates the male hormone, testosterone, and especially a certain fraction of testosterone, called dihydrotestosterone, that is associated with both the swelling of the prostate as well as higher rates of prostate cancer. Both human and animal studies have shown that men who eat a diet closer to the traditional human diet, which derives only 20 percent of its calories from fat, have lower rates of prostate problems in general, and prostate cancer in particular. On the other hand, those who eat more than 20 percent of fat in their diet have higher rates of prostate disease.

The second important factor is soy products, which contain genistein, a powerful anticancer phytoestrogen. Men who eat more soybeans, tofu, tempeh, soy milk, natto, shoyu, tamari, and miso all have lower rates of prostate cancer.

Yet another important factor is the intake of tomato products, especially cooked tomato sauce, which is rich in the carotinoid *lycopene*. Lycopene is part of the family of phytochemicals, which science is showing are powerful cancer fighters. Recent studies have demonstrated that lycopene is better absorbed by the body when tomatoes are cooked with a little bit of olive oil, a monounsaturated fat associated with lower rates of heart disease and cancer.

Stress plays a major role in the onset of prostatitis and cancer. Not only does it reduce urine flow from the bladder, but it also prevents blood and oxygen from flowing optimally to cells within the prostate gland. In the absence of adequate oxygen, nutrition, and immune cells, the prostate gland may become swollen and start to degenerate. Cells may mutate and form cancers.

Chinese medicine maintains that the kidneys provide qi to the prostate gland. To strengthen kidneys, eat beans, sea vegetables, white fish, barley, and avoid caffeine (especially coffee) and high-protein foods. Oriental medicine maintains that prostate problems are the result of excessive constriction or tightness within the pelvis. Relaxation or expansion of the pelvis results in more qi, blood, and lymph flowing to the gland.

The remedies provided below will provide both short-term relief and can serve as the basis for prevention of BPH, prostatitis, and prostate cancer.

REMEDIES

General Recommendations

- Reduce fat consumption. The best way to do that is to substantially reduce animal foods, especially red meat, dairy products, and eggs.
- Eat more soybean products.
- Eat tomato sauce with your pasta.
- Eat vegetables to obtain higher quantities of phytochemicals, such as genistein.
- Do more to relax and cope more effectively with stress.

(See recommendations for specifics, below.)

Foods to Eat

- Green, yellow, and orange vegetables are rich in carotenoids, bioflavonoids, and phytoestrogens.
- Tomatoes and tomato sauce, with small amounts of olive oil
- Make the diet rich in vegetables of all kinds. Each day, make the diet at least 60 percent vegetables to relax the body, especially the pelvis.
- Eat plenty of beans, especially soybeans and soybean products (such as tempeh, tofu, natto, shoyu, tamari, and soy milk, all of which contain genistein. (See foods that protect against cancer in the section on nutrition in Part III.)
- Whole grains, especially brown rice and barley
- Sea vegetables, especially nori, arame, wakame, and kelp
- Miso soup
- Pumpkin seeds are rich in vitamin E and reduce swelling of the prostate, especially when there is difficulty urinating.
- Vegetable juices, including celery, carrot, beet, and apple: Make fresh and drink one 8 oz. glass per day.

Foods to Avoid

- Reduce animal foods, especially red meat and whole milk products to reduce fat. Most days per week should be meatless and dairyless.
- Fried foods
- Refined carbohydrates
- Coffee weakens the kidneys and bladder and negatively affects the prostate.
- Excess protein weakens kidneys, bladder, and prostate.
- Sugar
- Meat
- Dairy products
- Poultry
- Alcohol
- Cigarettes

Herbs for Prostate

- Saw palmetto: tincture, 30–40 drops, twice daily; extract, 5–10 drops taken in water 4 times daily. Can be taken every hour during inflammatory stages.
- Pipsissewa: tincture, 25 drops, 3 times a day, in addition to drinking 3 cups of slippery elm tea daily.
- Mix together:

  1 part gravel root
  1 part plaintain
  1 part echinacea
  1 part parsley root
  ¼ part gingerroot
  1 part buchu
  ¼ part lobelia

Use one ounce of the herbs to one pint of water. Make a decoction and drink ½ cup, 3 times daily. Add honey to taste or put powdered herbs in #00 capsules and take 2, 3 times a day.

Homeopathy

Enlarged prostate:

- Sabal 6c: for difficult or painful urination, with spasms of bladder or urethra
- Baryta 6c: for frequent urge to urinate, slow stream, thin and underweight person
- Thuja 6c: for frequent, urgent desire to pass urine

Prostatitis: Take every two hours for ten doses.

- Sabal 6c: for enlarged prostate and if area around genitals feels cold; also if ejaculation is difficult or impossible
- Pulsatilla 6c: for thick, yellow discharge from penis; urgent need to urinate; lying on back makes condition feel worse
- Thuja 6c: for burning sensation at back of bladder, frequent urge to pass urine

Supplements

- Vitamin E: 100–400 IU/day
- Vitamin C: 100 mg/day

Exercise

- Walking daily
- Active aerobic sport that forces lower body to twist and turn
- Daily yoga, especially postures that stretch pelvic muscles
- Stretching exercise, especially before vigorous aerobic workout.

Mind/Body

- Daily meditation, prayer, or progressive relaxation to relieve stress
- Participate in any religious organization or service that strengthens faith.

Psoriasis

SYMPTOMS

Raised patches of red, inflamed skin, often appearing on the chest, knees, and elbows of the affected person. Sometimes the skin may be covered by white flakes or silvery scales.

WHAT IS PSORIASIS?

From Modern Western Medicine

Psoriasis tends to run in families, though no one knows why the disorder arises in the first place. The reason the skin forms raised patches is because the underlying cells reproduce ten times faster than normal, while the old cells remain unchanged and consequently go unshed. The result is that the new, live cells accumulate within limited areas, forming thick, raised patches that are often covered with dead, flaking skin.

Stress, physical illness, or some type of injury to the skin can trigger a flare-up of the condition. Sunlight or an ultraviolet lamp may reduce the symptoms in mild cases of psoriasis. Ointments containing coal tar or anthralin are used to treat moderate cases, while severe attacks are often treated with corticosteroid drugs, PUVA (a type of phototherapy), and forms of chemotherapy that are often used in the treatment of cancer.

From Traditional Medicine

Skin eruptions of all types are seen by traditional medicine as a way for the body to eliminate waste that is not being properly filtered by the kidneys, liver, and spleen. In some cases, toxins are being reintroduced into the bloodstream and lymph system from the wall of the large intestine.

The general approach to psoriasis is to reduce the level of toxicity in the diet and environment and to support the blood-cleansing and eliminative organs. In addition, the blood should be slightly alkaline, as opposed to acidic, which is often the case in people who suffer from skin disorders. The recommendations listed below will reduce toxicity and alkalize the blood.

WHO GETS PSORIASIS?

It occurs in about 2 percent of people in the United States and Europe and is probably less common among Blacks and Asians. It affects men and women equally. It usually appears between ages ten and thirty, but infants occasionally suffer from it. It also occurs in old age.

REMEDIES

Foods to Eat

- Miso soup alkalizes the blood.
- Whole grains
- Soybean products, such as tofu
- Vegetables, especially carrots, winter squash, pumpkin, leafy greens such as dandelion, beet, spinach, kale, chard, and watercress
- Mung beans, adzuki beans, chickpeas, lentils, and black beans (considered an herb for the kidneys)
- Cucumber slices, unpeeled
- Seaweeds: Sushi nori does not need to be cooked. It is widely available in natural food stores.
- Spirulina
- Foods rich in omega-3 and GLA fatty acids such as sesame seeds and unrefined sesame oil
- Black sesame seeds (an herb for the kidneys)
- Fish, especially low-fat white fish, such as haddock, cod, flounder, and scrod

Foods to Avoid

The following foods could be a source of food allergy:

- Citrus fruits
- Meat
- Wheat
- Eggs
- Dairy products

The following may also be contributing factors:

- Tomatoes
- Saturated and hydrogenated fats
- Sweets
- Alcohol
- Pastry
- Carbonated beverages
- Spicy foods

Herbs to Treat Psoriasis

- Burdock root: decoction or tincture, 20–40 drops, 2–4 times a day
- Common figwort: 1–3 ml of tincture, 1 or 2 times per day

Take any of the following blood-cleaning herbs:

- Dandelion root: tincture, 30–60 drops (½–1 tsp.), 2 times per day; infusion, steep 30 minutes and drink 3 cups daily; decoction, simmer 30 minutes, drink 6 oz., 3 times daily, hot or cold
- Goldenseal root: tincture, 20–30 drops, two times daily; infusion (powdered root), steep until cold, take 1–2 tsp., 3 times daily; decoction, simmer 15–30 minutes, take 1–2 tsp., 3 times per day
- Echinacea root: tincture, 20–30 drops, 3 times daily; fluid extract, ½–1 tsp., 3 times daily
- Yellow dock root: tincture, 5–30 drops, 2 times daily; fluid extract, ½–1 tsp., 2 times daily
- Red clover blossoms: tincture, 5–30 drops, 2 times per day; fluid extract, 2 tsp., 2 times per day; infusion, steep 30 minutes, take 1–2 oz., 2 times per day; powder, 5–10 #0 capsules (30–60 grains), 2 times per day

Physiotherapy

- Alternate hot and cold showers to stimulate circulation
- Castor oil packs (See the section on hydrotherapy and physiotherapy in Part III for recipe.)
- Wash the area with sarsaparilla tea or seawater; apply garlic oil or walnut oil; bathe in mineral water; add several cups of unrefined sea salt to bathwater. (To prepare garlic oil, soak several sliced, mashed cloves of garlic in 4 ounces of sesame oil for 3 days, then strain the oil by squeezing it through a cloth.)

Hydrotherapy

- Ocean swims and sun
- Colonics
- Enemas

Supplements

- Vitamin A: 15 mg per day
- Thiamine: 2.2 mg per day
- Riboflavin: 1.5 mg per day
- Niacin: 16 mg per day
- Vitamin B_6: 3.0 mg per day
- Folate: 400 mcg per day
- Vitamin B_{12}: 4.0 mcg per day
- Vitamin C: 80 mg per day
- Vitamin E: 44 mg per day
- Zinc: 14 mg per day

Rash

SYMPTOMS

Rash is a general term used to describe a collection of red spots or patches on the skin that are often itchy and inflamed. Sometimes accompanied by fever, a rash is a temporary condition that may last a few days, a week, or two weeks. It is rarely serious.

WHAT IS A RASH?

From Modern Western Medicine

A localized rash is restricted to a small area of the body. If it covers the entire body, it is referred to as generalized. Medical doctors describe rashes according to the characteristics of the spots: blistering, macular, nodular, papular, or pustular.

A rash is a sign of infection. In children, it is often a sign of infectious disease, such as chicken pox, measles, or scarlet fever. It may also be a symptom of bacterial infection (ringworm in children, for example) or athlete's foot (in adults).

Skin disorders, such as eczema and psoriasis, manifest as rashes. Other forms of rashes include purpura (a bleeding disorder with purplish red spots), lupus erythematosus (an autoimmune disorder), hives, and a toxic reaction to a drug.

From Traditional Medicine

Traditional medicine considers skin rashes as a discharge of toxins from within the system. The skin is an organ of elimination used by the body when toxins in the blood become excessive and overrun the blood-cleansing capacity of the kidneys, liver, and spleen. Usually, skin rashes occur when the kidneys are weak or overworked by an excessive amount of toxins taken in from the environment or the diet.

REMEDIES

Foods to Eat

- Miso soup
- Whole grains
- Lightly cooked vegetables
- Seaweed
- Mung beans

- Black beans
- Spirulina and chlorella
- Juices, such as celery, carrot, beet, and apple: Make them fresh and drink daily (to cleanse liver).
- Unprocessed food

Foods to Avoid

- Meat
- Dairy products
- Refined carbohydrates
- Sugar
- Fried foods
- Oily foods
- Sugar
- Processed foods
- Hot spices
- Coffee
- Tea
- Tobacco

Herbs for Rashes

Internally:

- Aloe: powdered root, ½–1 tsp. taken in capsules or steeped in a cup of boiling water; gel, 2 tsp. mixed in apple juice or water, 3 times a day
- Gromwell: 3–9 g
- Teas made from sassafras, dandelion, sarsaparilla, and burdock seed: Combine or use individually.

Externally:

- Impatiens: 1–3 g of the juice can be applied often
- Witch hazel: apply topically

Sinusitis

SYMPTOMS

Congestion and pressure in the interior passageways of the skull behind the nose, forehead, and cheeks. The congestion may result in a throbbing pain or a sinus headache. For some people, fever, runny or stuffy nose, loss of the ability to smell, and even a discharge of pus may result.

WHAT IS SINUSITIS?

From Modern Western Medicine

Sinusitis is an inflammation of the mucous membranes in the cavities or air pathways beyond the nose, cheeks, and forehead. It is caused by bacterial infection that usually develops during or after the onset of a viral infection, such as the common cold. Sinusitis may also arise from an infection of a tooth, water being forced into the sinuses, or from a blow to the face.

Medical doctors treat the infection with antibiotics, decongestant sprays, or steam inhalations. If the condition persists, surgery may be needed to open the blocked passageways.

From Traditional Medicine

Traditional medicine views the body holistically, so that blockages in one part of the body tend to create symptoms elsewhere. One of the axioms of Chinese medicine is that a symptom in the upper body is usually caused by an imbalance in the lower part, and vice versa. In the case of any sinus problem, including sinusitis, the problem has its origins in the intestines, which are blocked and unable to fully eliminate waste. The large intestine is lined with lymph vessels, which can reabsorb waste and recirculate it through the system. This occurs whenever the large intestine suffers from constipation or inadequate or inefficient elimination. Once the waste is reintroduced to the lymph system, the lymph becomes backed up, immune cells flood lymph nodes, and the lymph system in general becomes swollen and inflamed. The result is swollen glands (inflamed lymph nodes), tonsilitis, adenoiditis, and inflamed sinus tissue. If the large intestine continues to function in an inefficient and ineffective manner, it will create a chronic sinus condition, including sinusitis.

There are, of course, other ways to impair the lymph system and negatively affect the sinuses. An overly acidic diet causes the spleen to become imbalanced and swollen, which causes sinuses to become inflamed. The solution to sinusitis—and all sinus problems for that matter—is to support the function

Sinusitis

Four Paired Paranasal Air Sinuses

(named according to the bones in which they are found)

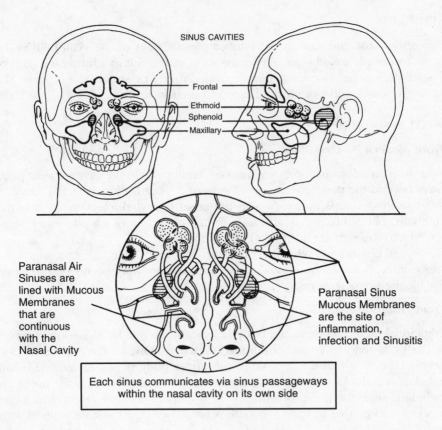

SINUS CAVITIES

Frontal
Ethmoid
Sphenoid
Maxillary

Paranasal Air Sinuses are lined with Mucous Membranes that are continuous with the Nasal Cavity

Paranasal Sinus Mucous Membranes are the site of inflammation, infection and Sinusitis

Each sinus communicates via sinus passageways within the nasal cavity on its own side

of the large intestine and spleen with a diet rich in fiber, vegetables, and alkalizing foods, such as miso soup.

WHO GETS SINUSITIS?

This is very common. Many people suffer an attack after every common cold.
It seems that once the tendency is established, reoccurrence is more likely
with each cold.

REMEDIES

General Recommendations

- See the section on constipation for improving bowel function.
- See the section on strengthening the large intestine, spleen, and lungs in
  Part IV.
- Boost immune function. See the sections on the immune system in Parts
  II and IV.

Foods to Eat

Start with a three- to five-day mucus-cleaning diet.

- Miso soup
- Whole grains: If constipated, make grains wet, with thick, soupy consis-
  tency. Add a teaspoon of freshly grated ginger, chopped carrots, and
  onions.
- A wide variety of vegetables, including leafy greens, roots, round veg-
  etables, and squash
- Fruit, such as grapefruit, lemons, and oranges for breakfast
- Carrot juice at midmorning
- Boiled or steamed onions for lunch
- Carrot juice at midafternoon
- Boiled or steamed onions for dinner

After the initial fast, enjoy the following foods:

- Fresh fruit
- Vegetable juice
- Garlic
- Radish
- Turnips (Chinese medicine uses turnips for lung imbalances such as
  sinus problems.)
- Raw salads: especially made of lettuce, cabbage, celery, cucumber, car-
  rots, and onions
- Boiled and steamed onions, often

- Tofu
- Whole grains
- Vegetables
- Seaweed

Foods to Avoid

- Coffee
- Tea
- Alcohol
- Spices
- Salt
- Sugar
- Tobacco

Herbs to Treat Sinusitis

- Tea made from goldenseal or mullein: Snuff a teaspoonful up each nostril several times a day.
- Garlic, chaparral, or echinacea tablets: 2 every 2 hours of one, or alternate them until the infection is gone. If using tincture, 20 drops every 2 hours.
- Any of the following natural laxatives: senna, cascara sagrata, or flaxseed

Hydrotherapy

- Boil two quarts of water, then turn the stove off and add fifteen drops of eucalyptus, peppermint, or some other volatile oil to the water. Cover your head and the pot of water with a towel and inhale through the nose and mouth several times. Do this two or three times a day.
- Alternate hot and cold compresses
- Nasal irrigations: beet root juice in ice-cold water, chlorophyll nasal douche, and lemon and water douche plus nasal spray

Supplements

- Vitamin A: 400 IU daily
- Vitamin B complex
  Thiamine: 1.5 mg per day
  Riboflavin: 1.8 mg per day
  Vitamin B_6: 2–10 mg per day
  Vitamin B_{12}: 2–10 mg per day
  Niacin: 20 mg per day
- Vitamin C: 100 mg per day

Sore Throat

SYMPTOMS

A sore throat is any pain, soreness, and raw sensitivity in the throat, which is especially painful or uncomfortable when swallowing.

WHAT IS A SORE THROAT?

From Modern Western Medicine

A sore throat is a common disorder that frequently accompanies the common cold, influenza, laryngitis, and viral infections, including those of childhood, such as chicken pox, measles, and mumps. Sore throat may be a symptom of streptococcus, which, if left untreated, can result in kidney disease or rheumatic fever.

Treatment includes gargling with salt water and, for adults, taking aspirin. A physician should be consulted if a sore throat persists for more than forty-eight hours, or if a rash develops with a sore throat.

From Traditional Medicine

A sore throat results when the body is attempting to eliminate accumulated toxins, especially from the lymph system and the intestinal tract. The most common dietary cause of a sore throat, especially in children, is dairy products and sugar consumption. A frequent underlying physical cause is constipation. When toxins remain in the large intestine, they are reabsorbed by the lymph system, which becomes backed up with waste and by-products of immune cell activity. Tonsils, pharynx, and larynx become swollen as a result. In general, treatment includes improvement of bowel function, lots of well-cooked, soft grains and vegetables, and rest.

REMEDIES

Foods to Eat

- Whole grains, especially brown rice, barley, and oats: Make grain a little wetter and softer for easier digestion.
- Green, yellow, and orange vegetables: Steam and boil.
- Kombu seaweed: Make soup stock from it or cut it up and cook with vegetables.
- Cucumbers, raw and whole, or cucumber juice
- Root vegetables, such as carrots, turnips, rutabagas, and parsnips
- Miso soup

- Lemon: dilute the juice with water. Cleanses liver.
- Radishes: Take a few slices 2 or 3 times per day or ½ cup radish juice daily. Radishes are contraindicated for those with cold and deficient conditions.
- Strawberries
- Watercress

Foods to Avoid

- Cold drinks
- Dairy products
- Sugar
- Coffee
- Tea
- Spices
- Salt
- Alcohol
- Cigarettes
- Animal fats

Herbs to Treat Sore Throat

- Goldenseal: Use with myrrh for sore throat. Use tinctures as throat swab; dilute for gargle.
- Garlic: 2 capsules with meals
- Marigold: Use tincture for throat swab.
- Alfalfa: Make tea by steeping one tablespoon seed or two ounces dried leaf in one quart boiling water. Have two to three cups per day. Or add the powder to soups and salads.

Physiotherapy

Gargles:

- Hot water and salt
- Hot water, lemon juice, and honey
- Hydrastis, myrrh, and water
- Sage tea
- Sage, cayenne, and honey
- Bayberry bark decoction

Chinese Medicine

Sore throat is a heat condition that is related to the lungs. See the foods sections above.

SPRAINS

SYMPTOMS

Symptoms of sprains are pain, swelling, and sometimes discoloration at a joint. Movement usually increases the pain. Muscle contractions and spasms may also occur.

WHAT IS A SPRAIN?

From Modern Western Medicine

A sprain occurs when a ligament between joints is stretched, sometimes with some degree of tearing. Sprains usually occur at the ankle, knee, back, or wrist. Sprains occur from trauma, usually the result of an accident.

From Traditional Medicine

While sprains occur from a traumatic incident that appears to be an accident, the underlying cause is actually an imbalance in the body's qi flow. The accident is an event that allows the body to restore harmony to the imbalanced area. The imbalance is either excessive qi that has been accumulating in that joint, in which case the accident provides an opportunity to release the excess energy; or deficient qi at the joint, in which case the accident allows the body to concentrate its healing energy on the joint and restore balance to that part of the body.

REMEDIES

- Rest
- Gentle overall body massage
- Physiotherapy, as described below

Herbs to Treat Sprains

- Arnica tincture: Apply topically 4–6 times per day.
- Witch hazel: Apply 1–30 drops of tincture to the sprain.

Homeopathy

- Arnica: Use for the initial shock of injury. Massage injured area with arnica oil or lotion, but only on unbroken skin.
- Bryonia: When injury is swollen, distended, and feels worse with movement, take internally.
- Ledum: When injured joint is cold and numb and there is much swelling, take internally.

- *Rhus toxicodendron* (after arnica): if joint is hot, swollen, and painful; "rusty gate" feeling; creaky on first movement; better when limbered up
- *Ruta graveolens* (use after arnica): for torn and wrenched tendons or ligaments, bruised periosteum (bone covering), if worse in cold and wet weather
- Symphytum can be taken internally or as a lotion. Take after arnica and *Ruta graveolens*, if necessary, for injury to sinews, tendons, and the bone covering.

Physiotherapy

First, apply ice as quickly as possible to reduce the swelling, minimize the pain, and speed healing. Keep ice applied for thirty minutes. Use ice throughout the time of recovery to reduce swelling. Keep extremities, such as toes and fingers, exposed and free to maximize circulation. If fingers or toes turn blue, unwrap and rewrap less tightly. Elevate the injured joint to prevent blood from accumulating at injured site. Allow greater mobility as healing occurs, usually within forty-eight hours.

Once pain is reduced, place the joint in hot water or apply moist, hot compresses to promote circulation and the removal of immune-related by-products. Slowly move the joint to promote circulation, but do not stretch or stress the joint beyond its comfortable limits of movement. Passive movement, in which the joint is moved without the use of the injured person's muscle activity, may be needed for some joints.

Reapply ice periodically throughout the day to prevent swelling and to speed healing.

After the joint has begun to heal and allows normal movement without pain, use muscle-assisted exercises. At first, use no weights; simply use the weight of the limb. Then, increase weight to one to two pounds, depending on the strength of the joint involved. Do not stress the joint. Be patient and allow the joint to heal over time.

All severe sprains should be checked for fracture.

Chinese Medicine

Tienchi ginseng is a very effective Chinese herb for injuries. The herb moves qi and is highly effective in the treatment of sports injuries. Dose is ½ to 3 g.

STAPHYLOCOCCAL INFECTION

SYMPTOMS

Staphylococcal infection is associated with symptoms that range from minor to severe to life-threatening. They can include pimples, boils, abscesses, furuncles, carbuncles, osteomyelitis, enterocolitic pneumonia, and bacteremia.

WHAT IS STAPHYLOCOCCAL INFECTION?

From Modern Western Medicine

These are infections brought about by the family of staphylococcus bacteria, perhaps the most common bacteria in existence. The bacteria appear under a microscope as grapelike clusters. They can cause a wide range of problems, from skin infections to serious internal disorders.

Present on the skin of most people, staphylococcal bacteria are generally harmless, but they can become trapped in sweat or sebaceous glands, causing skin infections such as pustules, boils, abscesses, sties, or carbuncles. The bacteria can invade the deeper tissues if the surface skin is broken. They often affect the mucous membranes of the nose, throat, and lungs, causing viral infections, including pneumonia.

Staphylococcal bacteria can also invade the mucous membranes of the vaginas of menstruating women, especially those who use highly absorbent tampons, where they can produce highly toxic by-products, which results in toxic shock syndrome. A different type of staphylococcus can cause urinary tract infections.

Other ways staphylococci can cause infection is through the use of an infected needle, which can result in septic shock, infectious arthritis, osteomyelitis, or bacterial endocarditis. Contaminated food may also transmit the bacteria.

From Traditional Medicine

Hygiene can play a role in the onset of staphylococcus infection, but a more important reason is a weakened immune system. Many clean and hygienic people contract the disease, while those with open cuts or sores can avoid infection. The underlying difference is often the relative strengths of the immune systems in question.

Staph infections are serious and often require medical care or supervision. In addition, immune-boosting activities help rid the body of the bacteria. The remedies provided below can assist in boosting the immune response and helping the body fight the disease.

REMEDIES

General Recommendations

- See the section on boosting the immune system in Part IV.
- See Part IV for a section on strengthening the lungs.

Foods to Eat

- Whole grains
- Green vegetables
- Miso soup
- Beans

Foods to Avoid

- Sugar in all forms, including fruit, honey, refined carbohydrates, and alcohol
- Meat
- Eggs
- Dairy products
- Oils

Herbs to Treat Staphylococcal Infections

- Honeysuckle: Used for infections and inflammations; broad-spectrum antimicrobial activity; dose is 9–15 g.
- Bear lichen is effective against most staphylococcus infections. Use 10–30 drops of tincture.
- Garlic: either in capsule form or chop up and swallow it raw with water

Hydrotherapy

- Remove dirt and foreign matter from all cuts and wounds and wash with soap and water and flush with hydrogen peroxide.
- Apply warm goldenseal tea compresses to firmly adherent crust.
- Flush with hydrogen peroxide and apply tea tree oil full strength.
- Repeat every two waking hours.
- Apply tea tree ointment at night. This is an antifungal agent. (Iodine and alcohol may kill bacteria, but they also destroy healthy cells and should not be used.) When the skin is very raw, as in the case of impetigo, do not use a tea tree oil application. Use 3 parts of castor oil to ½ part of eucalyptol. This is because the tea tree oil may cause burning or irritation.
- Expose to fresh air and sunlight.
- Change pillow covers, sheets, towels, and clothing daily to prevent reinfection and spreading infection to other family members.

Supplements

- Beta-carotene: 15–30 mg/day
- Vitamin C: 100 mg/day
- Vitamin E: 100–400 IU/day
- Zinc: 15 mg/day

STRESS

Stress is characterized by feelings of fear, dread, and anxiety, accompanied by a variety of physical side effects, including muscle tension; changes in heart rate, blood pressure, respiration, hormonal balance, metabolism, and immune function; and in elevations of adrenaline and norepinephrine. Chronic stress can cause numerous mental and physical disorders, including anxiety, depression, dyspepsia, palpitations, muscular aches and pains, depressed immune response, hormonal imbalance, and kidney disease.

WHAT IS STRESS?

Stress is another word for fear, often a low-level fear maintained chronically over time. Stress causes the instinctual flight-or-fight response, but in modern society neither of these options is always possible in the face of a stressful event. Very often, people feel they must endure situations without being able to fight or flee.

Many life-altering events, such as violence, internal conflicts, divorce, the loss of a job, the birth of a baby, or a change in residence can be stressful and sometimes lead to chronic stress. Post-traumatic stress disorder is a physiological response to an especially stressful event.

REMEDIES

Foods to Eat

- Whole grains promote the production of the brain neurotransmitter serotonin, which increases your sense of well-being.
- Green, yellow, and orange vegetables are all rich in minerals, vitamins, and phytochemicals, which boost immune response and protect against disease.

Foods to Avoid

- Coffee and other caffeinated beverages: If you are currently addicted to coffee, drink black tea; it has less than a third of the caffeine of coffee, and none of the harmful oils.
- Fried foods and foods rich in fat are very immune-depressing, especially when stress is doing that, as well.
- Reduce animal foods. High-protein foods elevate brain levels of dopamine and norepinephrine, both of which are associated with higher levels of anxiety and stress.

Exercise

- Aerobic exercise daily
- Walking in the woods, at the beach, or in a park
- Participate in a sporting event, such as tennis, basketball, volleyball, racquetball, softball, and many others.
- Ride a bicycle
- Yoga
- Tai chi chuan or some other form of martial arts

Hydrotherapy

Warm baths relax the muscles and slightly heat the brain. Soak for no more than fifteen minutes in water that is between 100° and 102° F.

Massage

Therapeutic massage, acupressure, shiatsu, or some other form of healing touch all reduce stress.

Supplements

The following list of supplements will help deal with the results of stress, and if taken in conjunction with efforts to deal with the cause, will be instrumental in the overall therapy.

- Beta-carotene: 15–30 mg per day
- Thiamine (vitamin B_1): 1.5 mg per day
- Riboflavin (vitamin B_2): 1.8 mg per day
- Niacin: 20 mg per day
- Vitamin B_6: 2–10 mg per day
- Vitamin B_{12}: 2–10 mcg per day
- Vitamin C: 100–500 mg per day
- Calcium: 1200 mg per day
- Magnesium: 400 mg per day
- Zinc: 15 mg per day

Herbs to Treat Stress

Drink chamomile tea often.

Mind/Body

- Exhale and breathe deeply.
- Drop your shoulders, relax, and rotate shoulders in small circles. Breathe deeply and exhale.
- Pray, meditate, and surrender.
- See a comedy and laugh.
- Adopt a pet.

- Listen to calm, peaceful music.
- Take a walk.
- Do progressive relaxation routines and meditations described in Part III.
- Talk to a friend or counselor.
- Do yoga.
- Tai chi chuan
- Biofeedback
- Psychotherapy
- Go fishing: guaranteed peace of mind.

Aromatherapy

Smell all the following aromatherapies and choose the one or combination of aromas that appeals to you the most.

- Lavender relaxes and relieves stress.
- Rosemary stimulates and sharpens the mind.
- Geranium reduces stress.
- Chamomile reduces stress.
- Sandalwood
- Juniper berry
- Sweet marjoram

STROKE

SYMPTOMS

Any of the following symptoms may occur: headache, dizziness, confusion, visual disturbance, slurred speech or loss of speech, difficulty swallowing, paralysis in one or more locations of the body, unconsciousness, coma, and death. Symptoms may take minutes, hours, or days to develop. Depending on where in the brain the stroke has occurred, those parts of the brain are damaged permanently, resulting in partial or total loss of function.

WHAT IS STROKE?

From Modern Western Medicine

Most strokes are caused either by atherosclerosis or high blood pressure. Atherosclerosis can cause a cerebral thrombosis, or the creation of a blood clot that blocks part or all of the blood supply from an artery to the brain. Without oxygen, a part of the brain suffocates and dies. Atherosclerosis can also cause a cerebral embolism, which is a piece of a blood clot that breaks free, floats downstream, eventually gets lodged in a vessel, and blocks blood flow to the brain, causing the death of tissue and a stroke. Hemorrhage occurs when a blood vessel ruptures, thus causing bleeding on the surface of the brain or within the brain tissues. The ruptured vessel no longer brings blood to the brain, causing the loss of oxygen to tissues, which results in a stroke.

Forty to 50 percent of strokes are caused by a thrombus; 30 to 35 percent are caused by an embolus; 20 to 25 percent are caused by a rupture of a blood vessel.

Small or tiny strokes are called transient ischemic attacks and usually result in a full recovery within twenty-four hours. These represent about a third of all strokes. Another third cause weakness and paralysis, known as hemiplegia. The final third are fatal.

From Traditional Medicine

The best approach to stroke from a traditional standpoint is to lower the fat in the diet and prevent the disorder. Strokes are the result of atherosclerosis, or cholesterol plaques clogging the arteries of the neck and brain; or from high blood pressure, which causes blood vessels in the brain to burst, causing a stroke.

WHO GETS STROKE?

In the United States, the overall incidence of stroke is about two people per thousand annually. The incidence rises steeply with age and is higher in men than in women.

REMEDIES

Foods to Eat

- Whole grains
- Omega-3 oils: Found in fish, these oils prevent the blood from forming clots.
- Rye: Have this in the form of good-quality rye bread. When all the bran and germ are kept intact, it has the capability of reducing and totally eliminating vessel and plaque calcification.
- Potatoes and sweet potatoes
- Squash
- Beans, peas, and soybean products such as tofu
- Green and yellow vegetables
- Round vegetables
- Root vegetables
- Mild spices and cooking herbs

Foods to Avoid

- Foods high in fat, especially red meat, dairy products, and eggs
- Sugar
- Nuts, nut butters, and seeds are all higher in fat.
- Salt: Allow about ½ teaspoon per day. Salt creates high blood pressure, a major cause of stroke.
- Alcohol
- Oil, which is liquid fat
- Tobacco
- Sulfur dioxide, often found in dried fruits: Sometimes restaurants use it to keep salad, uncooked vegetables, avocado dips, and shrimp from turning brown.
- MSG: Ask in Chinese restaurants if they use this. It's very high in salt.

Herbs to Treat Stroke

- Calamus helps restore brain tissue damaged by stroke. Dose: standard infusion or 3–9 g; tincture, 10–30 drops.
- Earthworm: 3.9 g or standard decoction
- Scorpion: powder, ½–1 g; decoction, 2–5 g
- Jack-in-the-pulpit: infusion, 1 tsp. in 1 cup of boiling water; formula, 1–6 g; tincture, 10–20 drops

Homeopathy for Stroke

First aid for stroke, if the person loses consciousness:

- Aconite 30c: if the person is very fearful
- Opium 6c: if the person has collapsed; face is dark and flushed; loud, "snoring" breathing; cheeks puff out as person exhales
- Arnica 6c: Once the person's condition is stable, give every 4 hours for up to 3 days.

Specific remedies to be given every fifteen minutes for up to ten doses during a stroke while medical help is being sought:

- Belladonna 30c: if the person's face is hot and flushed, if there is headache, if the eyes are wide and staring
- Nux vomica 6c: at first signs of attack, especially if brought on by a heavy meal or alcohol
- Aconite 30c: for a person who is panicky and afraid of dying once he or she realizes what is happening
- Opium 6c: In later stages, if the person is lapsing into consciousness, face is bluish and congested, and breathing is heavy and labored, take four times daily for up to two weeks immediately after a stroke.
- Arnica 6c to be taken four times daily for up to three weeks during recovery
- Baryta 6c: if the person is elderly and physically and mentally weak
- Gelsemium 6c: where main aftereffects are numbness and trembling, inability to speak, pain at back of head
- Lachesis 6c: if speech is very slow
- Hyoscyamus 6c: if speech is unintelligible, and person has a tendency to clutch private parts
- Aurum 6c: if the person is clearly depressed

Swollen Glands

SYMPTOMS

Swelling or discomfort in the neck (near the ears), throat, groin, or armpits, sometimes accompanied by sore throat or fever, are symptoms of swollen glands.

WHAT ARE SWOLLEN GLANDS?

From Modern Western Medicine

Swollen glands are actually enlargement of the lymph nodes, which is caused by the proliferation of white blood cells within the glands. The rapid multiplication of these cells occurs in the face of an antigen, or disease-causing agent, that is present systemically within the body. The activity of the white cells causes inflammation within the lymph nodes. Swollen glands are known medically as lymphadenopathy.

Swollen glands are a very common symptom and usually occur as a result of infection or allergic reaction. Swollen glands occur frequently in childhood.

In rare cases, swollen glands can be a symptom of lymphoma, Hodgkin's disease, leukemia, or a metastasis.

Treatments for swollen glands caused by infection usually include antibiotics or antihistamines for an allergy. In the case of cancer, radiation or chemotherapy is used.

From Traditional Medicine

The glands are a good early warning system that the body is being overloaded with toxins. Pollutants from the air, water, soil, and food all migrate into the body's tissue fluid, which exists like a giant lake that surrounds cells, or tiny islands. In addition to pollutants are bacteria and viruses that also occupy the tissue fluid. In its effort to cleanse the system of all of these toxins, the body circulates the tissue fluid into the lymph system. When these toxins become excessive, the immune system responds by creating more scavenger cells, such as macrophages and lymphocytes, specifically CD4 cells, which infiltrate the lymph nodes and attack the viruses, bacteria, and pollutants. Eventually, these antigens are neutralized and eliminated from the body, but before that happens, lymph glands swell. The body is sending a signal to you that it's time to clean up your act by eating a healing diet, getting gentle exercise and therapeutic massage, and taking appropriate herbal remedies to support the lymph system. These and other recommendations are made below.

REMEDIES

Foods to Eat

- Whole grains: Boil brown rice, ginger, carrots, and onion together in lots of water. Eat soupy.
- Leafy, green vegetables, such as collard, kale, and mustard greens
- Root vegetables
- Miso soup
- Sea vegetables, especially nori and arame
- Fish, preferably white fish, such as haddock, cod, flounder, and scrod
- Spirulina
- Chlorella

Herbs

- Goldenseal (blood cleanser): 30 drops, 2 times per day
- Echinacea (antibiotic): 30 drops, 2 times per day
- Milk thistle (liver cleanser): 15 drops, once a day

Supplements

- Magnesium: 400 mg per day
- Zinc: 15 mg per day
- Selenium: 70 mcg per day
- Beta-carotene: 15 mg per day
- Vitamin C: 100 mg per day
- Vitamin E: 100 IU per day

Exercise

- Gentle walking, daily
- Stretching exercise to release lymph from blocked areas
- Yoga

Physiotherapy

Take warm baths to relax the body, especially muscle tissues that are contracted and preventing lymph from moving freely.

TEETH AND GUM DISEASE

SYMPTOMS

Dental caries, also known as cavities, is the decay of teeth. Caries are caused by the acid created by bacteria that collect on the teeth. The acid gradually dissolves the enamel and dentin that coat the teeth, exposing the tissue below.

Periodontal disease manifests as *gingivitis,* or the inflammation of the gums that surround the teeth, and *pyorrhea,* which is the degeneration of the tissue—it becomes inflamed and swollen—and the bone that surrounds the teeth. Gradually, the gums recede from the teeth and the teeth themselves loosen. The disease can become chronic, making gums and teeth sensitive to various types of foods (sweets) and liquids (especially hot or cold liquids). Pus can also be discharged from the gums.

WHAT IS TEETH AND GUM DISEASE?

From Modern Western Medicine

In addition to dental caries, the most common condition affecting the teeth and gums is gingivitis (or inflammation of the gums). Gingivitis can lead to periodontitis (inflammation of the tissues that surround the teeth at their base), which is characterized by the gradual loss of the gums that surround the teeth. Dental caries and gingivitis can lead to more serious disorders, including dental abscess, granuloma, dental cyst, and periapical periodontitis.

Gingivitis is most often caused by poor oral hygiene. Plaque collects between the teeth and gums, fostering the growth of bacteria that lead to periodontal disease.

Periapical periodontitis is often caused when a cavity occurs below a filling; the tissues surrounding the cavity become infected and pus-filled. The area must be drained and cleaned; sometimes the tooth needs to be extracted, as well.

From Traditional Medicine

As virtually any dentist will attest, both tooth and gum disorders are caused by the typical American diet. Foods that are especially deleterious are those high in protein and refined foods, such as those devoid of fiber and rich in sugar. Traditional people around the world who eat diets rich in vegetables and grains do not suffer from tooth and gum diseases. Archaeological discoveries have demonstrated that even early humans had little sign of such disorders, in large measure because their diets had such a high quantity of vegetable foods.

Chinese medicine maintains that the gums are nourished by the liver. The more the liver is stressed by toxins, the greater the degeneration of the gums.

Recent studies suggest a link between osteoporosis and tooth and gum disease.

REMEDIES

Foods to Eat

- Raw fruits
- Raw and lightly cooked vegetables
- Nuts
- Whole, unrefined grains: Dried corn especially helps promote healthy teeth and gums.
- Green vegetables
- Sea vegetables
- Spirulina

Foods to Avoid

- Meat
- Sugar
- Soda
- Candy
- Refined grains
- Overcooked foods

Hydrotherapy

Massage gums with the following herbs:

- Eucalyptus oil: Massage once a day.
- Witch hazel: Massage once a day.
- Vitamin E: Massage once a day.

Gum rinse:

1 oz. hydrastis
1 oz. myrrh
1 pint water

Rinse three times a day.

Brush with baking soda to help stop gingivitis and pyorrhea.

Supplements

- Beta-carotene: 15–30 mg/day

- Vitamin B complex
    Thiamine: 1.5 mg per day
    Riboflavin: 1.8 mg per day
    Vitamin B_6: 2–10 mg per day
    Vitamin B_{12}: 2–10 mg per day
    Niacin: 20 mg per day
- Folic acid: 400 mcg per day
- Vitamin C: 100–500 mg per day
- Vitamin E: 100 IU per day; also apply topically to the gums.
- Zinc: 15 mg per day
- Calcium and magnesium in ratio of 2 to 1: calcium, 800 mg, and magnesium 400 mg per day

TEMPOROMANDIBULAR JOINT SYNDROME

SYMPTOMS

Symptoms of temporomandibular joint syndrome are headaches, pain and tenderness of the jaw muscles, and dull facial pain, especially around the area of the ear. Other symptoms include clicking or popping noises when the mouth is opened or closed, difficulty opening the mouth, jaws that "lock" or get stuck, or pain when yawning, chewing, or opening the mouth wide.

WHAT IS TEMPOROMANDIBULAR JOINT SYNDROME?

From Modern Western Medicine

Pain and other symptoms affecting the head, jaw, and face are brought about when the temporomandibular joints (jaw joints) and the muscles and ligaments that control and support them do not work together in a coordinated fashion.

Spasm of the jaw muscles, used to control chewing, is the most common cause. Most often, such spasms are brought on by habitual clenching and grinding of teeth, usually the result of emotional tension. Other factors can include an incorrect bite, which can place additional stress on the jaw muscles.

Temporomandibular joint problems (commonly referred to as TMJ) may also be caused by displacement of the joint as a result of jaw, head, or neck injuries. In rare cases, osteoarthritis is a cause.

Treatment is designed to reduce or eliminate the pain by taking the muscles out of spasm, and can include applying heat to the areas of the pain, taking muscle-relaxant drugs, massaging the muscles, eating soft, non-chewy foods, or using a bite splint (a device that fits over the teeth at night to prevent clenching or grinding). Counseling, biofeedback training, and relaxation exercises may also help.

The bite may also need to be corrected by selective grinding of teeth or by the use of braces or other orthodontic appliances. In severe cases, surgery on the jaw joint is required.

From Traditional Medicine

Problems related to the jaw and jaw muscles are seen in Oriental medicine as imbalances within the kidney, bladder, sex organs, and stomach meridian. The kidneys are seen as providing qi to the sex organs and, in general, as providing sexual energy and vitality. When sexual frustration builds, the qi can back up along the bladder meridian and manifest within the jaw muscles. (The bladder meridian, from the point where the inner eye joins the bridge of the nose, runs up over the top of the head, down the back, over the buttocks, along the backs

Temporomandibular Joint Disorder

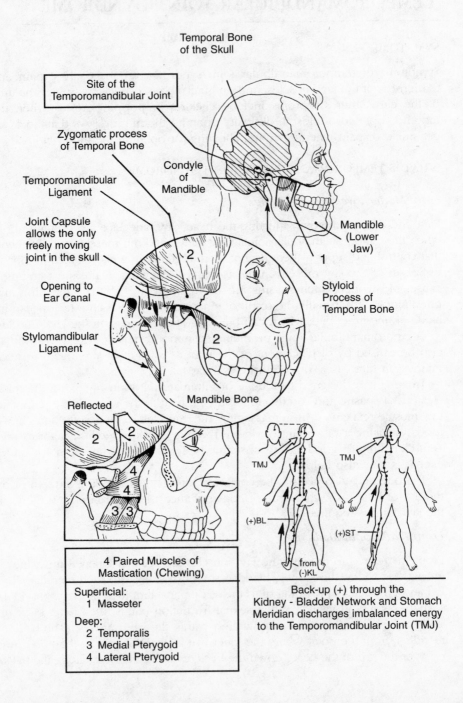

Temporal Bone
of the Skull

Site of the
Temporomandibular Joint

Zygomatic process
of Temporal Bone

Condyle
of
Mandible

Temporomandibular
Ligament

Joint Capsule
allows the only
freely moving
joint in the skull

Mandible
(Lower
Jaw)

Opening to
Ear Canal

Stylomandibular
Ligament

1

Styloid
Process of
Temporal Bone

Mandible Bone

Reflected

4 Paired Muscles of
Mastication (Chewing)

Superficial:
  1 Masseter

Deep:
  2 Temporalis
  3 Medial Pterygoid
  4 Lateral Pterygoid

TMJ

TMJ

(+)BL

(+)ST

from
(-)KL

Back-up (+) through the
Kidney - Bladder Network and Stomach
Meridian discharges imbalanced energy
to the Temporomandibular Joint (TMJ)

of the legs, and to the small toe on each foot.) The body, in its wisdom, sees the jaw as a place from which it can discharge excessive energy because the jaw is so active, either during eating, talking, or breathing. Grinding the teeth and over-working the jaw muscles at night is sometimes seen in children, especially when they are feeling frustrated with the parent of the opposite sex. In general, Oriental medicine—including both the Chinese and Japanese systems—views grinding the teeth and jaw-related problems as an expression of frustration, and oftentimes particularly sexual frustration.

The stomach meridian also runs along the jaw and provides qi to the jaw muscles. Excessive stomach energy, either from some type of stomach disorder or from anxiety or frustration, can also cause unconscious working of the jaw muscles, TMJ, and related symptoms.

Finally, grinding of teeth can be brought on by an infestation of parasitic worms in the digestive tract (see the chapter on Worms).

The remedies provided below can release the excessive energy that can be the cause of jaw-related problems.

REMEDIES

Foods to Eat

- Foods that are very soft and easy to chew
- Whole grains, especially barley, which strengthens kidneys, according to Chinese medicine; millet and sweet rice, to strengthen the stomach and stomach meridian
- Beans and bean products, such as tofu and tempeh, to strengthen kidneys, bladder, and sex organs
- Sea vegetables, such as arame, nori, kombu, and wakame to strengthen kidneys

Foods to Avoid

- Excessive amounts of salt. Never use salt at the table as a condiment; use salt only sparingly (a pinch) in cooking; and limit sodium-containing condiments, such as tamari, shoyu, and miso.
- Caffeine-containing beverages, such as coffee, tea, and cola drinks
- Spices or any food that upsets the stomach
- Pickled foods, which contain salt and upset the stomach
- Smoked foods, which contain salt and upset the stomach
- Sugar and foods containing sugar

Hydrotherapy

- Increase blood circulation to the area. Apply either moist heat or ice to the jaw, but don't interchange them (whichever one seems to relieve your symptoms the most is the one you should stick with).
- Massage the jaw briskly with a hot washcloth.

Miscellaneous

- Support your jaw with a mouth guard. This will keep your jaw steady and temporarily deal with your symptoms.
- Check your posture—when sitting or standing, your cheekbone should be over your clavicle and your ears should not be too far in front of your shoulders.
- When you feel a yawn coming, restrict it by holding a fist under your chin.
- When sleeping, put a towel under your back, a pillow under your knees, and a thin towel rolled up (to about the thickness of your wrist) under your neck.

Sleeping on your back is critical to overcoming TMJ. Place a beanbag on each side of your head to keep you from changing positions.

Physiotherapy and Massage

- Therapeutic massage
- Acupressure, especially along the spine, lower back, neck, and head area
- Acupuncture
- Yoga
- Meditation

THYROID DISORDERS (HYPOTHYROIDISM AND HYPERTHYROIDISM)

SYMPTOMS

Hypothyroidism can cause fatigue, weight gain, headaches, anemia, acne, eczema, chronic infection, psoriasis, menstrual disorders (including pain during menstruation), depression, poor circulation, and sensitivity to cold.

Hyperthyroidism (also known as Graves' disease) causes insomnia, weakness, sweating, hyperactivity, weight loss, sensitivity to heat, tremor, bulging of eyes, and frozen facial expression. The thyroid gland, found at the base of the neck, in front, often becomes enlarged and nodular. The heart may become overactive and enlarged, as well. High blood pressure (especially systolic pressure) and heart failure can occur.

In extreme cases, mental disorders can suddenly flare (such reactions are referred to as thyroid storms). These flare-ups can be brought on by stress, extreme emotions, infection, or surgery.

WHAT IS HYPOTHYROIDISM AND HYPERTHYROIDISM?

From Modern Western Medicine

Hypothyroidism occurs when the thyroid fails to produce adequate thyroid hormones. The underproduction of hormones is sometimes due to inadequate dietary iodine or when the thyroid is deformed or missing at birth.

Hashimoto's disease, an autoimmune disorder that destroys the thyroid gland, can also give rise to hypothyroidism. The thyroid may also not produce adequate thyroid hormone if the pituitary fails to produce sufficient thyroid-stimulating hormone.

The overproduction of thyroid hormones causes the gland to become overactive. The increase in thyroid is often caused when the pituitary gland produces excess thyroid-stimulating hormone, or when a cyst or nodule exists within the thyroid gland.

Common drugs for hypothyroidism are the synthetic thyroid hormones, levothyroxine and liothyronine, which can also reduce the size of the thyroid. Blood tests can help physicians determine how much thyroid hormone is needed.

As for hyperthyroidism, physicians may recommend the removal of the thyroid gland or the use of radioactive iodine therapy, which can stop the gland from functioning. In such cases, doctors then prescribe thyroid hormone.

From Traditional Medicine

For many with thyroid disorders, there are no adequate substitutes for taking synthetic thyroid hormones, which are generally safe and very effective. However, the person should take extremely good care of his or her health in addition by following a healthy diet and getting adequate exercise. The foods, herbs, and homeopathic remedies listed below can assist thyroid function.

REMEDIES

Foods to Eat

- Raw foods
- Unrefined, whole foods
- Whole grains
- Vegetables
- Sprouted seeds and beans
- Seaweed
- Garlic
- Radishes
- Watercress
- Seafood
- Egg yolks
- Wheat germ
- Mushrooms

Foods to Avoid

- Sugar
- Refined grains
- Caffeine
- Processed foods

The following foods contain goitrogens, which may inhibit iodine utilization, a common cause of hypothyroidism. Since these are very nutritious, be cautious in experimenting with their elimination.

- Kale
- Cabbage
- Broccoli
- Brussels sprouts
- Cauliflower
- Peanuts
- Kohlrabi
- Turnips

Herbs to Treat Thyroid

- Irish Moss: infusion, steep 5–15 minutes, take 2 oz., 2 or 3 times daily, up to 2 cups a day.
- Kelp (rich in iodine): fluid extract, 10 drops, 1 or 2 times daily; powder, 3–5 #0 capsules (10–30 grains), 1 or 2 times daily.

Homeopathy

For hyperthyroidism, take every hour for up to ten doses:

- Iodum 30c: for someone who is obsessive, feels very hot, can't stop hurrying, especially if he or she is dark-haired and dark-eyed
- Natrum mur 30c: for those with constipation, palpitations, and an earthy complexion
- Belladonna 30c: for flushed face and staring eyes
- Lycopus 30c: for pounding and racing heart and exothalmos (bulging eyes)

For hypothyroidism, take arsenicum (30c) every twelve hours for up to five days while seeking out a constitutional treatment with a licensed homeopathist.

Physiotherapy

These yoga exercises are specific to thyroid disorders: shoulder stand and plough.

Supplements

- Beta-carotene: 15 mg per day
- Vitamin B_1 (thiamine): 1.5 mg per day
- Vitamin B_2 (riboflavin): 1.8 mg per day
- Niacin: 10 mg per day
- Vitamin B_6: 2–10 mg per day
- Vitamin C: 100–500 mg per day
- Vitamin E: 100–400 IU per day
- Zinc: 15 mg per day

Tonsillitis and Adenitis

SYMPTOMS

Symptoms include fever, chills, sore throat, difficulty swallowing, and tender, swollen lymph nodes.

WHAT ARE TONSILLITIS AND ADENITIS?

From Modern Western Medicine

The infection and subsequent inflammation of the tonsils and adenoids. The condition occurs mainly in children. The tonsils are lymph glands, and part of the lymph system. Inside these glands are immune cells that help to protect the upper respiratory tract against infection. When the lymph system becomes overburdened, the tonsils become infected by the microorganisms they fight. Tonsillitis, or the swelling of the tonsils, is most common in children under nine.

Consult a physician if the above symptoms continue for more than twenty-four hours. Among the most common treatments are bed rest, plenty of fluids, pain-killing drugs, antibiotics, and the surgical removal of the tonsils.

From Traditional Medicine

The tonsils and adenoids become inflamed when the blood or lymph vessels become overburdened with toxic waste or bacteria, caused by an imbalanced diet that includes excesses of artificial ingredients, refined foods, sugar, and dairy products. The lymph system tries to eliminate these waste products, but when they are in excess—and temporarily overwhelm the lymph and immune systems—they cause the swelling of lymph glands. Especially important in the treatment of swollen tonsils and adenoids is to encourage bowel elimination (see Constipation in Part II and The Lymph System in Part IV). Other causes include the overuse of drugs to suppress the common cold, and antibiotics, which eliminate friendly flora and weaken large intestine and immune functions.

REMEDIES

Foods to Eat

- Whole grains
- Vegetables, especially the green leafy variety
- Carrots and carrot juice, which clear acidic blood conditions such as tonsillitis

- Miso soup
- Seaweed
- Vegetable protein, such as beans and tofu
- Hot water, lemon, and honey tea
- Citrus fruit
- Boiled or steamed onions with natural soy sauce (a few drops) for flavor

Foods to Avoid

- Sweets
- Highly processed foods
- Dairy products
- Flour products
- Oily foods, such as fried foods and nut butters
- Refined foods
- Wheat (in the case of food allergy)

Herbs to Treat Tonsillitis

- Baptisia: half an ounce of the root boiled for 10 minutes in a pint of water. Take one tablespoon every three or four hours. If nausea or sick feelings result, lower the dose. For children, give half or less according to size and age. Standard infusion 3–9 g.
- Gotu Kola: 6–15 g per day
- Garlic: 2 capsules three times a day

Homeopathy

Try the following remedies. If there is no improvement within twenty-four hours, consult a physician or homeopath. Give every two hours for up to ten doses during acute attack.

- Belladonna 30c for raw throat, high fever with delirium, staring eyes, and bright-red tonsils
- Apis 30c for sore throat without thirst, tender neck region and sensitivity to pressure, and swollen and shiny uvula
- Hepar sulph 6c for chilliness, irritability, and unreasonableness, for someone who hates undressing or leaving warmth of bed, says pains in throat feel like splinters or fish hooks, or pus from tonsils tastes unpleasant.
- Mercurius 6c if tonsils are dark red, swollen and sore, if tongue is swollen, if glands in neck are swollen and tender, if breath smells foul, or if there's copious saliva.
- Phytolacca 6c if throat pain extends up to ears, neck glands are swollen, tonsils are dark red, hot, and swollen, or if throat feels rough and constricted.

- Lycopodium 6c if infection starts in right tonsil and moves to left, or if child has high fever and feels most ill between 4 and 8 A.M.

Physiotherapy

- Gargle with:
  Hydrastis (goldenseal), myrrh, and glycothymoline. (Mix 1 oz. of the two herbs (as alcohol tincture) with 16 oz. of glycothymoline.) Gargle daily four to six times.
  Hot water, lemon and salt: Gargle three times a day
  Lemon juice
  Chlorophyll
- Throat sprays or swabs:
  Hydrastis
  Myrrh
- Throat pack: Soak a small towel in ice-cold water. Wrap around throat and pin. Leave on 1–3 hours. Repeat two times per day and at night.

Supplements

- Beta-carotene: 15–30 mg per day
- Vitamin B complex: 25–50 mg per day
- Vitamin C: 100–500 mg per day
- Zinc: 15–30 mg three times per day.

TOOTHACHE

SYMPTOMS

Pain, oftentimes acute and severe, is caused by a single tooth or teeth or gums.

WHAT IS TOOTHACHE?

From Modern Western Medicine

Most toothaches are caused by dental caries (or decay), but a fractured tooth or a deep, unlined filling may also cause inflammation and pain of the gums and teeth (see Periodontitis). Sometimes toothache can be caused by sinusitis pain, which is being transferred to a molar and premolar.

Analgesic drugs are used to provide temporary relief until one sees his or her dentist.

From Traditional Medicine

Dental caries are yet another diminution of health caused by the modern diet, rich in refined sugars, grain products, artificial ingredients, and protein, all of which can increase the acid content of the mouth, rob the body of minerals, and bring on tooth decay.

The natural remedies below can be used to diminish pain and strengthen gums and nerves until a dentist can be seen.

REMEDIES

Foods to Eat (high in calcium)

- Seaweeds
- Raw carrots (for teething children)
- Leafy green vegetables
- Sardines
- Amaranth grain (a soft grain)
- Parsley
- Watercress and turnip greens
- Garbanzo beans

While in pain, eat grains and vegetables prepared in tamari or miso broth, which is soothing and relaxing to the entire body.

Foods to Avoid (these inhibit calcium absorption)

- Sugar
- The nightshades: spinach, chard, beet greens, tomatoes, potatoes, eggplant, and bell peppers
- Coffee
- Soft drinks
- Protein excesses, especially meat
- Alcohol
- Cigarettes
- Excess salt

Hydrotherapy

- Oil of cloves: Drop a little directly on the tooth and gum, or put it on a piece of cotton and pack it next to the ache. (Do not use with homeopathy, as this could have a counteracting effect on remedies.) Very effective.
- Rub an ice cube into the V-shaped area where the bones of the thumb and forefinger meet for about five to seven minutes, on the same side of the body that the toothache is on. This works by sending rubbing impulses along the same nerve pathways that the toothache pain would normally travel on. Since the pathways can only carry one signal at a time, rubbing outweighs the pain. Usually highly effective.
- Rinse the mouth vigorously with body-temperature water; this will dislodge any trapped food that might cause toothache.
- Floss gently to get little bits of food out from between your teeth.
- Pour some whiskey over the sore tooth. Your gums will absorb the alcohol and numb the pain.
- Rinse with salty water after each meal and at bedtime.

Herbs

- The following formula will improve the condition of teeth:

  1 part Horsetail
  1 part Oat straw
  1 part Kombu seaweed or Kelp powder
  ⅓ part Lobelia

Simmer each one ounce of formula in one pint water for twenty-five minutes and drink ½ cup two to three times a day. At the end of every three weeks, stop for one week. If this is taken every winter, there will be noticeable improvement.

Homeopathy

These remedies are to relieve discomfort while waiting to get to a dentist. They can be given every five minutes for up to ten doses.

- Plantaga 6c: if tooth is very nervy, is aggravated by cold air and the slightest pressure but feels better when eating; if teeth generally feel sensitive, as though they are exposed, or mouth is full of saliva
- Coffea 6c: if toothache is made worse by heat and hot food and relieved by applying ice
- Chamomilla 6c: if pain is unbearable, and is made worse by cold air, warm food and drink, and by coffee at night
- Staphisagria 6c: if severe toothache is aggravated by cold air, food, and slightest pressure; if there is a drawing or tearing pain; if the cheek is red and swollen; if a bad tooth is black and disintegrating
- Pulsatilla 6c: if pain is unbearable, especially with hot food or drink, and is relieved by cold water; if the person is not thirsty at all; if it feels better in open air
- Arnica 30c: for pain after a filling or extraction
- Apis 30c: if gums feel tight and swollen, or toothache burns and stings

ULCER (STOMACH, OR PEPTIC)

SYMPTOMS

The primary symptom of an ulcer is usually a gnawing pain or burning sensation in the stomach. Other symptoms can include nausea, vomiting, loss of appetite, belching, or a noticeable increase in appetite (a sign of a duodenal ulcer, one that occurs in the first stage of the small intestine). With duodenal ulcers, eating causes a temporary relief of the pain, but it recurs a few hours after a meal.

WHAT IS A PEPTIC ULCER?

From Modern Western Medicine

A peptic ulcer is a wound in the stomach, esophagus, duodenum, or some other area of the small intestine, brought about when the mucus lining of the stomach is eroded and the stomach's digestive juices, including hydrochloric acid and pepsin, eat away at the tender tissue beneath the protective mucus layer. Other highly irritating substances may also wear away this mucus lining and expose the tissues below to hydrochloric acid and other digestive secretions. These include alcohol, cigarette smoke, coffee, tea, bacteria, and nonsteroidal anti-inflammatory drugs (including aspirin and ibuprofen).

Physicians use a variety of treatments for ulcers, including antacids (which reduce the amount of acid in the stomach), drugs such as sucralfate, which help to form a protective coat over the ulcer, and antibiotics to kill bacteria that eat away at the stomach's protective mucus lining.

Stress, which increases production of stomach acid, may also play a role in the onset of ulcers. Therefore, controlling stress is essential.

From Traditional Medicine

Diet and lifestyle play central roles in the onset of ulcers. The modern diet, rich in fat, refined carbohydrates, coffee, tea, tobacco, sugar, alcohol, spices, and fried foods, all increase production of stomach acids. Many common drugs, such as aspirin, also promote stomach acids, as do many salted, pickled, and smoked foods. Since these foods make up the bulk of the Western diet, there is little wonder that so many millions of people suffer from stomach disorders and particularly ulcers.

In addition, milk products can increase stomach discomfort and exacerbate ulcers and pain for people who are lactose intolerant. Lactose, the sugar found in milk, requires the enzyme *lactase*, which is produced by the body to digest milk products. Approximately forty percent of Eastern Europeans, seventy percent of African Americans, and most Asians are lactose intolerant.

REMEDIES

The following foods to eat and avoid, as well as the lifestyle recommendations listed below, are designed to help strengthen the stomach and prevent stomach disorders.

Patterns of Eating

- Eat four to six small meals through the day, rather than three larger meals. This will place less stress upon the stomach.
- Do not overeat.
- Chew each mouthful thirty-five to fifty times each. The more you chew, the less stress you put upon your stomach.
- Minimize fat. Foods rich in fat increase stomach acid and the likelihood of stomach disorders.
- Eat protein and starchy foods in separate meals.
- Proteins, fats, and starches combine best with green and non-starchy vegetables.
- Eat alkalizing foods, such as those that contain small amounts of salt, first, as opposed to those containing fat, protein, or sugar.
- Eat fruit and sweetened foods alone, immediately after a meal.
- Eat melons alone because they digest very quickly.
- Avoid drinking fruit juice for at least two hours after eating a meal containing starch and four hours after a meal containing protein.
- Avoid excessively cold drinks.

Foods to Eat

- Whole grains, cooked with a pinch of sea salt to alkalize them
- Barley, which treats indigestion from starchy food stagnation or poorly tolerated mother's milk in infants
- Apple, which inhibits growth of ferments and disease-producing bacteria in the intestines
- Ginger. Eat ginger freshly grated in tea, or in capsule form, or chew a small piece. Studies have shown that ginger settles the stomach and overcomes nausea.
- Grapefruit peel moves and regulates spleen-pancreas digestive energy and is good for getting rid of gas.
- Lemon and lime, especially for those who eat a high-fat, high-protein diet, alleviates flatulence and indigestion.
- Umeboshi plums, sometimes called "Japanese Alka-Seltzer." Take one plum or half-teaspoon of umeboshi paste. It will cure most dyspepsia in ten minutes.
- Carrots treat indigestion, excess stomach acid, and heartburn.

Use soothing, mucilaginous foods and preparations:

- Soups
- Congees of oats, barley, or rice
- Honey-water
- Flaxseed, soaked
- Banana
- Avocado
- Tofu
- Soy milk
- Goat milk, soured
- Spinach
- Cucumber
- Cabbage, especially raw cabbage juice, taken on an empty stomach immediately after juicing
- Cereal grass, microalgae, and liquid chlorophyll

Foods to Reduce or Avoid

- Coffee, tea, and other caffeinated beverages
- Meat (rich in fat)
- Milk products, which contain fat and lactose
- Eggs (rich in fat)
- Poor-quality oils (all oils are liquid fat)
- Sugar
- Spicy foods
- Fried foods
- Alcohol
- Mints, which have been shown to create regurgitation of stomach juices and heartburn
- Excessive salt
- Vinegar
- Citrus fruit
- Plums

Chemicals to Avoid

- Limit over-the-counter medications, including aspirin. The anti-clotting effects of aspirin can promote bleeding of the stomach, inflammation (or gastritis), and bleeding ulcers.
- Avoid ibuprofen and other nonsteroidal anti-inflammatory medicines, which also contribute to stomach distress, especially for those with existing stomach problems.

Homeopathy

- Bryonia: if your stomach feels heavy after eating and is sensitive to touch; if moving makes you feel worse; if you have bitter rising and may vomit
- Carbo vegetabilis: if even the plainest food causes gas and belching about one-half hour after eating; if any indulgence causes a headache; if there is a craving for fresh air
- Chamomilla: if indigestion follows a fit of anger and irritability; if the stomach is distended with gas and cramping; if your mouth has a bitter taste; if you have flushed cheeks and an aversion to warm drinks
- Ignatia: if you are tense and nervous and crave food that doesn't agree with you; if you have rumbling in the bowels and sour belching; if you have a tendency to take deep breaths or sigh frequently
- Nux vomica: for the hard-driven type who overindulges; if you experience heartburn, belching, or bloating of the abdomen a few hours after eating; if you are constipated

Herbs to Treat Ulcer

- Licorice root tea
- Slippery elm tea
- Marshmallow root
- Red raspberry leaf tea
- Chamomile tea

Chinese Medicine

- Acupuncture to strengthen stomach meridian and the organ itself

Body/Mind

- Progressive relaxation exercises
- Meditation
- Prayer

Aromatherapy

- Rosemary
- Lavender
- Chamomile
- Pine

Vaginal Discharge (Vaginitis)

SYMPTOMS

Symptoms of vaginitis are discharge of mucus, irritation, redness, intense itching, odor, and pain during sex.

WHAT IS VAGINAL DISCHARGE?

From Modern Western Medicine

Most women experience mucous discharge from the vagina during the child-bearing years, especially as part of their menstrual cycle. The use of the birth control pill can affect the mucous membranes of the vagina and increase or decrease the discharge. However, mucous discharge may be abnormal if it is excessive, yellow or green, odorous or offensive in smell, and causes irritation or itching. Vaginitis (inflammation of the vagina) is among the most common causes of vaginal discharge and is often accompanied by itching of the vagina and the vulva.

From Traditional Medicine

Vaginal discharge is the body's attempt to rid itself of toxins, especially those accumulating in a woman's sex organs. It is among the most common problems affecting women today, largely because women's hormonal health has been compromised in the West by diet and lifestyle factors that stimulate the ovaries and encourage higher production of estrogen at an early age.

The primary problem facing women is the rich American diet, which encourages hormonal disorders in several ways. First, the diet is loaded with fat, which stimulates fat cells to produce estrogens. The fat and the lack of fiber combine to foster the growth of intestinal bacteria (clostridia varieties) that are able to convert bile acids into estrogenlike hormones.

The high-fat, highly refined American diet also allows estrogens that are produced by the body to circulate numerous times inside the body. Normally, the liver places a chemical on estrogens that prevents them from circulating more than once, but anaerobic intestinal bacteria are able to remove this compound and thus allow estrogens to keep circulating in a woman's body. These hormones stimulate hormone-sensitive tissues, especially those in the breast, uterus, and vagina.

In addition, many women take the birth control pill, which adversely affects hormonal health.

The best approach to regain the health of the female organs is to eat a diet that is rich in complex carbohydrates and fiber and low in animal fats and proteins. *The New England Journal of Medicine* reported that vegetarian women eliminate two to three times more estrogen in their feces than nonvegetarians. This, of course, promotes hormonal health; it occurs simply because vegetarian women eat diets that are low in fat and have an abundance of fiber.

REMEDIES

Foods to Eat

- Miso soup
- Whole grains
- Sprouts
- Green, leafy vegetables
- Cabbage
- Black and white sesame seeds
- Adzuki beans (will dry damp conditions)
- Kombu/kelp
- Chives (strengthen kidneys, treat dampness)
- String beans
- Clams
- Mussels
- Unsweetened cranberry juice
- Garlic
- Onions

Foods to Avoid

- Sugar
- Meat
- Coffee
- Dairy products
- Fruits
- Refined carbohydrates
- Alcohol

Herbs to Treat Vaginal Discharge

Take two myrrh/goldenseal capsules every two hours.

Douches

- Mix together equal parts of the following:

  Goldenseal
  Red raspberry
  Echinacea
  Slippery elm

Make a strong infusion using one ounce to a pint of distilled water; strain. Add one teaspoon of apple cider vinegar. Douche in morning and try to retain liquid for five minutes (incline position).

- Tea tree oil: 1 tbs. to 1 qt. warm water, twice a day
- White oak bark or bayberry bark: 1 ounce per 1 pint of water daily
- Apple cider vinegar: 2 tbs. to 1 qt. warm water, twice a day
- Daikon leaf hip bath

Supplements

- Vitamin A: 5000 IU per day
- Vitamin B_1 (thiamine): 1.5 mg per day
- Vitamin B_2 (riboflavin): 1.8 mg per day
- Niacin: 20 mg per day
- Vitamin B_6: 2–10 mg per day
- Vitamin C: 100–500 mg per day
- Vitamin E: 100–400 IU per day
- Zinc: 15 mg per day
- Garlic: 2 tablets, 3 times per day

VISION PROBLEMS

WHAT ARE COMMON PROBLEMS WITH VISION?

From Modern Western Medicine

Most visual disorders arise from errors of refraction, or the failure of the eye to focus light properly on the optic nerve, which is a postage-stamp-sized group of nerves at the back of the eye. The cause of these problems are mis-shapen eyeballs; either they are too long (in the case of nearsightedness or *myopia*) or too short (in the case of farsightedness or *hyperopia*). Distortions in the shape of the eye prevent the eye from focusing images properly on the optic nerve.Both problems can be corrected with glasses or contact lenses.

After the age of forty, the lens of the eye can lose flexibility and cause problems focusing on nearby objects, a condition called *presbyopia*. Reading glasses are usually prescribed by an ophthalmologist, or an eye doctor. If there are two or more refractory problems, bifocals or trifocals may be needed.

Another common problem affecting the eyes, especially among the elderly, is cataracts, or the gradual hardening of the lens. The lens becomes increasingly opaque, as cloudlike images start to appear. Vision is blurred and hazy; halos appear around lights, and the person may have difficulty seeing at night. Eyeglasses may compensate, but surgery is often recommended to replace the damaged lens with a plastic implant.

For people sixty years and older, the small areas at the center of the retina where cells detect light and color—a group of cells called the macula—can degenerate, making the ability to see fine details difficult, if not impossible. Straight lines or details begin to appear wavy or distorted. Peripheral vision usually remains, however. Laser surgery can sometimes be helpful.

Glaucoma is a disorder in which the pressure within the eye increases and, in the process, damages blood vessels that supply the retina and optic nerve. An early sign of glaucoma is the gradual loss of peripheral vision, but a routine eye test can determine if the intraoccular pressure is increasing. Medication can control and reduce the pressure within the eye, but sometimes laser surgery is necessary.

From Traditional Medicine

Chinese medicine maintains that the eyes are nourished by the liver; the liver meridian runs through the tissues surrounding the eyes and brings qi, or life force, to the entire area. When qi is diminished to the eyes, distortions begin to occur, including myopia, hyperopia, cataracts, and glaucoma. All forms of eye disorders are therefore seen as a liver imbalance and treated by restoring qi to the area around the eyes.

Of all the organs in the human body, the liver has the greatest regenerative powers. More than half of the liver can be impaired and the organ can still heal and regenerate, given the right conditions. The foods listed below will enhance liver function and allow the organ to heal itself.

Finally, pioneer scientist Nathan Pritikin, creator of the Pritikin diet and exercise program, maintained that glaucoma and cataracts occur because the tiny vessels within the eye become blocked with atherosclerosis, the result of a diet excessively high in fat and cholesterol. In order to improve vision, Pritikin recommended significant reduction of animal foods to reduce fat and cholesterol. The recommendations listed below are consistent with Pritikin's advice.

REMEDIES

General Recommendations

- See the section on the liver in Part IV for ways to enhance liver function.
- Avoid eating three hours before bed so that the liver has time to regenerate in the evening and at night, without having to work hard at assisting digestion.
- Two days a week, drink lemon water instead of breakfast. Chinese healers maintain that moderate amounts of sour taste strengthen and purify the liver.
- Do not overeat.
- Get plenty of exercise and rest.
- Do the eye exercises listed below for myopia and hyperopia.

Foods to Eat

- Raw vegetables, especially sprouts and green, leafy vegetables
- Orange and yellow fruits and vegetables such as carrots, winter squash, pumpkins, cantaloupes, and apricots
- Black sesame seeds
- Soybeans
- Dried, unripe raspberries (for blurred vision)
- Parsley
- Fish
- Whole grains
- Tofu
- Almonds and sunflower and sesame seeds

Foods to Avoid

- Fried foods
- Meat

- Poultry
- Eggs
- Refined grain products
- Sugar
- Dairy products
- Nuts (except almonds)
- Coffee
- Chocolate
- Alcohol

Exercise

Do the following exercise several times per day. Hold your index finger up to the level of your mouth, at a distance of about two feet in front of your mouth. Focus on a detailed object, poster, or work of art at a distance of ten to twenty feet. Hold the focus for ten seconds. Now, shift your focus to the top of your index finger. Hold the focus on your finger for ten seconds. Shift your focus again to the object at a distance. Hold the focus for ten seconds. This is two repetitions of this exercise. Do at least ten repetitions, at least three times a day. The exercise strengthens the eye muscles and restores the eye's ability to make accurate refractions.

Homeopathy

See a licensed homeopath for constitutional treatment.

For glaucoma, take 30 c of belladonna every fifteen minutes for up to ten doses when symptoms start. This remedy also treats blurred vision and pain in one eye, which are made worse by bright light.

Supplements

- Beta-carotene: 15–30 mg/day may prevent onset of cataracts.
- Vitamin C: 500 mg/day to prevent cataracts

WARTS

SYMPTOMS

Usually, there are no other symptoms.

WHAT ARE WARTS?

From Modern Western Medicine

Warts are caused by the papilloma virus, of which there are thirty types. A wart is a contagious, harmless growth that forms on the skin or mucous membranes. Warts appear only on the uppermost layer of skin. They have no roots, seeds, or branches. Sometimes, capillaries appear as black dots within the wart. There are several types of warts. Common warts, which are hard, irregular or round, with a firm exterior, flesh-colored to brown, grow up to one-quarter inch in diameter. Common warts often appear on the hands, face, knees, and scalp. Flu warts are flat-topped and flesh-colored. They appear on the wrists, the backs of the hands, and the face, and they may itch. Digitate warts are dark-colored growths with fingerlike projections. Filiform warts are long, slender growths that appear on the eyelids, armpits, or neck, often on people who are overweight and middle-aged. Plantar warts appear on the soles of the feet. Genital warts are pink, cauliflower-shaped growths that appear on the genitals of men or women. Genital warts require medical attention because the infection can spread between partners. Condoms can prevent transmission.

Most warts usually last between six and twelve months, then disappear without any treatment. The exceptions are plantar warts, which can be painful underfoot, and genital warts, which are highly contagious.

Several treatments exist for the removal of warts. Liquid nitrogen freezes warts, causing them to fall off. Corrosive salicylic acids are also used, as is surgery.

From Traditional Medicine

As viral infections, warts are a sign that the immune system has been weakened and that immediate repair of the immune system must begin. Proper diet and immune boosters must be undertaken. (See the section on immune boosters in Part IV.)

REMEDIES

Foods to Eat

- Miso soup
- Whole grains

- Lots of raw, fresh vegetables
- Seaweeds, especially nori
- Burdock
- Garlic
- Alfalfa sprouts (good for plantar warts)

Foods to Avoid

- Refined grains
- Sugar
- Caffeinated beverages
- Spicy foods
- Oily foods
- Chemicalized foods

Herbs to Treat Warts

- Alfalfa: To make tea, steep 1 tablespoon seed or 2 ounces dried leaf in 1 quart boiling water. In powder form, add to soups and salads.
- Buttercup: Apply juice of leaves and flowers directly to warts.
- Bloodroot: Apply ointment.

Homeopathy

- Thuja: Apply tincture twice daily and cover with plaster. Protect surrounding skin.

Physiotherapy

- Garlic: Apply thin section over wart as a continuous poultice.
- Vitamin E: Apply 400 IU capsules three times per day and cover with a Band-Aid. May take two months.
- Vitamin A (miscellized): 25,000 IU applied topically three times per day and night; cover. Especially useful in plantar warts.
- Salicylic acid: Apply two to three times a day. Protect surrounding skin.

Supplements

- Beta-carotene: 15 mg per day
- Vitamin B_1 (thiamine): 1.5 mg per day
- Vitamin B_6: 2–10 mg per day
- Vitamin C: 100–500 mg per day
- Vitamin E: 100–400 IU per day
- Zinc: 15 mg per day

WORMS

SYMPTOMS

The presence of worms may trigger no recognizable symptoms, or may cause local irritations, especially at the anus. Worms may also cause weakness, fatigue, lack of vitality, grinding of teeth at night, loss of appetite, irritability, frequent colds, brittle and hard fingernails with ridged longitudinal lines, anemia, and loss of weight.

WHAT ARE WORMS?

From Modern Western Medicine

Several types of parasitic worm and their larvae can live inside human intestines, blood, the lymphatic system, bile ducts, or organs, such as the liver. Worms are more common than many people realize, and can live within the system for years without a person realizing it. Worms can cause severe reactions, including chronic and debilitating illnesses.

Two main classes of worms are most common: roundworms, which have long, cylindrical bodies; and the platyhelminths, which have flattened bodies. The platyhelminths are further subdivided into the cestodes (tapeworms) and trematodes (flukes).

Worms can be transmitted to humans via undercooked or infected meat, soil, water, and contact with other people—especially children—who have been infected themselves.

The diagnosis of a worm infestation can be easily eradicated with antihelmintic drugs.

From Traditional Therapy

Drug therapy is usually rapid and effective, while dietary measures are usually much slower, but can be helpful in preventing reinfestation. As with any infection, worms will develop best if immune function is weakened. Those people who eat diets of refined carbohydrates and sugar are going to be more susceptible. Therefore, increasing the immunity of the host is invaluable in dealing with this long-term.

REMEDIES

Foods to Eat

- Miso soup
- Whole grains
- Raw brown rice: have on an empty stomach for breakfast. Chew very well. (Continue for a few weeks in case eggs continue to hatch.)

- Mugwort tea: have two or more hours after the last meal of the day.
- Leafy green vegetables
- Green cabbage
- Pumpkin seeds
- Garlic
- Onions
- Figs
- Raw pineapple

Foods to Avoid

- Sugar
- Refined carbohydrates
- Dairy products
- Pomegranate

Herbs to Treat Worms

- Wormwood (for pinworms, roundworms): take 1 teacup infusion morning and evening
- Wormseed: this is useful with tapeworms. Use small doses frequently, ½ to 1½ grains.
- American wormseed, Jerusalem oak (for roundworms, hookworms, tapeworms): Children take 20–30 grains powdered seeds or 3–10 drops oil. Adults take 1–2 tsp. powdered seeds or 10–20 drops oil.
- Pomegranate (for pinworms, roundworms, tapeworms): decoction of root bark used
- Bitterwood: enema or decoction. Use wood and bark. 1 tbs. to 1 cup water; boil 30 minutes. Dose: 1 tsp. in 1 cup water one to two times per day.
- Corsican tea: especially for pinworms and roundworms

Homeopathy

The following are for pinworms. Take three times daily for up to fourteen days. See homeopath if no improvement.

- Cina 6c: for itchy bottom; if child is irritable, picks nose, grinds teeth, is very hungry, or has dark rings under the eyes
- Teucrium 6c: for itchy bottom and itchy nose; if it's worse in evening; if you are restless in sleep, or there is crawling sensation in the rectum after passing stools
- Santonium 6c: a standby remedy if above remedies fail

Physiotherapy

- Garlic clove inserted rectally at night
- Garlic foot compresses at night

WOUNDS, CUTS, ABRASIONS

WHAT ARE WOUNDS?

From Standard Western Medicine

Wounds are injuries caused by trauma and damage to tissues. All wounds should be placed in ice-cold water immediately to stop the bleeding, reduce the chance of inflammation, and speed recovery. Thoroughly clean cuts in cold water and wash away all dirt and foreign objects. Bandage appropriately and keep the injury clean.

REMEDIES

Foods to Eat

- Miso soup
- Seaweeds
- Grains, boiled so that they are soupy
- Green, orange, and yellow vegetables for their antioxidant content

Foods to Avoid

- Sugar
- Refined foods with artificial ingredients
- High-fat foods, which diminish circulation

Herbs to Treat Wounds

Topical treatments:

- Aloe vera juice and/or comfrey juice
- Vitamin E: to accelerate healing and reduce scarring
- Tea tree oil: to prevent infection; reapply every two to three hours.

Internally:

- Arnica: take frequently.

Supplements

- Beta-carotene: 15–30 mg per day
- Vitamin C: 100–500 mg per day
- Vitamin E: 100–400 IU per day
- Zinc: 15 mg per day

YEAST INFECTIONS (CANDIDIASIS)

SYMPTOMS

Yeast infection, or candidiasis, manifests in a wide array of symptoms, depending on the severity of the infection, where the yeast has infiltrated, and the immune system's response. Common symptoms include the following:

- Recurrent vaginal infections
- Fatigue
- Depression
- Inability to concentrate
- Constipation or diarrhea
- Gas
- Bloating
- Abdominal pain
- Muscle or joint pain
- Headaches
- Allergies
- Skin rashes
- Nail fungus
- Menstrual problems
- Prostatitis
- Hypoglycemia
- Hyperactivity
- Athlete's foot

WHAT ARE YEAST INFECTIONS?

From Modern Western Medicine

The most common form of yeast is *Candida albicans,* which is the bacteria that causes candidiasis. Yeast infections commonly turn up in the mouth and vagina, where they manifest as sores, discharge, and infections. In health, *Candida albicans* is kept in check by competing bacteria that live throughout the digestive tract and the mucous membranes throughout the body. Unfortunately, these friendly bacteria commonly are destroyed by antibiotics. In the absence of such friendly bacteria, the *Candida albicans* flourishes and spreads.

Candida can be diagnosed as a patch of broken or scaly skin, a fungal rash (sometimes appearing on the fingernails or toenails), or the discharge from such patchy skin. Once diagnosed, physicians usually prescribe antifungal drugs. The drugs usually clear up the infection, but it often recurs, sometimes as a result of reinfection by a sex partner. Treatment of both partners is preferred. The condition can be exacerbated by birth control pills, which should be stopped once candida has been diagnosed.

From Traditional Medicine

Though yeast infections have been a problem since the time of Hippocrates, never before have they plagued humanity so intensely as they do today. Most women, at one time or another, suffer from yeast infections, or candidiasis.

In health, the body's immune system and bacterial environment keep candida in check, preventing it growing into a disease state. However, a whole host of antagonists have weakened the body's defenses, starting with antibiotics, which science is now showing weakens the immune system; a diet devoid of immune-supporting nutrients; a lack of dietary fiber, which promotes intestinal health; the absence of healthful fermented foods; and sufficient fresh air and exercise, which also support immune response. Under such conditions, candida can flourish.

Nystatin is an antifungal drug commonly prescribed by physicians to treat candidiasis. Foods such as garlic will also kill yeast. So, too, do oxygen therapies, such as hydrogen peroxide taken orally.

Such therapies cause die-off symptoms that may provide irritating or sometimes disturbing side effects, such as dizziness, irritation of mucous membranes, temporary inflammation, forgetfulness, and other symptoms that are commonly associated with yeast infection.

REMEDIES

Foods to Eat

- Miso soup: Cook slightly to reduce effect of fermentation.
- Raw, saltless sauerkraut
- Seaweed
- Whole grains (Although whole grains contain a lot of carbohydrates, the fiber and protein components help reestablish proper bowel function.)
- Tofu
- Seeds
- Nuts
- Beans, especially adzuki beans, which dry damp conditions; and mung beans, which are detoxifying
- Chlorella microalgae
- Vegetables
- Fish
- Onions
- Garlic

Foods to Avoid

- Sugars promote the growth of yeast.
- Refined carbohydrates also promote yeast growth.
- Meat
- Dairy products tend to aggravate the infection.
- Yeast and yeast-containing products, which are found commonly in bakery products, vitamins, alcohol, beverages, cereals, condiments, dairy products, mushrooms, and various meats
- Limit potatoes, sweet potatoes, squash, wheat, and corn.
- Eggs
- Fruit or fruit juice
- Alcohol, especially white wine

Herbs to Treat Yeast Infections

- Garlic: one fresh clove, two or three times a day (Swallow with water if chewing is too difficult.)
- Taheebo inner bark tea (antifungal): 1 cup infusion four times per day
- Tea tree oil: Use topically on local nail fungus patches. Add 1 tbs. water-soluble tea tree oil to 1 cup hot water and soak nail for 20–30 minutes, 1 or 2 times per day. Do this for 30–60 days.
- Aloe vera juice: 2 oz., 4 times per day
- Pau d' arco: tincture, 30–40 drops taken in water, 3 times daily; tea, 3 times daily; or 2 capsules, 3 times daily (Scientific research has proven the herb kills yeast infection.)
- Goldenseal: tincture, 30 drops, twice daily (Pregnant women should avoid taking goldenseal because it contains berberine, a chemical that may be toxic during pregnancy.)
- Usnea: tincture, 30 drops, twice daily

Physiotherapy

Hydrogen peroxide, taken orally, should be monitored by a physician, naturopath, or other health counselor experienced in the use of hydrogen peroxide therapies.

Supplements

Make sure they are yeast-free.

- Vitamin A: 5000 IU per day
- Vitamin B_1: 1.5 mg per day
- Vitamin B_2: 1.8 mg per day
- Niacin: 20 mg per day
- Vitamin B_6: 2–10 mg per day
- Vitamin C: 100–500 mg per day
- Vitamin E: 100–400 IU per day

PART III

HEALING TOOLS, DISCIPLINES, AND PRACTICES

AROMATHERAPY AND ESSENTIAL OILS

Aromatherapy uses fragrance to create relaxation, resolve inner conflicts, and assist healing. The fragrances themselves are drawn from plants in the form of essential oils. Each of these oils is pregnant with its own distinct odor, stimulating an array of emotional, psychological, and physical responses. Some arouse, excite, create alertness, or heighten sensuality; others relax, cool, and soothe.

In one way or another, all of them play on the mind in subtle yet powerful ways, creating a symphony of moods, depending on the fragrance used. Proponents say that the emotional and psychological states give rise to physical responses—changes in pulse rate, respiration, perspiration, and immune response—which in turn can heal the body.

The use of fragrant oils to heal goes back 4,000 years to the Egyptians and was later used by both the Greeks and the Romans. It has only recently begun to catch on again, and this time in a big way. Elizabeth Taylor and Princess Diana are only two of its more glamorous proponents.

Essential oils are concentrated, volatile liquids derived from the leaves, barks, roots, flowers, resins, or seeds of some 700 plants. They are produced principally by steam distillation and are sold in small quantities, typically an ounce or less. Because essential oils are so potent, only a few drops are needed to treat most conditions.

Herbalists and aromatherapists apply essential oils topically, usually after dilution, through massage, compresses, or by adding them to a bath. Essential oils are also inhaled by dispersing a few drops in liquid that is then sprayed in a mist or evaporated to create steam. Essential oils are rarely taken orally, and then only with the supervision of a knowledgeable practitioner. They affect the psyche by influencing mood, emotions, and sexual arousal or relaxation, and influence the body by promoting the healing of wounds, clearing lung congestion, and relieving pain.

The secret of aromatherapy lies in human experience—that is, how we relate fragrance to specific experiences, even those odors that were present in a forest, a meadow, or a room that we failed to consciously notice, but we recorded nonetheless on an unconscious or subliminal level. But it goes beyond that. Aromatherapy lies as much with the experience of the plant as it does with your experiences of life. Each plant responds to the sun, the moon, the earth, and the rain in specific ways.

The rosemary flower, for example, is nestled deeply among its branches, close to the earth, and sends out a strong and stimulating fragrance to the entire plant. The flower has a kind of charisma all its own. It draws the sun toward itself, like a magnet, and then radiates its odors outward. Thus, rosemary offers the same characteristics to those who use it as an essential oil: it is said to stimulate, invigorate, and awaken the entire organism. It also imparts an earthy allure, drawing life toward you. For these reasons, rosemary is often found in morning lotions, day creams, or skin cleansers.

Traditionally, it has been used as a purifying, warming, and decongesting herb, as well. Lavender is just the opposite. Its flower lifts away from the plant, "almost like a cloud or a dream," says Christine Murphy, president of Weleda, one of the companies that makes essential oils. "Lavender leaves you feeling relaxed and light. It's wonderful after a stressful day."

Aromatherapists examine how each plant behaves in nature to discover the effects of its essential oils. Below is a list of popular and evocative essential oils commonly used in a wide variety of natural body care products.

Arnica. The plant itself grows high in the mountains, where the sun is pure and the air clean. It has been used traditionally as an herb for bruises and other injuries. It promotes healing, creates warmth, stimulates circulation, and moistens the skin. It arouses, restores vitality, and awakens.

Cassia, a tree that grows in India and Southeast Asia, is exotic, seductive, warming, and relaxing.

Chamomile or **Camomile.** One of the most widely used herbs and essential oils, chamomile soothes, relaxes, refreshes, and calms the overall condition. It is used as an analgesic, anti-inflammatory, antispasmodic, nervine, and sedative.

Clove is a colorless, aromatic, concentrated liquid prepared from the flowering buds of a tropical evergreen tree. Rubbed on gums, clove relieves toothache pain and has antiseptic and anesthetic properties. Clove is also used externally to disinfect minor wounds and scrapes, reduce warts, and alleviate skin problems like scabies and insect bites. Taken internally (by diluting a few drops in a cup of water), it may help eliminate intestinal gases and control vomiting and nausea. The dried herb is a spice used in cooking, and the oil is used for flavoring everything from cigarettes to candy. Undiluted clove oil is potentially toxic in large doses. It can sting the gums, so is often diluted before it is used on teeth or skin. Avoid taking clove during pregnancy.

Coriander warms, relaxes, deodorizes, and soothes.

Eucalyptus. One of the oldest traditional herbs, eucalyptus has been used to purify and decongest the lungs, as well as cool the overall condition. The essential oil has the same effects on the skin: it cleanses, purifies, and soothes and heals blemishes. It has a dispersing effect; it also enhances breathing. The oil is noted for its antibacterial and antiviral effects. Applied topically, it helps relieve pain and inflammation, promote wound healing, and reduce muscle spasms. Eucalyptus also combats sunburn, blisters, and sprains, and repels insects. It is inhaled to loosen mucus and treat asthma and bronchitis. Drops can be used in the bath or diluted with a carrier oil and applied by massage. High concentrations of eucalyptus can irritate the kidneys when taken internally or irritate the skin when used externally.

Geranium is seductive and sensual. It refreshes, lifts moods, and invigorates.

Heather is a purple English evergreen shrub recommended for those who need emotional self-sufficiency and tranquility. People who appear self-absorbed and overtalkative are often lonely and seek contact with others in a dysfunctional way. Heather helps the soul to become self-fulfilled rather than self-absorbed.

Lavender is relaxing, relieves stress, is analgesic, antispasmodic, nervine, and sedative. Lavender is prepared from the leaves and blue flowers of a Mediterranean shrub (*Lavandula officinalis*). The fragrant essential oil has analgesic, antiseptic, anti-inflammatory, and immune-boosting effects. Lavender may be inhaled to help induce sleep, alleviate stress, and reduce depression and nervous tension. The essential oil is also applied topically to heal wounds, sprains, insect bites and stings, athlete's foot, muscular aches and pains, and earaches. As an herb, lavender has traditionally been used to treat coughs and the common cold. The oil is mild enough to be applied full strength and is often recommended for use on children. (Lavender oil should not, however, be taken internally.) As an herb, lavender is usually sold dried or in concentrated drops.

Madia is a mandalalike wildflower that closes its petals during the heat of the day. It is recommended for those who are easily distracted, unable to concentrate, or who feel listless. Madia assists in precise thinking and concentration, and thus is recommended for students and writers who may have trouble focusing.

Marjoram is considered analgesic, antispasmodic, nervine, and sedative.

Olive trees grow and produce fruit under the intense Mediterranean sun. Olive warms and soothes, creates circulation, and contains a certain fiery quality.

Peppermint refers to both an herb and an essential oil derived from the leaves of a garden perennial (*Mentha piperita*) that has long been used to make digestive remedies. In tea form, peppermint is still widely used to relieve upset stomach, heartburn, nausea, diarrhea, and flatulence. The essential oil contains menthol, a medicinally active alcohol that exhibits significant antiseptic, anti-inflammatory, and astringent powers. The oil is sometimes diluted and taken internally for the same conditions treated by the dried herb, as well as for shock, asthma, travel sickness, fainting, and dizziness. The essential oil is also applied externally for itchy skin, hemorrhoids, toothaches, muscle aches, and insect bites. Peppermint oil may irritate some people's skin if applied undiluted or in high doses. The oil is also a good insect repellent and a popular flavoring agent in foods, candies, chewing gum, and toothpastes. Peppermint comes dried or as tea bags, extracts, and essential oil.

Pine. The tree remains unaltered by the most severe winters or harshest summers, and therefore provides one of nature's greatest examples of constancy, stability, and duration in the face of life's vicissitudes. Pine is used to stimulate these same qualities, to balance the breathing, and refresh and stimulate the entire organism. As an herb, pine is used to decongest the lungs and arouse sensuality.

Red chestnut is an English tree that grows to heights of 50 to 75 feet and produces rosy pink flowers. The flower essence is intended for worrisome individuals who live in fearful anticipation of problems for friends or family members. It assists in attaining inner peace and calm trust in the unfolding of life.

Tea tree, a pale yellow essential oil made from the aromatic leaves of an Australian tree (*Melaleuca alternifolia*), is one of the premier natural remedies for bacterial, viral, and fungal skin conditions, including athlete's foot, nail infections, and mouth sores. It is also effective for treating injuries (including burns, cuts, and scrapes), bites and stings, and for repelling insects. Tea tree is a popular ingredient in skin creams, shampoos, throat lozenges, toothpastes, deodorants, and other body care products. It is nontoxic and can be safely applied directly to the skin without being diluted. Don't get it in the eyes, though.

Tiger lily is grown in the Sierra Nevada foothills and is striking in its orange color and dramatic form. It balances many masculine traits and is also indicated as a toner for women during menopause. It assists in the ability to shift from competitive, aggressive behaviors to those that are more inclusive and cooperative.

Wintergreen helps to warm and relax muscles when rubbed into the back.

Yarrow has long been regarded as a strengthener. It is recommended for people who are hypersensitive to environmental factors or who feel extremely vulnerable to others. It assists in creating an inner strength and stability.

All of these essential oils have been used traditionally as healing herbs. Consequently, they influence the body directly, as medicinal compounds, as well as create their own atmospheres.

Essential oils are worth studying and experimenting with, especially on occasions when you want something a little different in the day or night. They can also be applied either before or after placing a steaming towel over the face, which allows them to penetrate more deeply into the skin.

When experimenting with these and other body care products, be conscious of how the product affects you. We all respond individually to odors and other body care products. There are no universal applications here, which can make the products more fun.

NUTRITION

In the past thirty years, nutrition has gone from being a dull, overlooked science to one of the most exciting areas of health care. The reason, simply, is that scientists are discovering that to a great extent, the foods we eat each day determine the rate at which we age and whether or not we become ill. Even more, an increasing body of evidence is demonstrating that diet plays a key role in the recovery from disease. More and more, scientists are finding that food is highly effective medicine.

Of course, that's an old message—a message, in fact, that goes back to the time of Hippocrates. Perhaps that's what is so exciting about the times in which we live. We are witnessing the possible integration of science and traditional medicine, between the new worldview and the old. As scientists delve ever deeper into the workings of atoms, cells, and micronutrients, they find the scientific basis for the wisdom offered by our ancestral healers. Little by little, science, in effect, is validating the ancient medicine. (See the section on immune boosting in Part IV of this book.)

In a way, we have come full circle in our understanding of nutrition. In the early 1900s, the only diseases thought to be related to nutrition were nutritional deficiency diseases, such as scurvy (from lack of vitamin C) and pellagra (from a lack of nicotinic acid). This belief gave rise to the need for fortification of foods, which became a routine part of food processing in the 1950s.

In the 1970s, scientists recognized that nutritional deficiencies were rare, indeed, highly unlikely in a well-nourished person. The more ominous threat to health was an excess of fat, cholesterol, and refined foods, which were devoid of important nutrients and fiber. With that recognition, medical science de-emphasized the micronutrients and instead began to focus attention on the macronutrients, namely fat, protein, and carbohydrates. Special attention was paid to the relationship of fat and cholesterol (the latter is not a nutrient, but a sterol) to heart disease and cancer. Soon, it was discovered that fat is a causal factor in the creation of heart disease, cancer, diabetes, and other serious illnesses.

Then came the late 1980s and 1990s, when scientists became aware of the effects of micronutrients on how the body ages and becomes ill, a process known as oxidation or free radical formation. Free radicals occur when atoms break down, or decay, and in the process lose electrons. Since there must be the same number of electrons as protons for an atom to remain stable, these imbalanced atoms steal electrons from their neighbors. Soon, a mad rush of thefts takes place, as atoms steal electrons from other atoms. Ultimately, such thefts cause the breakdown of molecules, cells, and tissues, causing the body to age. Free radical formation also causes such diseases as atherosclerosis and cancer. In fact, it has now been established that oxidation, or free radical formation, is the cause of more than sixty major illnesses, including heart disease, cancer, and cataracts.

Remarkably, a group of food substances called antioxidants stop the process of free radical formation by donating electrons to these imbalanced atoms. Antioxidants restore balance to atoms and molecules and stop the decay of cells, tissues, and organs. In the process, they slow the progress of aging and illness. They also boost immune function.

As antioxidants were being discovered, so, too, were groups of nutrients that scientists realized were essential in the body's fight against cancer. Groups of these newly discovered anticancer nutrients had names like indoles, flavonoids, and phytoestrogens (also called phytochemicals). Whatever their names, it soon became obvious that they were essential to the prevention of malignancy. Such discoveries shifted the focus back to micronutrition, but did not cause a de-emphasis upon macronutrients, especially fat, because fat is a major cause of free radical formation, which triggers the onset of disease. Thus, the old focus on micronutrition and the relatively modern understanding of macronutrients achieved an integration.

The new research is not without its dark side, however. Anyone who follows the newspaper reports about the health-promoting effects of vitamins C or E may wonder if they shouldn't just skip food altogether and take vitamin and mineral supplements instead. A deeper look at the science is proving otherwise. According to Elinor Levy, Ph.D., professor of immunology at Boston University, the best way for most people to get these immune boosters is through food. Nutrients work in harmony with one another, said Dr. Levy. Often, the availability and usefulness of one nutrient depends on the presence of another. The relationship between vitamins C and E is a good example. Vitamin C has been found to help regenerate vitamin E. Without vitamin C, there are lower levels of vitamin E.

Food not only provides a wide variety of nutrition, but also provides that nutrition in appropriate quantities that the body has been trained to handle. Take zinc, for example. At the lower doses found in food, zinc is a powerful immune booster. But taken in doses that are common in pill form—60 to 100 milligrams, for example—zinc depresses immune function.

Finally, scientists point out that food possesses many mysterious substances that science may never fully understand. The more food is studied, the more scientists appreciate its enormous complexity. Food contains nutrients, cancer-inhibiting enzymes, and subtle chemical factors that help to make nutrients available to the body. This gives food qualities that no pill could match.

"Take beta-carotene, for example," said Dr. William Pryor, a pioneer antioxidant researcher and director of the Biodynamics Research Institute at the University of Louisiana at Baton Rouge. "Actually, beta-carotene is one of hundreds of chemicals called *carotenoids* that color food. A single vegetable can contain many carotenoids, and beta-carotene may be the least powerful immune booster among them. We simply don't know what the other carotenoids do yet."

As with every other aspect of our lives, nutrition requires balance. Traditional Oriental, Greek, and American healers have always recognized the need for balance in life. The more scientists discover about food, the more this view is being supported.

Here's a review of some of the most recent scientific findings and how you can use food to fight disease, especially cancer and heart disease. The foods listed below will improve the quality of your life and perhaps make it longer, too.

FIRST, STAY FOCUSED ON THE BIG PICTURE

While there is an ever-increasing emphasis upon individual nutrients, scientists find that people with the best health follow a diet made up largely of grains, fresh vegetables, beans, and low-fat animal products. One of the best examples of the effects of such a diet on health is the Chinese.

In 1990, Cornell University scientists reported the results of a long-term study in which the diets and disease patterns of 6,500 Chinese were examined. The study revealed that the Chinese diet, which consists largely of whole grains, vegetables, and very small amounts of animal food, protects against virtually all the common degenerative diseases, including heart disease, cancer, osteoporosis, diabetes, and high blood pressure.

The cancers that are most common in the West—namely, those of the breast, colon, and prostate—are rare in those regions of China where the traditional diet is eaten. That diet looks nothing like the American diet, which is rich in fat, animal protein, refined foods, and relatively low in grains, fresh vegetables, beans, and fruit.

The Chinese obtain only 7 percent of their protein from animal foods; Americans get more than 70 percent of their protein from animal sources. Animal protein has been linked to cancer and osteoporosis.

Most Chinese do not consume dairy products, yet osteoporosis also is rare in China. Interestingly, the Chinese consume only half the calcium Americans do. They get their calcium almost exclusively from plant food, such as leafy, green vegetables.

The Chinese eat 20 percent more calories than Americans do, but obesity is rare among the Chinese. The reason for the difference: Chinese people eat only a third as much fat as Americans and twice the complex carbohydrates from grains and vegetables. Complex carbohydrate foods are easily burned as fuel or consumed by the body to produce heat. In other words, they are not readily converted into fat.

THE IMPORTANCE OF BLOOD CHOLESTEROL

The Chinese blood cholesterol levels are also uniformly low. They range from 88 mg/dL to 165 mg/dL, nearly half of what Americans average, which is from 155 mg/dL to 274 mg/dL.

Blood cholesterol is a good indicator of illness. There are some regional dietary differences in China. In places where a higher fat and cholesterol diet is consumed, the disease rates are also higher. We think of blood cholesterol as related only to heart disease, but in fact cholesterol level is related to all degenerative illnesses, because high cholesterol prevents oxygen from going to cells.

"So far we've seen the plasma cholesterol is a good predictor of the kinds of diseases people are going to get," Dr. T. Colin Campbell, biochemist at Cornell and organizer of the study, told the *New York Times*. "Those with higher cholesterol levels are prone to the diseases of affluence—cancer, heart disease, and diabetes," said Dr. Campbell.

After reviewing the evidence, Dr. Campbell summarized his thoughts this way: "We're basically a vegetarian species and should be eating a wide variety of plant foods and minimizing our intake of animal foods."

Scientists maintain that the healthiest blood cholesterol is under 180 mg/dL, and an ideal blood cholesterol level is below 160 mg/dL.

THE FIRST PRIORITY: REDUCE FAT

Americans, on average, eat 80 to 100 grams of fat per day—the equivalent of almost a whole stick of butter! Saturated fats are found in animal foods—red meat, dairy products, and eggs—as well as a handful of vegetable foods, such as olives, coconuts, and palm-kernel oils. Other experts recommend even less fat and saturated fat intake.

Such quantities of fat have been shown to elevate your risk of heart disease, cancer, diabetes, and other degenerative diseases. William Castelli, M.D., director of the Framingham Heart Study, recommends that people limit fat intake to no more than sixty-seven grams per day, with only a third of that coming from saturated fat.

Two ways you can do just that are:

Replace Meat with Grains and Fish

One way to lower your fat intake is to consume more whole grains, fresh vegetables, fruit, and low-fat fish. Three ounces of very lean ground beef, for example, has 70 milligrams of cholesterol, 5.4 grams of saturated fat, and 13.8 grams of total fat, while a three-ounce serving of scallops contains 45 milligrams of cholesterol, 0.13 milligrams of saturated fat, and 1.2 grams of total fat.

Eat Cholesterol-Lowering Oils

Many fish, such as haddock, cod, flounder, and salmon, also contain omega-3 polyunsaturated oils that have been shown to lower blood cholesterol. (See recommendations below.)

FIBER: PROTECTIVE AGAINST CANCER, HEART DISEASE, AND OTHER ILLNESSES

For decades, studies have been showing how a diet rich in fat and low in fiber directly correlates to a higher incidence of cancers of all types, especially colon, breast, and prostate cancer. Scientists have found that fat consumption and a lack of fiber from whole grains, vegetables, and fruit combine to create the perfect intestinal environment for colon cancer. A high-fat diet causes an increase in the body's production of bile acids, which are used to help digest fat. The more fat in the diet, the more the body secretes bile into the intestinal tract. Together, the fat and bile deplete oxygen levels in the intestines and create the ideal conditions for anaerobic bacteria, which proliferate in oxygen-deprived conditions. These anaerobic bacteria convert bile acids into powerful carcinogens, which trigger the onset of malignancy.

The lack of fiber slows intestinal transit time—the amount of time it takes for waste to move through the intestinal tract and then be eliminated from the body. As intestinal transit time is delayed, the intestines are exposed to toxins that would otherwise be eliminated more rapidly. These toxins also add to the unhealthful conditions within the digestive tract.

Dr. Denis Burkitt, who studied the diets and health of African tribes, discovered that, because of their high-fiber diet, the African people have little or no incidence of intestinal cancer. Other studies have shown that cholesterol in the bowel increases tumor growth.

A high-fiber diet has been shown to be protective against heart disease, as well. Fiber binds with cholesterol in the intestinal tract and thus causes it to be eliminated from the body in greater quantities.

High-fiber diets have also been associated with lower blood levels of estrogen and lower breast cancer rates.

CANCER FIGHTERS ON YOUR PLATE

Research has consistently shown that diet plays a major role in both the cause and prevention of cancer, especially the most common cancers—those of the breast, colon, and prostate. Diets that raise your risk of cancer are rich in fat and low in fiber, antioxidants, and certain minerals.

In a recent study, scientists compared the eating habits of forty-one people who contracted colorectal cancer with those who remained healthy and concluded that those who got the cancer ate foods that were richer in fat, protein, and carbohydrates and lower in fiber, calcium, and phosphorus than those who remained cancer-free.

When the scientists looked closer at eating habits and disease patterns, they concluded that those who ate diets richer in fiber and calcium were less likely to get colon cancer, while those who ate diets higher in total fiber were less likely to get rectal cancer. (Published in *Cancer*; April 15, 1992.)

NUTRIENTS THAT FIGHT BREAST CANCER

Research is supporting the theory that certain nutrients in fruits and vegetables—especially fiber and antioxidants—protect women against breast cancer. When researchers compared two groups of women—one with breast cancer and another group without the disease—they found that those who did not contract the illness ate significantly more vegetables, fruits, and fiber.

Researchers at the State University of New York compared the eating habits of 310 women who had breast cancer with 316 women free of the illness. The difference in their eating patterns, said the researchers, was that the women who did not get cancer ate diets richer in fiber, folic acid, carotenoids, and vitamin C, all derived from their increased intake of vegetables and fruit. The researchers theorized that the antioxidants, especially, provided protection against the disease.

THE CABBAGE FAMILY

These include broccoli, cabbage, kale, brussels sprouts, collard greens, and mustard greens. Such vegetables contain a group of compounds called indoles, which may prevent tumor-causing estrogen from targeting the breast, according to researchers at the National Cancer Institute. In animal studies, they've been shown to switch on enzymes that prevent exposure to carcinogens.

Broccoli, as well as other cruciferous vegetables, are also rich sources of another cancer fighter called sulforanphane. Sulforanphane has been called a "major and very potent" trigger for detoxifying tissues and blood and for promoting production of cancer-preventive enzymes, according to research published in the *Proceedings of the National Academy of Sciences* (89, 1992).

Additional green, yellow, and orange foods rich in phytochemicals and other cancer fighters include citrus fruit, carrots, parsnips, squash, celery, and parsley. "To harness anticarcinogenic activity, a combination of these vegetables would probably work best," said Dr. Herbert Pierson, a leading cancer researcher formerly of the National Cancer Institute.

SOYBEANS AND SOYBEAN PRODUCTS

Soybeans and soybean products, such as tamari, miso, and soy sauce, contain a newly discovered compound called genistein. Genistein prevents blood vessels from attaching to tumors, which prevents tumors from obtaining essential oxygen and nutrients to survive (*Proceedings of the National Academy of Sciences*; April 1993).

According to Michael Wargovich, M.D., professor of medicine at Texas University's M. D. Anderson Cancer Center in Houston, soybeans also contain a substance called protease inhibitor, which interferes with cancer cell proliferation at both the early and later stages of development.

GARLIC

Garlic promotes health in a wide variety of ways. For starters, it improves the ability of the liver to metabolize and neutralize carcinogens that would otherwise produce cancer cells and tumors, said Dr. Wargovich.

Garlic stimulates the liver to more effectively identify these poisons and turn them into harmless, water-soluble compounds, added Dr. Wargovich. Garlic also encourages a variety of detoxifying enzymes to be produced by the body, some of which directly attack cancer cells and tumors. Studies have found that the rates of stomach and colorectal cancers are lower among those who have high garlic consumption. Scientists speculate that garlic may block the tumor-promoting effects of a certain group of fatty acids, called prostaglandins, which are hormonelike substances in the body. Prostaglandins may encourage tumor growth when they go unregulated. The sulfur compounds found in garlic—the most widely known is allicin—are responsible for promoting the body's detoxifying activities. Allicin is most effective when eaten raw, but researchers at the National Cancer Institute say that garlic has health-promoting effects when eaten cooked, as well. Consequently, scientists are recommending that garlic be used both raw and cooked.

Many of these sulfur chemicals are also found in onions, though apparently in smaller quantities.

"It seems that the stronger the food—and in the case of garlic, that means the smell—the stronger the health-enhancing effects are," said Dr. Wargovich.

Eat it raw and cooked. Eat parsley with raw garlic to counteract the smell.

FOODS RICH IN B VITAMINS

B vitamins strengthen immune cells, increase their number, and help to regulate hormones. Good sources are whole grains, such as brown rice; broccoli; leafy greens, such as collard and kale; beans and peas; potatoes, nuts, green peppers; and fruit.

WHITE FISH AND SALMON

These include haddock, cod, flounder, fluke, and scrod. Fish oils can increase the activity of white blood cells, which detect and attack foreign cells. They have been shown to prevent metastasis in early stages of cancer and to lower cholesterol.

WHAT YOU CAN DO

Ten Ways of Protecting Yourself Against Disease

1. Eat whole grains and whole grain products daily. Whole grains include brown rice, barley, oats, millet, corn, and wheat, and whole grain products include bread, pasta, and whole grain flour products. Whole grains are rich in complex carbohydrates for stable and long-lasting energy. They contain minerals, such as zinc and selenium, which boost immune response. They provide protein. They also offer many essential vitamins, including vitamin E, an antioxidant and immune booster. Finally, whole grains provide an abundance of fiber, which promotes intestinal health.

2. Eat at least two vegetables per day. Vegetables are rich in vitamins, minerals, and fiber. Many contain beta-carotene, an immune enhancer and antioxidant. You should vary your vegetables, but the ones to emphasize are:

- Leafy greens, such as collard greens, mustard greens, kale, and cabbage. These are loaded with vitamins and minerals, especially calcium. A cup of cooked collard greens contains 320 milligrams of calcium; a cup of milk contains 300 milligrams of calcium, plus fat, cholesterol, steroids, antibiotics, and lactose.
- Broccoli, brussels sprouts, and onions: Broccoli and brussels sprouts are rich in beta-carotene and vitamin C, both antioxidants and immune boosters. Onions have been shown to protect against stomach cancer and other cancers.
- Squash: All the squashes are rich in beta-carotene and strengthen the immune system. They also contain fiber.
- Roots, especially carrots, are rich in beta-carotene.

3. Get the majority of your protein from beans and whole grains, and restrict your animal foods to those that are low in fat. All the essential amino acids are located in beans, grains, and vegetables. Beans are also rich in minerals, complex carbohydrates, and fiber. Meanwhile, eat low-fat animal foods, such as the white meat of poultry, fish, and skim milk products.

4. Eat sea vegetables, such as wakame, arame, hijiki, nori, and spirulina. These are rich sources of trace minerals (including zinc, iron, magnesium, manganese, and selenium), which are essential to immune function; some are abundant sources of antioxidants; they also contain sodium alginate, an im-

portant tissue and blood cleanser (see the section on the immune system in Part IV).

5. Eat health-protecting specialty foods, such as shiitake and reishi mushrooms, miso, tamari, and shoyu; and garlic. Shiitake and reishi mushrooms have been shown to have a wide array of immune-strengthening properties (see above). Miso, tamari, and shoyu repopulate the intestines with friendly oxygen-producing bacteria that promote nutrient uptake and a healthy intestinal environment. They also alkalize the intestines, which mitigates against the spread of disease. Garlic is antifungal and immune-enhancing.

6. Eat organic foods. Pesticides, which have been shown to cause cancer and liver, kidney, and blood disease, must be dealt with by the immune system. As pesticides increase in our tissues, the immune system becomes weakened, allowing other carcinogens and pathogens to affect our health.

7. Eat sweets that are less refined and part of a whole grain food, such as oatmeal cookies sweetened with apple juice or barley malt, or cakes sweetened with apple juice or rice syrup. At the same time, minimize or avoid white sugar. Sugar dramatically raises insulin levels, which prevents fat stores from being burned. The more sugar and fat in your diet, the more you will burn sugar and store fat, thus causing weight gain. Sugar also robs the body of essential minerals and vitamins because it stimulates cells to function (sugar is a fuel) without offering the raw materials—such as vitamins and minerals—for the cells to do their work. Sweets found in whole foods provide nutrients as well as fuel, which promotes healthy cell metabolism.

8. Don't smoke. Tobacco is a major free radical producer.

9. Get regular exercise, such as walking, bicycling, and sports. All promote excellent circulation, which brings oxygen and nutrients to cells. Studies have shown that cells in oxygen-deprived environments become cancerous.

10. Seek balance in life. Stress is a major factor in the onset of disease. There will always be problems; let's find ways to put them in perspective and enjoy life.

CHINESE MEDICINE

No one knows how old the Chinese medical system is. It is thought to have been fully codified somewhere between 2,500 and 3,000 years ago when the book *The Yellow Emperor's Classic of Internal Medicine* is believed to have been first produced.

The Chinese medical system is based on a philosophical system that unifies the human being with nature in the largest sense, that is, with both the heavens and the earth. Humanity is the product of the interaction between these two great archetypes, heaven and earth, and as such never loses direct contact with both of these spheres throughout life. That unifying thread that exists among heaven, earth, and each human being is a living energy, called the life force, or qi. Heaven and earth combine to create qi, which flows through the human being, maintaining our health and leading each of us to our destiny.

At the root of all Chinese thinking is the recognition that all reality is composed of paradox, or opposites. There is no such thing as a singular condition of good or bad, for example. Everything has front and back, left and right, up and down, good and bad. Human life is a struggle to balance opposites and to create harmony, peace, and health. All illness arises from imbalance, or a condition in which there is an excess of something in a person's life: weakness, strength, wealth, poverty, a particular food or drink, a particular kind of thinking. Something dominates the other factors in life and causes imbalance, which gives rise to disease.

Health is a state of balance and wholeness, the Chinese say. Health is a condition in which all the parts of the human psyche find their place of balance and harmony within each of us. In such a condition, we are able to fully understand and love ourselves, under all conditions. Thus, we are able to understand, utilize, and express all that we are. In the process, we are able to understand and embrace everyone else in life.

Health begins by establishing harmony between opposites. To do that, we must understand that all of life is based upon paradoxical opposites, or what the Chinese refer to as yin and yang.

YIN AND YANG: THE ENDLESS CREATION OF OPPOSITES

From the Chinese point of view, all change is made possible through the interaction of opposites, or the archetypal forces of yin and yang. Yin and yang, which are implicit in all things, including each of us, causes the attraction or repulsion of objects, making movement and change possible. The medium of change is an underlying energy implicit in all of life, a living river of energy, called *qi* or *chi*. This life energy of qi imbues the material world, including each of us, and causes all things to change and evolve.

A crude analogy for life energy would be electricity, which is made possible by the attraction of positive and negative poles of a magnet. Magnetic forces pull electrons from atoms and put them into motion as a stream of electricity. Like the poles of a magnet, yin and yang attract or repel, causing life energy to flow in one direction or another.

Yin represents the condition of things when they contract or are passive, cool, wet, and slow-moving. Yin is the female principle, the negative pole of a magnet. The earth is yin, as is the moon. So, too, are autumn and winter, when the energy of the seasons declines and become less active. Nighttime is yin. The northern climates are yin, and the farther north you go, the more yin the conditions become—that is, cooler, quieter, and less active. Space is yin. Things in a relaxed state are yin. Thus, rest, sitting, and sleep are all yin. A warm bath causes the body to become more relaxed or yin.

Yang represents the condition of things when they expand, become active, fiery, hot, dry, and fast-moving. Yang is the masculine principle, the positive pole of a magnet. Heaven is yang, as is the sun. So, too, are spring and summer, when the energy is rising, blossoming, expanding, and active. Daytime is yang. The southern climates are more yang—that is, warmer, more fertile, bursting with life. Time is yang. Things in an active or fiery state are yang. Stressful conditions are considered more yang.

Health is a state of balance between yin and yang. Therefore, stressful conditions are harmonized by yin things, such as rest, warm baths, and walks in the forest or by the ocean. Daytime, which is active and demanding and yang, is balanced by nighttime, which is more relaxing, peaceful, and yin.

All reality is made up of opposites, or yin and yang. All physical objects are composed of left and right (yang and yin, respectively), up and down (yang and yin), and inside and out (yin and yang). Even the earth is composed of its four directions, each a manifestation of yin and yang—south: yang; north: yin; west: yin; east: yang. Together, yin and yang balance each other and make physical reality possible.

Yin and yang cause the movement of qi, or the life force, but each of us is responsible for maintaining the flow of that life force within our life and physical body. Our behavior determines the degree to which the life force flows through us, whether we imbibe the life force abundantly or engage in behaviors that diminish the flow of qi within us.

We control the qi in the body by our thinking, daily activity, dietary patterns, exercise habits, and our emotional condition. Each of these areas of life causes us to be in a state of balance or excessive contraction or excessive expansion. For example, fear causes muscle contraction. When muscles contract, they prevent the optimal flow of blood and lymph, which means that cells are deprived essential oxygen, nutrients, immune cells, and proteins. When lymph is blocked, waste accumulates in tissues, causing the basis for disease. Chronic fear causes these conditions to be maintained over time, which means that fear can be the basis for disease. The same is true of anger or hysteria or any other extreme emotional state. Blood, lymph, and qi flow optimally in a balanced emotional condition.

ACUPUNCTURE: PATHWAYS OF HEALING

According to the Chinese system, qi flows through the body in fourteen distinct patterns, known as meridians. When qi flows abundantly through these meridians, the body receives optimal amounts of life force. Consequently, the organs function to their peak efficiency, which means that the body has abundant energy and vitality, is able to eliminate waste products, and maintains a strong immune function. It sustains health and wards off disease. When qi is diminished in one or another part of the body, the organ or tissue begins to function less efficiently, which means that the organ is easily fatigued and waste products accumulate. These include carbon dioxide, cellular debris, environmental pollutants, and free radicals, or the breakdown of cells. The body becomes less effective at eliminating toxins and carcinogens from the diet. Fat and cholesterol accumulate in tissues, arteries, and cells. Free radicals become more numerous, causing aging, degeneration of cells and tissues, and ultimately triggering a life-threatening disorder, such as heart attack, stroke, or cancer.

The end result of this process is a disease that Westerners believe is the actual problem. However, when seen from the Chinese perspective, the disease is the end result—the fruit, you might say—of a long process of degeneration that began with the diminution of the life force, or qi. The Chinese maintain that if qi flow is restored, health can be restored as well. Therefore, Chinese healers treat disease by boosting the flow of qi to the diseased part of the body. They particularly focus their healing efforts on certain organs and tissues, which may have deficient or excessive qi, and try to bring these organs into balance.

Among the primary tools Chinese healers use to boost qi flow is acupuncture. Since Western science has no unifying theory for the human body nor of health and illness, the notion of qi flow is extremely foreign. Therefore, there is no basis in the Western mind for understanding how acupuncture might work. Western scientists have demonstrated the effectiveness of acupuncture in the laboratory using animals and humans. Despite the remarkable results of acupuncture, no Western theory exists for how it might work. Part of the problem is orthodox medicine's rejection of the Chinese medical model, which explains acupuncture theory.

Acupuncture theory maintains that in addition to the fourteen distinct channels of energy that pass in orderly patterns throughout the body, there are thousands of tiny points on these meridians that serve as portals of energy, and even as generators of qi. These acupuncture points can be stimulated with needles or with the use of pressure (as with acupressure) to promote the flow of qi along the meridian to specific organs or tissues of the body. Healing occurs when qi flow is increased or balanced in specific parts of the body.

Recently, new research at American universities has demonstrated that electromagnetic energy does indeed flow along these discreet meridian lines, just as the Chinese have been saying, and by stimulating acupuncture points, the electromagnetic energy that flows along these lines is increased.

Among the leaders in this field of research is Robert Becker, M.D., an orthopedic surgeon and former professor at the State University of New York (SUNY). Becker, author of the book *Cross Currents: The Perils of Electropollution; The Promise of Electromedicine* (Jeremy P. Tarcher, 1990), has demonstrated that physical healing is associated with an increase in electromagnetic energy flowing to diseased or injured parts of the body. He and his colleagues have attached sensitive electrodes to the body and measured increased electromagnetic charges flowing along meridian lines after a specific acupuncture point has been stimulated. Becker has shown that a variety of techniques can boost the body's underlying electrical currents, which in turn strengthens the body's healing functions, including the immune, endocrine, and nervous systems. Included among these techniques are acupuncture, certain dietary practices, and therapeutic touch.

In his book *Cross Currents,* Dr. Becker reports: "We found that about 25 percent of the acupuncture points on the human forearm did exist, in that they had specific, reproducible, and significant electrical parameters and could be found in all subjects tested. Next, we looked at the meridians that seemed to connect these points. We found that these meridians had the electrical characteristics of transmission lines, while nonmeridian skin did not."

Becker and others have shown that the immune system is strengthened by boosting the electromagnetic energy that flows along these meridians.

STAGES OF MOVEMENT: THE THEORY OF THE FIVE ELEMENTS

Energy moves throughout the body in a precise pattern, according to the Chinese, much like the integrated circuitry of a computer. This pattern of energetic movement takes place in the human body and throughout nature. For the Chinese, the pattern is really how change occurs. Energy is moving from one stage to the next in a very orderly way. The theory can be applied to any aspect of nature: the seasons, for example, or the human body. In the case of the body, the energy moves in a continuous circuit, a kind of loop, unifying all the organs and making them mutually interdependent. The Chinese called this pattern of this energetic movement the theory of the five elements.

The theory of the five elements is one of the fundamental healing tools of traditional Chinese medicine. It dates back some 2,500 years to the first book of medicine, *The Yellow Emperor's Classic of Internal Medicine.* The Chinese used the concept of the five elements in virtually every aspect of life, from understanding the stages of change to restoring balance within the body and

The Theory of the Five Elements

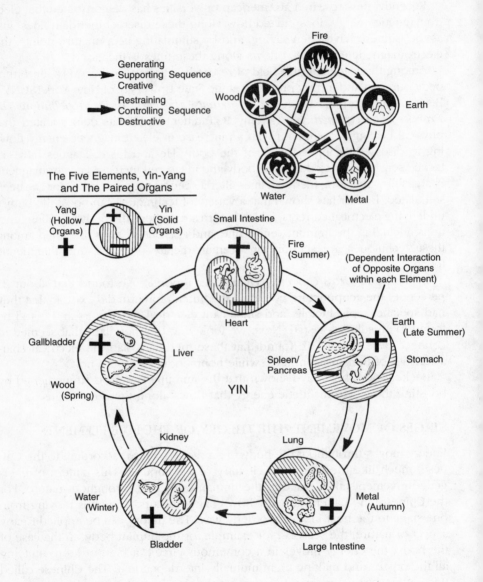

The Five Elements and The Seasonal/Daily Cycles

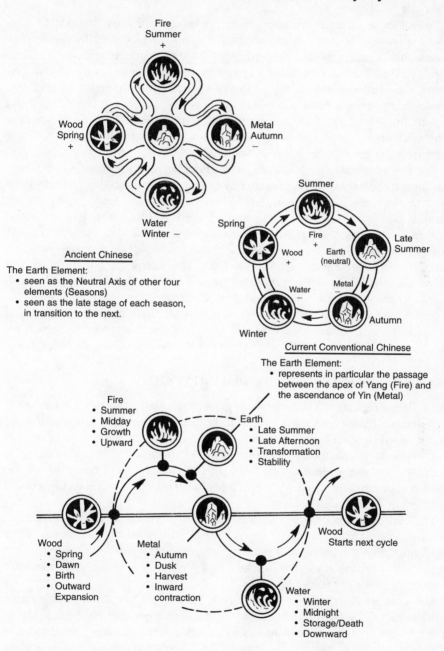

Fire
Summer
+

Wood
Spring
+

Metal
Autumn
−

Water
Winter −

<u>Ancient Chinese</u>

The Earth Element:
- seen as the Neutral Axis of other four elements (Seasons)
- seen as the late stage of each season, in transition to the next.

Summer

Spring

Fire
+

Wood
+

Earth
(neutral)

Late
Summer

Water
−

Metal
−

Winter

Autumn

<u>Current Conventional Chinese</u>

The Earth Element:
- represents in particular the passage between the apex of Yang (Fire) and the ascendance of Yin (Metal)

Fire
- Summer
- Midday
- Growth
- Upward

Earth
- Late Summer
- Late Afternoon
- Transformation
- Stability

Wood
- Spring
- Dawn
- Birth
- Outward
  Expansion

Metal
- Autumn
- Dusk
- Harvest
- Inward
  contraction

Wood
Starts next cycle

Water
- Winter
- Midnight
- Storage/Death
- Downward

derstanding the stages of change to restoring balance within the body and healing it of disease.

The Chinese viewed change as taking five steps, or movements. The Chinese expression of the five elements is *wu xing,* which literally means *five movements.* Unfortunately, Western scholars didn't understand the Chinese system and instead of calling the Chinese system the theory of the five movements, they called it the theory of the five elements, reducing it to primitive suspicion and prescientific thought.

Actually, the Chinese are among the most sophisticated the earth has ever witnessed, and their philosophical approach to life has been worked out over thousands of years under rigorous scrutiny.

The five elements (we'll use the more familiar term) represent five stages that are characteristic of all change. As a tool for healing, the Chinese used the five elements to understand and chart how the life force, or qi, moves through the body. The body is an integrated whole, unified by an ever-present flow of energy that is itself joined with the creator of the universe. As a living energy, the life force has all the characteristics of the human body and mind. Indeed, the Chinese see the life force as creating the human body and maintaining its life by supporting the physical body with what it needs most: energy to sustain all its biological and psychological functions.

Rather than describe the five elements in all their permutations, which would require a whole book, we will give you the short version, which relates to the Chinese use of food to promote the health of specific organs.

ORGAN PAIRS, SEASONS, AND HEALING FOODS

The Chinese recognized that certain organs have related functions, such as the liver and gallbladder, or the kidneys and bladder. They also saw that the life force flowed in such a way that certain organs were unified and far more dependent upon one another than others were. The health of the stomach, for example, was dependent upon the health of the spleen. The health of the heart was dependent upon the small intestine. This contributed to their belief that certain organs were paired.

The early sages coupled organs as related and joined them with a particular element in nature, such as wood or fire, and a particular season. They maintained that the element of nature represented the nature of the particular organ pair, and the season was when that pair of organs received the most amount of qi, or life force.

The Chinese discovered that during each season, a particular set of organs was nourished by the life force to a far greater extent than the other organs of the body. This meant that the organ pair that received the optimal amount of energy during that particular season had a great opportunity to be healed. Conversely, if one abused that particular organ pair during that season, it also had a greater likelihood of manifesting a symptom.

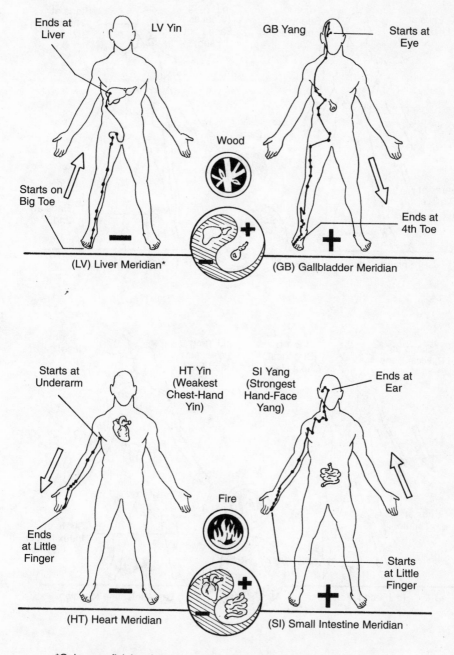

Ends at Liver

LV Yin

GB Yang

Starts at Eye

Wood

Starts on Big Toe

−

Ends at 4th Toe

(LV) Liver Meridian*   +   (GB) Gallbladder Meridian

Starts at Underarm

HT Yin (Weakest Chest-Hand Yin)

SI Yang (Strongest Hand-Face Yang)

Ends at Ear

Fire

Ends at Little Finger

−

Starts at Little Finger

(HT) Heart Meridian   +   (SI) Small Intestine Meridian

*Only superficial pathways are shown/applies to both sides of the body

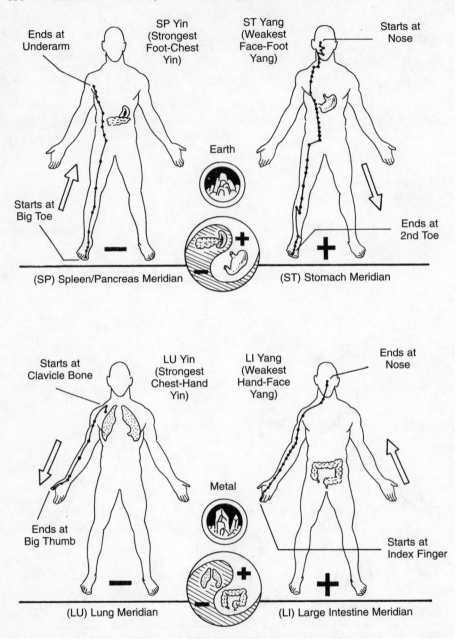

Ends at Underarm

SP Yin (Strongest Foot-Chest Yin)

ST Yang (Weakest Face-Foot Yang)

Starts at Nose

Earth

Starts at Big Toe

Ends at 2nd Toe

(SP) Spleen/Pancreas Meridian

(ST) Stomach Meridian

Starts at Clavicle Bone

LU Yin (Strongest Chest-Hand Yin)

LI Yang (Weakest Hand-Face Yang)

Ends at Nose

Metal

Ends at Big Thumb

Starts at Index Finger

(LU) Lung Meridian

(LI) Large Intestine Meridian

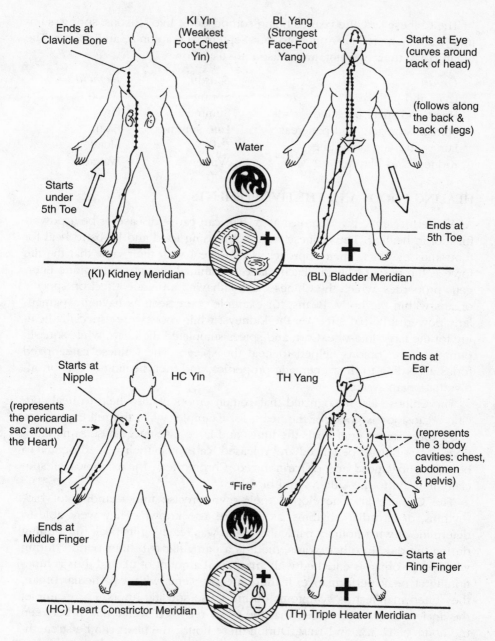

Ends at Clavicle Bone

KI Yin (Weakest Foot-Chest Yin)

Starts under 5th Toe

Water

(KI) Kidney Meridian

BL Yang (Strongest Face-Foot Yang)

Starts at Eye (curves around back of head)

(follows along the back & back of legs)

Ends at 5th Toe

(BL) Bladder Meridian

Starts at Nipple

HC Yin

(represents the pericardial sac around the Heart)

Ends at Middle Finger

"Fire"

(HC) Heart Constrictor Meridian

Ends at Ear

TH Yang

(represents the 3 body cavities: chest, abdomen & pelvis)

Starts at Ring Finger

(TH) Triple Heater Meridian

(These two Meridians have no corresponding visceral structures; compare with Fire Network)

The Chinese saw the year as being composed of five seasons: spring, summer, late summer (late August to late September), autumn, and winter. The organ pairs, their element, and season are as follows:

Organ	Season	Element
Liver and gallbladder	Spring	Wood
Heart and small intestine	Summer	Fire
Spleen, stomach, and pancreas	Late summer	Earth
Lungs and large intestine	Fall	Metal
Kidneys and bladder	Winter	Water

HEALING FOODS AND THE FIVE ELEMENTS

As Western science has demonstrated, diet can cause disease or be a powerful tool in healing. The Chinese have been using food and herbs to heal for thousands of years. Their approach is consistent with their view that the life force is the basis of health. Each plant and animal has its own unique energetic properties, which the Chinese saw as having a unique effect on specific organs within the body. Beans, for example, were seen as having a particularly powerful herbal effect on the kidneys, while roots were especially healing for the large intestine. Corn and spices stimulated the heart, while squash, pumpkin, and onions helped to heal the spleen. The Chinese categorized foods according to their energetic properties, and their healing effects on individual organ systems.

The Chinese also recognized that certain emotions also help to heal specific organs: joy is good for the heart, for example, while the full experience and expression of grief heals the lungs and large intestine. These same emotions, if not fully experienced and released, can cause their related organs to become imbalanced and disharmonized. Chronic fear, for example, is especially harmful to the kidneys and bladder.

The Chinese also developed their own precise understanding of biorhythms, or circadian rhythms, as they are also known. They were able to determine at what hours a particular organ was reaching its peak functioning during the day. In other words, there is a particular two-hour period during which each organ is enriched with an optimal amount of qi, and thus is functioning at peak performance. If there are problems with a particular organ, they often manifest as symptoms during these specific hours. For example, the ancient sages maintained that the heart received additional qi between the hours of 11 A.M. and 1 P.M. During these hours, the heart can be strengthened significantly. But if there is heart disease, the symptoms will tend to manifest in the morning hours, and become more intense as the time moves closer to 11 A.M. The reason is simply that with the ever-increasing qi building within the heart, the organ itself is under increasing stress as the time builds toward a peak near noon. And indeed, as any cardiologist will tell you,

The 14 Chinese Meridians

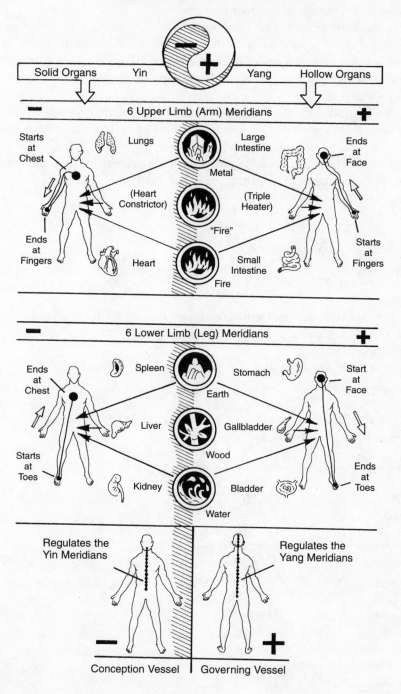

builds toward a peak near noon. And indeed, as any cardiologist will tell you, most heart attacks occur in the morning hours.

Just as there are peak hours, so too are there low periods in which each organ is receiving the least amount of qi during the day. For example, the heart receives the least amount of qi twelve hours earlier, at 11 P.M. Symptoms can manifest as well during the hours when the energy flowing to a particular organ wanes.

In order to heal individual organs, Oriental healers created acupuncture, acupressure, and offered a vast armamentarium of foods, herbs, and even specific tastes that were used to restore health.

The five element theory, the organ pairs, their related natures, elements, seasons, emotions, time of day they are being most stimulated, and their related healing foods are as follows:

Wood

Nature: tree (strong rising energy)
Season: spring
Organs: liver, gallbladder
Color: green/blue
Emotion: anger (anger and irritability injure the liver; when balanced, excellent tolerance)
Sound: shouting
Flavor: sour (mildly sour things stimulate the liver/gallbladder)
Head part: eyes
Sense: vision
Time of day receiving most abundant energy: gallbladder: 11 P.M. to 1 A.M.; liver: 1 A.M. to 3 A.M.

Foods that enhance the wood element:

Wheat	String beans
Oats	Carrots
Rye	Lima beans
Broccoli	Green lentils
Parsley	Split peas
Lettuce	Summer squash
Alfalfa	Zucchini
Grapefruit	Limes
Plum	Quince
Green apple	Orange
Sour cherry	Lemon
Avocados	Sauerkraut

Fire

Nature: fire (peak rising energy)
Season: summer
Organs: heart and small intestine
Color: red stimulates the organs and helps to heal them.
Emotion: joy, when balanced; hysteria, when excessive
Sound: laughing
Flavor: bitter and slightly burnt (such as the edge of toast)
Head part: tongue
Sense: smell
Time of day: heart: 11 A.M. to 1 P.M.; small intestine: 1 P.M. to 3 P.M.

Foods that enhance the fire element:

Corn	Chicory
Popcorn	Dandelion
Amaranth	Red lentil
Asparagus	Shrimp
Brussels sprouts	Spices
Chives	Raspberry
Endive	Persimmon
Okra	Chocolate (caffeine)
Scallions	Apricot
Guava	Strawberry
Beer	Wine (red)
Coffee	Tobacco

When fire is excessive, the person is often overly emotional and given to hysterical outbursts; reduce fire foods, especially spices. When there is a lack of joy and poor circulation, increase fire foods and reduce water foods.

Earth

Nature: soil (very stable)
Season: late summer
Organs: stomach, spleen, and pancreas
Color: yellow
Emotion: sympathy, compassion, understanding
Sound: singing and humming
Flavor: sweet
Head part: mouth (inside, especially saliva)
Sense: taste
Function: imagination; ideas
Time of day: spleen/pancreas: 9 A.M. to 11 A.M.; stomach: 7 A.M. to 9 A.M.

Foods that enhance the earth element:

Millet'	Sweet corn
Squash	Parsnips
Acorn	Rutabaga
Hubbard	Collards
Buttercup	Chard
Butternut	Artichoke
Hokkaido	Cantaloupe
Spaghetti	Banana
Pumpkin	Honeydew
Shiitake mushrooms	Papaya
Apple, sweet	Dates
Figs	Tangerine
Orange, sweet	Raisins
Tangelo	Sweet grapes

Herbs: licorice; anise
Nuts: almonds, pecans, macadamia
Fish: salmon, tuna, swordfish, sturgeon
Sweeteners: maple syrup, yinnie rice syrup, barley malt

Sugar, sweet wines, and other highly sweet foods will injure the earth element. Among the symptoms of a troubled spleen are indigestion, gas, acidic stomach, and heartburn.

Remedy: Reduce or eliminate all sweet foods, especially sugars; eat more alkalizing foods, such as umeboshi plum or pickles. Chew food thoroughly, thirty-five to fifty times per mouthful, minimum. Swallow saliva. Two or three drops of shoyu in kukicha (bancha) tea is recommended to settle the stomach.

Metal

Nature: cool, strong descending energy
Season: fall
Organs: lungs, large intestine
Color: white
Emotion: grief
Sound: weeping quality, especially in voice
Flavor: pungent
Head part: nose
Sense: touch
Time of day: lungs: 3 A.M. to 5 A.M.; large intestine: 5 A.M. to 7 A.M.
Function: establishing rhythm and order in daily life; controls animal
  nature

Foods that enhance the metal element:

Brown rice	Celery
Sweet rice	Chinese cabbage
Potatoes	Gingerroot
Mochi	Turnips
Cabbage	Garlic
Cauliflower	Turnip greens
Daikon radishes	Cucumber
Onions	Watercress
Mustard greens	Radishes
Cinnamon	Dill, fennel, nutmeg, thyme
Horseradish	Black pepper

Fish: cod, haddock, herring, scrod, flounder, halibut, perch

When the large intestine is disorderly, slightly increase metal foods, wood foods, and water foods; decrease or eliminate sugar and alcohol. Chew very well, 50 to 100 times per mouthful.

Water

Nature: beginning ascent; upward energy; highly flexible; moving forward constantly
Season: winter
Organs: kidney, bladder
Color: black, brown, dark blue
Emotion (psychological nature): the will; perseverance
Sound: groaning
Flavor: salty
Head part: ears
Sense: hearing
Time of day: bladder: 3 P.M. to 5 P.M.; kidneys: 5 P.M. to 7 P.M.

Kidneys nourish sexual vitality and sex organs.

Foods that enhance the water element:

Barley	Buckwheat
Adzuki beans	Burdock
All other beans	Blackberries
Beets	Blueberries
Dulse	Purple grapes
Arame	Watermelon
Irish moss	Black raspberries
Kelp	Chestnuts
Nori	Wakame
Kombu	Hijiki

Tempeh, considered a metal food, will have a strengthening effect on kidneys and sex organs when fried and eaten occasionally.

Salty foods, especially:

Pickles
Tamari and shoyu
Miso
Tekka
Gamasio
Fish: Bluefish, crab, lobster, caviar, scallops

When kidneys are troubled, reduce or eliminate fat and cholesterol foods; use only small amounts of salt in cooking (a pinch); avoid salt as a condiment; avoid salty foods; eat more water foods. Avoid sugar and reduce earth foods.

CONCLUSION

The Chinese model for healing represents a very different type of thinking from that which we are used to in the West, yet more and more Westerners are turning to Chinese medicine and acupuncture for relief from disease. Most of us are more interested in whether or not the system works rather than how it works. Nevertheless, the reasons are important, because it challenges us to reexamine our worldview and to question if there isn't more to healing—and to life—than what we currently perceive.

EXERCISE

The first thing you need to know about exercise is that a little bit goes a long way. You do not have to become a well-trained athlete to benefit from exercise. Nor should you drive your body too hard. The greatest benefit comes from moderate exercise. That does not have to be any more than thirty to forty minutes of walking four or five times per week. That's all.

Walking is an aerobic exercise, meaning that it increases the amount of oxygen that flows to cells throughout the body. There are many forms of aerobic exercises—walking, running, bicycling, swimming, tennis, basketball, cross-country skiing, and jumping—and many benefits from these exercises. All increase the flow of oxygen to your heart, brain, and other organs.

They also improve the efficiency of your heart, which means that your heart pumps more blood per beat. By causing the heart to beat faster, exercise causes the heart's beating action—the expansion and contraction—to become more coordinated. In this way, the heart is able to take in more blood during its expansive phase, or diastole, and pump greater quantities of blood in the contractive phase, or systole. The net effect of this is to give the heart more time in between beats, and therefore more time spent resting. The average man's heart beats at a rate of seventy-two beats per minute, the average woman's at seventy-six beats per minute. As heart rate slows down, the time between beats is extended. The difference between sixty and ninety beats per minute is that, at sixty beats, the heart rests twice as long between beats.

Exercise raises HDL (the good cholesterol) levels, which significantly reduces your risk of heart disease and stroke. Exercise lowers blood pressure, too. It does this in part by opening blood vessels throughout the body and by creating new blood vessels to accommodate the increased amount of blood flowing to cells.

Exercise reduces the stickiness between blood platelets, which causes sludging of the blood and diminishes blood flow. (Exercise will not lower your cholesterol level or reverse atherosclerosis, however; only your low-fat, low-cholesterol diet will do that.)

Studies have shown that moderate exercise boosts the immune system and protects against cancer. Any exercise that involves the legs, such as walking or bicycling, improves circulation because the leg muscles act as auxiliary pumps. They are the body's secondary hearts. Their expansion and contraction causes blood to be pumped through the vessels and back to the heart. This substantially reduces the burden on the heart.

Exercise also improves circulation to the brain and helps to dissolve blood clots throughout the body that might otherwise cause a heart attack or stroke. Exercise increases the body's demand for fuel and thus burns stored calories,

Exercise: The Muscular System

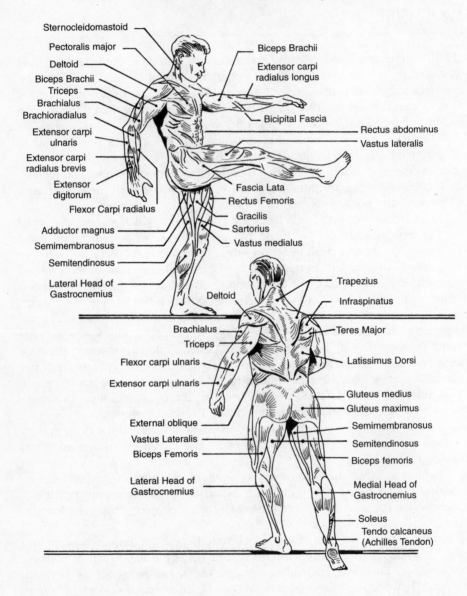

which, of course, means fat. Thus, it reduces weight. It also stretches muscles and speeds elimination of carbon dioxide, uric acid, and other waste products now stored in your tissues.

Exercise strengthens bones in two ways: first, it increases bone growth and mass; second, it strengthens muscles; stronger muscles take the stress off bones. Exercise has been shown to decrease the number of bone fractures and prevent osteoporosis.

Muscles and bones that are not exercised begin to atrophy. One of the major causes of osteoporosis is a sedentary lifestyle, or the lack of exercise.

IT MAKES THE MUSCLE BETWEEN THE EARS STRONGER, TOO

The benefits of exercise to the mind are also well documented. The natural high runners talk about is the secretion of beta-endorphins in the brain. These morphinelike chemicals cause a deep sense of well-being and are a natural antidote to depression and anxiety. Beta-endorphins are produced after only twenty minutes of running or brisk walking.

THE GREATEST EXERCISE OF ALL

"I have met but one or two persons in the course of my life who understood the art of walking, that is, of taking walks—who had a genius, so to speak, for sauntering," noted Henry David Thoreau in his essay "Walking."

Humans were built to walk. It is the best exercise there is and it is free for the taking. It should not even be called exercise, for exercise is a modern word that separates us from the joy of this, a human's most natural means of locomotion. For those who are not handicapped, walking is a blessing.

Still, walking is a wonderful exercise, and a half hour's worth of walking conditions the entire body. With arms swinging and legs stepping freely according to your own pace, you are exercising your muscles, heart, and respiratory and circulatory systems without even thinking of the fact that you are exercising. Walking seems to lighten the load; it provides perspective while it works off the tension generated by stressful thoughts.

Walking in nature is the ideal because the trees and plants pump out so much oxygen and provide a healing and relaxing atmosphere. The calm of nature is infectious. It soothes the body and mind; walking in nature provides a kind of massage for the soul.

If you cannot walk in a local park or wood, you can still lose yourself on the city streets or by trekking around your own block. Walk at a brisk pace, but do not go beyond your capacity. Rest whenever you need to, and follow by taking up a pace that is comfortable. Walking briskly is not jogging or running. Brisk walks are those that maintain a pace just beyond a comfortable stroll. As your conditioning improves, you can increase your speed. Start out slowly and work up to a faster pace as you gain conditioning and confidence.

WALKING MAY WELL EXTEND YOUR LIFE

In November 1989, the *Journal of the American Medical Association* reported a study conducted by the Institute for Aerobic Research in Dallas in which 13,344 men and women were followed for eight years to determine what effect, if any, fitness had on mortality rates. The participants were divided into five groups, from least fit to most fit. The least fit did no exercise at all; the second level only walked; the next three levels participated in various sports or physical fitness programs. The fifth group, for example, were marathoners. Fitness was measured by having each participant walk on a treadmill. People were categorized into levels of fitness according to how well they performed on the treadmill test.

After eight years of following the participants, the scientists discovered that death rates were dramatically higher among the least fit—the people whose only exercise was to get up from the couch to flip the television channels around. Naturally, the scientists expected that the greatest difference in mortality would exist between the first group (the nonactive people) and the marathoners, since they would be the most fit.

What they found, however, was surprising. The greatest difference in mortality rates existed between the people who were least fit and those who were in the next, or second level of fitness, the people whose only exercise was to walk four or five times per week. When the scientists compared the first and second groups, they found that the death rate was three times higher among the least fit than those in the second level of fitness. They found only small differences in mortality rates between the second, third, fourth, and fifth groups. In other words, the scientists discovered that a small amount of exercise—walking—created enormous differences in health and longevity.

"Even modest amounts of exercise can substantially reduce a person's chances of dying" of heart disease, cancer, and other illnesses, reported the November 3, 1989, *New York Times*.

"This is a hopeful message, an important message for the American people to understand," Dr. Carl Caspersen of the Federal Centers for Disease Control told the *New York Times*. "You don't have to be a marathoner. In fact, you get much more benefit out of being just a bit more active. For example, going from being sedentary to walking briskly for a half hour several days a week can drop your risk dramatically."

GET CHECKED OUT BEFORE YOU START A PROGRAM

Before you begin any type of demanding exercise program, you should know the condition of your health, especially your cardiovascular system. That requires blood pressure, cholesterol, and EKG tests. People who are moderately obese or have high cholesterol, hypertension, smoke cigarettes, have abnormal EKGs, or a history of heart disease should have a medical checkup. Also, change your diet to lower fat and cholesterol before you begin any type of strenuous exercise program. The more fat and cholesterol in your diet, the greater your risk of heart attack or stroke. That risk increases as you exercise, especially for people who take up running, basketball, or some other competitive sport.

A SIMPLE TEST TO SEE IMPROVEMENT IN YOUR CONDITIONING

Exercise experts tell us that there's a simple self-test to assure you that you are exercising enough to improve your conditioning. The self-test is as follows:

Conditioning improves when your heart beats at 80 percent of your maximum heart rate, per minute. You can find out your maximum heart rate by subtracting your age from 220. If you are 40 years old, your maximum heart rate would be 180. Eighty percent of that would be 148 beats per minute. Any exercise that gets your heart rate up to 148 beats per minute is causing you to improve your muscular and cardiovascular conditioning.

An easier test—and one that is safe—is that you should be able to carry on a conversation while you are walking. If you can't talk while walking, rest and stop exerting yourself to that level. People who are not in good health should avoid stressing their heart unduly. However, any type of walking, even strolling, will be enough to improve your health.

The beauty of walking is that very few people go beyond their capacity. Consequently, walking rarely causes any real discomfort or serious side effects. For example, heart attacks while walking are rare but are much more frequent while running.

WEIGHT TRAINING

Weight training is no longer for body builders alone. According to research done at MIT, people well into their nineties can benefit by using weights, either the small hand weights or various equipment, such as Nautilus. The benefits from weight training include stronger muscles, stronger and more flexible ligaments and tendons, stronger bones and greater bone density (thus preventing osteoporosis and other skeletal injuries), increased rate of metabolism (which causes greater weight loss, even while resting), increased stamina and strength, and higher HDL levels (which protect against heart disease and stroke).

TEN IDEAS FOR STARTING AN EXERCISE PROGRAM AND KEEPING IT GOING

1. Make your intention clear. All you're looking for is fun. Remember that the best exercise is fun. Unless your intention is to become a highly conditioned, competitive athlete, your true goal is to enjoy your life. Being fit is a way to better enjoy your body and your life in general. Becoming fit shouldn't be painful or unpleasant. We all are little children at heart and the last thing

we want to do with our leisure hours is torture our bodies. Such things rarely last, as most of us have learned at one time or another. Instead, eat well and have fun. Your appearance will improve dramatically, without effort, and the glow of your smile will attract friends and lovers from near and far.

2. Pick a safe place and time to walk and do it at least four times a week. It's free, it doesn't require a partner, and the only equipment you need are some comfortable shoes and loose clothing.

3. Walk with a friend. Walking is cheap therapy. Walk with your spouse, friend, or lover and get to know each other better. Also, someone from your neighborhood might love to get into a routine of walking at a particular hour of the day.

4. Take up dancing. Aerobic dancing was the craze during the 1980s and is still available to nearly everyone. Begin slowly, and gradually increase the level of intensity as your conditioning improves. Do not tax yourself excessively, especially in the beginning.

5. Join a club. Lots of towns have organized nature walks and hiking clubs. Walking with others is a chance to make new friends and have fun while you are exercising. Consult your local recreation department for organizations that provide regular walking clubs or hiking programs. Join the YMCA or YWCA. The YMCA or YWCA provides everything from swimming to basketball to volleyball to hiking. Call the Y or drop by and talk to the nice people there about the programs being offered and see what works for you. Private instructors offer ongoing classes in yoga, stretching, and other forms of exercise. These clubs and classes are usually very inexpensive and are great ways to socialize while you exercise. Consult the newspaper or your town's recreation department for the whereabouts and times for such classes.

If you can afford it and you are sufficiently fit, join a fitness, racquetball, tennis, or golf club or take lessons in one or another of these sports.

6. Ride a bike. One of the greatest and most enjoyable exercises you will ever experience on this earth is bicycling. It is highly aerobic. It can also be a very demanding conditioning program. People are advised to start out slowly and gradually work up to greater distances or hillier terrains.

Before you buy a bicycle, talk to someone who knows bikes. Tell him or her where you will be riding most of the time—in parks, on paved roads, or off the road. The bike shop person will fit you correctly for a bike, depending on your height and weight. Once you've got a bicycle, start out on flat terrain and avoid hills or irregular surfaces until you've grown stronger and more accustomed to riding.

Bicycling is addictive; once you get into the habit of bike riding, you'll be out every morning or evening, weather permitting, of course.

7. If not a two-wheeler, then ride a stationary bike. Stationary bikes are among the most popular forms of exercise available today. One of the benefits of a stationary bike is that you don't have to look where you are going. People who use stationary bikes often listen to music or self-help tapes, watch television, or meditate themselves into tranquillity.

8. Avoid competitive games, especially if you are out of shape. If you are new to exercise, it's wise to avoid competitive games because people often forget themselves in the heat of battle. The consequence for many is a fatal heart attack. If you take up tennis or some other strenuous game, see a physician first and engage in some other less strenuous exercise program, such as brisk walking, to improve your conditioning before you engage in any competitive sport.

Beginning tennis players should spend a few weeks volleying and allowing the body to get used to the demands of exercise. Volleying will condition your heart and body and will be lots of fun. Also, begin each session with a set of warm-up exercises, especially stretching.

People who are out of shape can enjoy a variety of exercises grounded in Oriental philosophy, such as do-in, a self-massage technique, or tai chi chuan, a martial art that is performed as a beautiful and graceful dance. Classes are provided for these and other meditative exercises in many cities and towns. Consult your Yellow Pages, or call your recreation department or an adult education department at a local college.

9. Before you begin, warm up. It only takes ten minutes to flex and stretch your muscles and joints, but it will protect your body from injury and make it easier for you to walk or exercise longer.

10. Begin slowly, and gradually increase your pace. Start off at a leisurely pace. Don't go running off to the races, lest you burn out before you even begin. Keep in mind that you are trying to enjoy yourself. As your body adapts to the exercise, gradually increase your pace. This protects you against injury and will diminish pain (such as angina or leg pain). When you feel angina pain, ease up or stop walking altogether. Rest awhile and continue.

Remember that when you finish your exercise, you should feel better than you did when you started, not worse. There are lots of ways to be physically fit, and most of them can be fun. In fact, the only way to be fit is to maintain your program consistently, and the only way to maintain consistency is to enjoy yourself.

A GUIDE TO SUPPLEMENTS

There is growing debate over the use of supplements and their effects on health. Recent research reported in the *New England Journal of Medicine* and elsewhere has demonstrated that supplements, especially those in high doses, may not provide protection against certain diseases and may even increase the vulnerability of some people to cancer.

On the other hand, other studies have shown that when supplements have been used in small doses—enough to reach the recommended daily allowances (RDA)—they had significant immune-boosting effects. In the interests of protecting your health, we have taken a conservative approach in this book. We have recommended that large doses of supplements not be used. Rather, when taking a supplement, we urge people to take a dose closer to the RDA, or the amount you would get in a healthy and balanced diet.

In making this decision, we have also taken into account several factors and talked to some of the more preeminent scientists in the fields of nutrition and disease prevention. Allow us to list some of our reasons for asking our readers to take smaller doses of vitamins, minerals, and other supplements.

First, throughout this book, we have tried to provide a traditional approach to healing. The use of vitamin and mineral pills is a very modern phenomenon, taking place largely in this century. No one knows as yet what effects taking large doses of vitamins and minerals have on the human body. The preliminary research is mixed at best, but important studies have suggested ominous possibilities.

The most troubling report came when the *New England Journal of Medicine* (330:1029–1035, 1994) reported that cigarette smokers who took supplements of vitamin E and beta-carotene actually had higher rates of lung cancer than those who avoided the supplements. Conversely, the study reported that those men who smoked cigarettes but got these same vitamins from a diet richer in vitamin E and beta-carotene than the controls actually had lower rates of cancer. A follow-up letter to the *New England Journal of Medicine* stated the obvious conclusion nicely. Said the writer: One may draw the conclusion from this study that "it is better to obtain nutritionally active substances such as vitamin E and beta-carotene from the grocery store than from the pharmacy."

Renowned cancer researcher Bruce Ames, Ph.D., at the University of California at Berkeley, agreed. Ames pointed to the plethora of nutrients that are included in foods that also boost immune function and fight cancer. Many of these nutrients have not been well understood, nor are they available in supplement form. Said Ames: "What is clear is that fruits and vegetables contain many necessary micronutrients in addition to antioxidants, some of which can also prevent mutations. Folic acid, for example, is required for the synthesis of the nucleotides in DNA. Inadequate intake has been shown to cause chromosome breaks and increased cancer and birth defects. . . . Folate deficiency may be a risk factor for myocardial infarction [heart attack]. Niacin is required for making poly(ADP-ribose), a component of DNA repair. Other micronutrients are also likely to be part of our defense systems."

In short, an emphasis upon supplements as a panacea or even as a healthful drug may be misplaced, simply because we know so little about individual nutrients and their synergistic effects at this point.

"Take beta-carotene, for example," said Dr. William Pryor, a pioneer antioxidant researcher and director of the Biodynamics Research Institute at the University of Louisiana at Baton Rouge. "Actually, beta-carotene is one of hundreds of chemicals called *carotenoids* that color food. A single vegetable can contain many carotenoids, and beta-carotene may be the least powerful immune booster among them. We simply don't know what the other carotenoids do yet."

In this book, we have tried to emphasize food, herbs, and other natural remedies, without leaving out the use of supplements, which can still play an important role in healing. A good guide to the use of supplements may be a study published in the British medical journal *The Lancet* (November 11, 1992), in which scientists used supplements to boost the immune systems of patients sixty-six years old and older.

The seniors were divided into two groups, one of which was given a placebo (a pill containing some calcium and magnesium), while the experimental group was given supplements containing the following nutrients:

- Vitamin A (400 IU)
- Beta-carotene (16 mg)
- Thiamine (2.2 mg)
- Riboflavin (1.5 mg)
- Niacin (16 mg)
- Vitamin B_6 (3.0 mg)
- Folate (400 mcg)
- Vitamin B_{12} (4.0 mcg)
- Vitamin C (80 mg)
- Vitamin D (4 mcg)
- Vitamin E (44 mg)
- Iron (16 mg)
- Zinc (14 mg)
- Copper (1.4 mg)
- Selenium (20 mcg)
- Iodine (0.2 mg)
- Calcium (200 mg)
- Magnesium (100 mg)

Both groups were followed for one year. The researchers found that the supplemented group had significantly fewer infections and sick days during that year than the placebo group. The supplemented group suffered a total of twenty-three sick days, as compared to forty-eight sick days recorded by the placebo group. Blood tests revealed that the supplemented group had stronger immune responses to antigens and a greater number of circulating macrophages and other immune cells.

Moreover, these benefits were accomplished on relatively small doses of nutrient supplementation. As the researchers point out, "It is important to note that large-dose supplements were not used; indeed, very large doses of many micronutrients may impair immunity."

With that in mind, we encourage you to experiment with supplements, but do it in small amounts.

SUPPLEMENT GUIDE

ACEROLA is the tart, cherrylike fruit of a small tree (*Malpighia glabra*) of the West Indies and adjacent areas, used by supplement makers for its high concentration of vitamin C. It is also called Barbados cherry and Puerto Rican cherry. Most vitamin C supplements fortify acerola-derived vitamin C and other natural sources of vitamin C with synthetic vitamin C. It is sold in tablet form.

BETA-CAROTENE is a vegetable-based precursor to vitamin A widely taken for its antioxidant, wound-healing, vision-enhancing, and cancer-preventing properties. It is an antioxidant and a highly effective immune-booster. Studies have shown that beta-carotene makes immune cells (such as macrophages) more effective against infection, heart disease, and cancer. It increases the number of CD4 and natural killer cells and boosts production of antibodies. It is as effective as preformed, meat-based vitamin A, yet is safe and nontoxic (unlike vitamin A in high doses). Beta-carotene is found in high concentrations in dark green, leafy vegetables and orange and yellow fruits and vegetables. It is the most bioavailable of the several related carotenoid plant pigments that act as precursors to vitamin A. It's sold as tablets and capsules. (See the description of vitamin A.)

BIOFLAVONOIDS are plant compounds found in citrus fruits; dark green, leafy vegetables; and other typically vitamin C–rich foods. Bioflavonoids play an important role in healing capillaries and helping the body form collagen, which holds body tissue together. The bioflavonoids are also known collectively as vitamin P, or flavonoids. Some of the most common ones include hesperidin, quercetin, and rutin. They are found in high concentrations in certain herbs like ginkgo, hawthorn, and bilberry. Bioflavonoids exhibit a broad range of antioxidant activity and are taken to treat nosebleeds, bleeding gums, and a tendency to bruise. They are sometimes prescribed for allergies, viruses, and inflammations. Often combined in supplements with vitamin C, they're typically found in tablet and capsule form. Studies have shown that flavonoids play a key role in protecting people against the effects of environmental toxins, especially air pollutants. They also protect against cell mutations and cancer.

BORON is a trace mineral found in legumes and some fruit. Boron may be necessary to help prevent bone loss and osteoporosis, possibly by working in conjunction with other bone builders like calcium and magnesium. There is also evidence that it helps prevent arthritis. Boron is often combined with other minerals in tablets and capsules.

BREWER'S YEAST is the dried, pulverized cells of a yeast (*Saccharomyces cerevisiae*) that is taken as a supplement principally because it is high in trace minerals, protein, and a number of the B vitamins. It is so named because it is a by-product of beer making and is similar to (though usually somewhat lower in nutrients than) nutritional yeast, which is grown specifically for human consumption. Brewer's yeast is high in substances known as skin respiratory factor and glucose tolerance factor and thus shows promise in the treatment of wounds, burns, skin problems, and type II diabetes. It is a different form of yeast from that which causes yeast infections (*Candida albicans*) and is not thought to cause yeast-related conditions. It is sold in the form of powder, flakes, and capsules.

CALCIUM is a well-known mineral nutrient that plays an important role in a variety of essential bodily functions, including building bones and teeth, transmitting nerve messages, regulating heartbeat, and coagulating blood. The adult RDA is 800 to 1200 milligrams. It is recommended in the treatment or prevention of osteoporosis, heart disease, problems of menopause, and certain cancers. Taken before bed, calcium may have a slight sedating effect. Supplements are derived from a variety of sources, including dolomite, oyster shells, and bonemeal. It is also produced in different chemical forms, with calcium citrate and calcium carbonate noted for being highly absorbable. Calcium is often combined with magnesium and other minerals. It is available as tablets, capsules, and liquids.

CHOLINE is a nutrient that some nutritionists now consider to be a B-complex vitamin (though no RDA has been established). It plays a role in the metabolism of fats, the working of the nervous system, and the production of neurotransmitters that affect mood and emotions. Choline is synthesized in the body and is present in high concentrations in lecithin, a fatty acid found in egg yolks and soybeans. Choline is necessary for the healthy functioning of cells, nerves, and the brain, and deficiencies have been linked to certain neurologic disorders such as Parkinson's disease and tardive dyskinesia that are characterized by convulsive muscular movements. It may help protect against heart disease and Alzheimer's disease. Choline has been known to cause side effects like depression when taken in large doses. It is available as tablets, capsules, and liquids. (See the description of lecithin in the section on essential fatty acids.)

CHROMIUM is a trace element found in brewer's yeast, organ meats, whole grains, cheese, and nuts. There is no established RDA. In the body, chromium is involved with insulin production and protein synthesis. It works with insulin to promote the metabolism of fats and carbohydrates, including glucose (blood sugar). Chromium deficiencies can cause difficulties in regulating blood sugar. Supplementation of 200 micrograms daily can benefit some type II (adult-onset) diabetics and people suffering from hypoglycemia. Chromium's effects on blood sugar can also spill over to affect fat metabolism and blood cholesterol levels. It thus may help prevent heart disease. Chromium is often combined with cysteine, niacin, and other nutrients to assist in metabolism of blood sugar. It comes in tablets and capsules.

FOLIC ACID, also known as folate and folacin, is a B-complex nutrient that plays a role in the production of red blood cells, DNA synthesis, and protein metabolism. Women in the earliest stages of pregnancy must be sure to get sufficient quantities, since folic acid is necessary for the fetus to develop nerve cells. The name *folic* is derived from the same Latin root as the word *foliage,* and the nutrient is found in highest concentrations in leafy, green vegetables like spinach, chard, and kale. Legumes, root vegetables, brewer's yeast, wheat germ, whole grains, fruits, and liver are also sources of folic acid. The adult RDA is 180 to 200 micrograms. Deficiencies are common throughout the world, partly because the vitamin is easily lost in the refining, cooking, and storing of foods. Symptoms of a deficiency include anemia and neurological problems. Folic acid is used therapeutically to treat cervical dysplasia (a precancerous condition in women), depression and anxiety, and fatigue.

GERMANIUM is a trace mineral and natural element found in soil and in some foods. The mineral itself appears to have limited effects on human health but was recently developed by Japanese researchers into a synthetic organic compound (known as Ge-132 or Ge-Oxy 132) with promising medical applications. The organic compound improves oxygenation of tissues and restores normal function of immune-boosting cells. It may help prevent cancer, relieve pain, and combat viral infections, as well as improve circulatory and mental problems and reduce allergies. It is relatively nontoxic, though the FDA has warned against potential kidney damage from long-term use. Germanium comes in powders, granules, tablets, and capsules.

IRON is a trace element found in meat, poultry, fish, nuts, sunflower and pumpkin seeds, whole grains, and dark green, leafy vegetables. The adult RDA is 10 to 15 milligrams. Iron aids in energy production and is necessary for proper immune function. It is part of the hemoglobin that helps carry oxygen in the bloodstream to tissues throughout the body. It is used therapeutically to treat fatigue and depression, due both to iron-deficiency anemia and other causes. It has also been shown to benefit certain inner ear dysfunctions and learning disabilities. The body readily stores iron, and too much can be toxic or cause cardiovascular disease. Excess iron can also be countereffective, for instance, by causing fatigue, fostering bacterial growth, or compromising the immune system. Most nutritionists now recommend that iron supplementation be undertaken only if an iron deficiency has been clinically demonstrated. Iron is available in liquid formulas, capsules, and tablets.

MAGNESIUM is an essential major mineral found primarily in leafy, green vegetables; soybeans; and nuts and seeds. The adult RDA is 280 to 350 milligrams. Magnesium is required for strong, healthy bones and is concentrated in the body in the bones and teeth. It is important to a variety of other bodily processes: It helps keep cells electrically stable and, with calcium, regulates the body's energy levels and maintains normal heart function and nerve transmission. A magnesium deficiency can cause muscle tremors, convulsions, and possibly psychiatric problems. Supplements are used to treat premenstrual syndrome (PMS), high blood pressure, anxiety, osteoporosis, fatigue, and diabetes. Some therapists use magnesium supplements to treat convulsions in pregnant women. Supplement makers often combine magnesium in a one to two ratio with calcium. Recent research has shown that people with heart disease who take magnesium supplements may increase their risk of suffering a heart attack. People with heart disease, therefore, should avoid magnesium supplements.

NIACIN (vitamin B₃) helps the body produce energy, metabolize fats and carbohydrates, and manufacture fatty acids and sex and adrenal hormones. A deficiency causes pellagra, characterized by rough, cracked skin and diarrhea. Niacin is found in high amounts in brewer's yeast, peanuts and other legumes, sesame seeds, whole grains, fish, and meats. The RDA is 19 milligrams. Therapeutically, it is used in the treatment of schizophrenia, high blood pressure and high blood cholesterol, arthritis, Raynaud's disease, and lack of blood circulation to the extremities. It comes in two forms, nicotinic acid and niacinamide. The latter is sometimes referred to as *flush-free* niacin, since, unlike nicotinic acid, niacinamide taken in excess of 50 to 100 milligrams at one time won't cause a temporary flushing of the skin. Doses in excess of 250 milligrams daily should be monitored by a physician.

SELENIUM, a trace mineral and powerful antioxidant, is needed by the body in minute amounts. The adult RDA is 50 to 75 micrograms. Selenium is found in fish and in plants that have been grown in selenium-rich soil. High soil levels have been linked to low cancer rates of local people, and low soil levels to higher rates. Selenium may also be beneficial in the prevention of heart disease and immune-deficient conditions. It helps protect the body against harm from heavy metals and environmental toxins, and inhibits aging-related processes. It is also used to treat acne and may play a role in the production of sperm. Selenium is potentially toxic in high doses. It comes in tablets and capsules.

SILICON is an essential trace mineral found in plant fiber and hard water. It has only recently begun to gain scientific recognition for its role in the formation of bones, teeth, nails, cartilage, and connective tissue, where the highest levels in the body are found. The FDA has not established an RDA, although it admits there is substantial evidence that silicon is essential to health. The mineral can prevent buildup of cholesterol-laden lesions in the heart and may protect against aluminum poisoning. It is found in high concentrations in the herbs horsetail, nettle, and alfalfa. Silicon is toxic if inhaled (as silica dust, a by-product of semiconductor production), but no adverse effects are reported from consuming silicon supplements. It is frequently combined with other nutrients in formulas for hair, skin, and nails. It comes in tablets and capsules.

VITAMIN A is a fat-soluble micronutrient essential for healthy vision, cell reproduction, wound healing, immunity, and other crucial bodily functions. The U.S. RDA is 5000 IU. Vitamin A is also a potent antioxidant. Studies have confirmed that it can help treat or prevent cancer and that it improves resistance to infection. Vitamin A derivatives are used to renew aged skin and treat acne. In its preformed state, it is found in highest concentration in meats, though the plant-based precursor, beta-carotene, is as effective and totally nontoxic. Taking high doses of preformed vitamin A can allow it to accumulate in the body and cause adverse health effects. It comes in tablets and capsules. (See the description of beta-carotene.)

VITAMIN B$_6$ is a B-complex micronutrient, also known as pyridoxine, that boosts immunity, protects against nervous disorders, helps produce red blood cells, and plays an important role in hormone balance. Vitamin B$_6$ is an antioxidant. It causes the proliferation of lymphocytes and antibodies, especially when confronted with a disease-causing agent. The adult RDA is 1.5 to 2.2 milligrams. Vitamin B$_6$ is concentrated in meats and whole grains. It may help regulate eye pressure, alleviate fatigue, and cure carpal tunnel syndrome. It is an important vitamin for healthy bioelectric functioning of the central nervous system and plays a role in the metabolism of the neurotransmitters norepinephrine and acetylcholine, which may inhibit certain types of seizures. Vitamin B$_6$ also helps maintain a proper balance of sodium, potassium, and magnesium. Daily dosages in the 500 milligram range may be toxic for some people. It comes in tablets and capsules.

VITAMIN B$_{12}$, or cobalamin, unlike the other water-soluble B vitamins, is actually stored well in the body. The adult RDA is 2 micrograms. Vitamin B$_{12}$ is found in animal products like meat, milk, and eggs. Vegetarian sources can provide some vitamin B$_{12}$ (principally tempeh, sea vegetables, brewer's yeast, and mushrooms), but are unreliable, and strict vegetarians are at risk of deficiency. Vitamin B$_{12}$ aids in energy production from fats and carbohydrates and in the production of amino acids. It also plays a role in nerve building; deficiency causes neurological problems and confusion, depression, and memory loss. Vitamin B$_{12}$ deficiency in the elderly has been linked to Alzheimer's disease. Supplementation of this vitamin helps treat fatigue (even with no evidence of a deficiency), depression, and infertility. Some conditions respond only to injected vitamin B$_{12}$, available from medical practitioners. Vitamin B$_{12}$ comes in capsules.

VITAMIN C, or ascorbic (from *antiscurvy*) acid, is the most widely taken vitamin in supplement form. The adult RDA is 60 to 95 milligrams. Studies have shown that 100 milligrams to 500 milligrams of vitamin C cause lymphocytes to react more vigorously to disease-causing agents. Those same amounts also cause immune cells to boost production of antibodies. Other research has demonstrated that people who eat optimal amounts of vitamin C—obtaining these amounts exclusively from vegetable and fruit sources—have lower rates of cancer and heart disease than those who do not get adequate amounts. It is concentrated in certain fruits and dark green, leafy vegetables. It is frequently used to boost the immune system and reduce the symptoms of colds, asthma, and allergies. It also strengthens blood vessels, helps the body resist infection, and plays a crucial role in the healing of wounds, broken bones, and surgical operations. It can be made into a paste and applied topically to kill viruses that cause warts and other skin problems, to relieve pain and inflammation of burns and stings, and to lessen the risk of infection. Vitamin C supplements are inexpensive, widely available, and nontoxic (though pregnant women should avoid megadoses in the 3 to 6 gram range). It comes in powders, tablets, and capsules.

VITAMIN E, also known as tocopherol, is a powerful antioxidant nutrient that protects the body against the harmful effects of free radicals, which are unstable particles in the body that have been implicated in problems ranging from cancer to the effects of aging. The RDA is 30 IU. Food sources include vegetable oils, wheat germ, nuts, seeds, and whole grains. Vitamin E helps eliminate exercise cramps and nighttime leg cramps. Applied topically (break open capsules), it boosts the healing of burns, canker sores, and diaper rashes, and prevents scarring. It is sold as a liquid and in dry and oil-filled capsules. Research has shown that vitamin E is one of the most powerful nutrients against atherosclerosis, the underlying cause of heart disease. It also protects the body against the normal age-related decline of the immune system. Vitamin E boosts the body's production of CD4 cells, natural killer cells, and certain antibodies. It may also promote virility.

WHEAT GERM OIL is the liquid expelled from the highly nutritious embryo of the wheat kernel. A rich source of vitamin E, the oil is taken internally and applied like vitamin E to burns and skin conditions. Wheat germ oil may also promote the body's use of oxygen and thus have a positive effect on performance, endurance, and overall vitality. It comes in liquids and oil-filled capsules.

ZINC is a trace mineral essential for proper wound healing, male sexual potency, immunity, liver detoxification, and numerous other bodily functions. The adult RDA is 12 to 19 milligrams. Zinc is a powerful immune booster. It significantly boosts the body's immune response against all forms of viral and bacterial infections. Zinc is essential to a healthy thymus gland, which is where immature immune cells are trained to recognize pathogens and environmental poisons. It is especially important to children whose immune systems are just developing. Conversely, excesses of zinc can be immune depressing. Studies have shown that people taking greater than 100 milligrams per day of zinc experienced impaired immunity and greater risk of infection. Pregnant women, especially, should avoid excesses of zinc. Zinc is naturally high in animal foods, oysters, whole grains, and nuts. Its potential therapeutic applications include acne and other skin diseases and injuries, colds, infertility, eye disorders, ulcers, and alcoholism. It is often taken before and after surgical operations to speed recovery. Zinc is frequently combined with copper, selenium, and other minerals and vitamins. It is nontoxic, though dosages of 2 grams may cause gastrointestinal irritation and vomiting. It comes in lozenges, tablets, and capsules.

Amino Acids: The Basis of Protein

Amino acids are the building blocks of protein molecules. The body makes proteins from twenty amino acids, eight of which—isoleucine, leucine, lysine, methionine, phenylalanine, threonine, tryptophan, and valineare—are termed *essential* because they cannot be synthesized by the body and therefore must be obtained through diet or supplements. Amino acid products come in single and *branched-chain,* or mixed, forms as powders, capsules, and liquids.

Single amino acids include the essential ones as well as others like taurine and arginine, which are taken for their effects on brain neurotransmitters and other cell functions. Taking single amino acid supplements for an extended period of time may cause an imbalance in the function of other amino acids.

BRANCHED-CHAIN, or mixed, amino acids may help in recovery from hangover and are widely taken by bodybuilders for muscle bulking. There is also some evidence of a positive effect on amyotrophic lateral sclerosis, a degenerative nerve disease, but most therapeutic applications of amino acids are for single amino acids like lysine, tyrosine, tryptophan, and taurine. Over the long term, too much protein in the form of amino acid supplements may be toxic to the liver and kidneys.

ARGININE is an amino acid that has become a popular muscle-building supplement due to its possible ability to increase the body's production of growth hormone. It may help in the treatment of male infertility by boosting sperm counts among men with low levels of active sperm. It may also have a positive effect on the immune system. Arginine has an antagonistic effect on the amino acid lysine. Supplements and foods rich in this nutrient, like chocolate, peanuts and other nuts, various seeds, and peas, may promote the growth of the herpes virus, so they should be avoided by people with active cold sores or genital sores. Arginine is sold in capsules.

LYSINE is an essential amino acid. As a supplement, nutritionists use it primarily to help prevent and treat conditions caused by viruses of the herpes family, including cold sores, shingles, and genital sores. Studies confirm that it reduces the severity of symptoms and frequency of outbreaks of cold sores. Dietary sources of lysine include beans, dairy products, potatoes, and brewer's yeast. Lysine may increase blood cholesterol levels. It comes in capsules.

PHENYLALANINE is an essential amino acid that stimulates production in the brain of the neurotransmitters dopamine and norepinephrine, which have an energy-boosting effect on the body. It is taken as a supplement (in the form of L-phenylalanine) to help treat depression and (as D-phenylalanine) to control chronic pain. It also seems to enhance the pain-relieving effects of acupuncture. Some studies show a beneficial effect on people with Parkinson's disease. L-phenylalanine should be avoided by people with high blood pressure. Phenylalanine may also cause stimulant-like side effects, including insomnia and anxiety. Both forms should be avoided by people with phenylketonuria, a genetic disorder of phenylalanine metabolism. A mixture of the two forms is sold as DL-phenylalanine or DLPA. It comes in capsules.

TAURINE is found in high levels in fish and egg proteins. In the body, it is concentrated in the brain, where it plays a central role in regulating the nervous system and coordinating electrical activity. Though not an amino acid that plays a role in protein synthesis, taurine is intimately connected with the minerals sodium, potassium, calcium, magnesium, and zinc, all of which also affect brain metabolism. Its main therapeutic use (at dosages of about 1500 milligrams per day) is in epilepsy management, although it may also protect the eyes against cataracts, alleviate symptoms of alcohol withdrawal, reduce blood pressure, and lower the risk of gallstones. High levels may cause depression or other adverse effects. It comes in tablets and capsules.

TRYPTOPHAN, an essential amino acid, is currently banned by the FDA as a food supplement. It was formerly taken as a sleeping aid. It is naturally found in a variety of foods, including whole grains, beans and legumes, and some nuts and seeds. Tryptophan is the precursor of the brain neurotransmitter serotonin, which acts as a natural sedative, pain reliever, and mood enhancer. Serotonin elevates mood and boosts feelings of well-being. Deficiencies of serotonin have been tied to depression and sleep-related problems. Studies at the Massachusetts Institute of Technology have demonstrated that a single meal of whole grains, grain-flour products, and beans boost brain levels of serotonin within minutes of consuming the food. Consistent consumption of these foods increase serotonin levels over time. Tryptophan supplements were removed from U.S. markets by the FDA in November 1989, when consumption was tied to a rare blood abnormality that caused thirty-eight deaths. The ill effects may have been caused by product contamination rather than tryptophan itself.

TYROSINE is an amino acid taken to help relieve depression. Like phenylalanine, it helps the brain to produce the natural painkilling, energizing, and mood-boosting chemicals dopamine and norepinephrine. It is taken to help relieve anxiety and emotional lows associated with PMS, and it may play a role in the treatment of drug detoxification and Parkinson's disease. It should be avoided by anyone who suffers from high blood pressure. It comes in capsules.

EFAs: The Fats You Must Eat

Essential fatty acids (EFAs) are fats that are needed by the body but not manufactured by it and thus must be obtained through the diet. They are sometimes collectively referred to as vitamin F.

EFA supplements are usually derived from the oil of cold-water fish like herring and bluefish, and from the oil of the seeds of certain plants including rape (canola oil), flax, hemp, borage, evening primrose, and black currant. Important EFAs include the omega-3s (such as eicosapentaenoic acid [EPA] and docosahexaenoic acid [DHA], and alpha-linolenic acid, a plant oil–derived EPA/DHA precursor) and omega-6s (gamma-linolenic acid [GLA]). In the body, EFAs act to strengthen cell membranes and promote the growth of muscles and nerves. They are used therapeutically to thin the blood, inhibit clotting, improve cholesterol profiles, and thus help prevent heart disease. EFAs also have natural anti-inflammatory effects that are potentially useful in the treatment of arthritis, allergies, and asthma. Supplements may need to be refrigerated. They are sold as liquids and in capsules.

BORAGE OIL is a vegetable oil derived from a blue-flowering plant (*Borago officinalis*) that is also used as an herb in Europe, primarily to restore adrenal function, alleviate PMS, and counter inflammation. The oil is taken as a supplement because it is one of the few natural sources of gamma linolenic acid (GLA). This may help in the prevention or treatment of heart disease, arthritis, skin problems, and PMS. Borage oil may also stimulate the growth of hair and nails. It has a soothing effect when applied topically to the skin. It comes in liquids and capsules.

DOCOSAHEXAENOIC ACID (DHA) is an omega-3 essential fatty acid primarily found in the oil of cold-water fish, such as salmon, bluefish, herring, mackerel, and tuna. Studies indicate it is capable of thinning blood and lowering blood fat and cholesterol levels. It may have therapeutic applications for heart disease, inflammatory conditions like arthritis, and psoriasis. Taken in excess, DHA can reduce blood-clotting capability. It often has vitamin E oil added to prevent rancidity. It comes in liquids and capsules.

EICOSAPENTAENOIC ACID (EPA) is an omega-3 essential fatty acid found primarily in the oil of cold-water fish, such as salmon, herring, bluefish, mackerel, and tuna. It usually occurs with DHA and has similar effects on the body; it reduces inflammation and lowers blood fat and cholesterol levels. It may help in the treatment of arthritis, allergic reactions, heart disease, and skin conditions. Taken in excess, it can reduce blood-clotting capability. It comes in liquids and capsules.

EVENING PRIMROSE OIL (EPO) is a fatty liquid extracted from the seeds of a yellow-flowering willow family plant (*Oenothera biennis*) that is a richly endowed source of the omega-6 essential fatty acid GLA. It is produced primarily in Great Britain and is a popular remedy in Europe. It is taken therapeutically, as are other essential fatty acids, to help prevent heart disease, arthritis, and inflammatory conditions. It is also used to treat skin problems and relieve symptoms of PMS. Technically, its use is still experimental, but few side effects have appeared. Since the late 1980s, EPO has been the subject of a regulatory dispute between the FDA and importers, who have had some shipments seized as an unapproved food additive. Nevertheless, it is still available as a liquid or in capsules.

FISH OILS are the fatty liquids expressed from certain cold-water fish (including salmon, mackerel, sardines, bluefish, herring, and tuna) that are a rich source of omega-3 essential fatty acids. As supplements, they are taken to thin the blood and inhibit clotting, improve cholesterol profiles, and strengthen cell membranes. They also have a natural anti-inflammatory effect. Fish oils are now being used therapeutically to help treat or prevent diseases including arthritis, heart disease, allergies, and asthma. They come in liquids and capsules.

GAMMA LINOLENIC ACID (GLA) is a biologically active omega-6 essential fatty acid found in significant quantities in oils derived from only a few plants, including evening primrose, hemp, borage, and black currant. Studies indicate it has potential therapeutic use in the prevention or treatment of heart disease, arthritis, skin problems, and PMS. GLA may also stimulate the growth of hair and nails. It comes in liquids and capsules.

LECITHIN is a fatty acid naturally found in certain foods such as egg yolks and soybean oil. It is taken as a supplement mainly to protect against heart disease, increase longevity, and improve memory. Lecithin is an important natural source of choline, sometimes considered one of the B-complex vitamins, and a nutrient necessary for the healthy functioning of cells, nerves, and the brain. Lecithin may help to lower cholesterol levels. It also helps to strengthen nerve sheaths and thus can play a role in the treatment of multiple sclerosis. Lecithin is a mild antioxidant. It is nontoxic; side effects from pure choline are much more common. The food industry adds lecithin to products such as mayonnaise to act as an emulsifier, thickener, or stabilizer. Lecithin is available in liquids, granules, and capsules. (See the description of choline, in the section on vitamins and minerals.)

Probiotics: Microorganisms for Life

PROBIOTICS are a category of dietary supplements consisting of beneficial microorganisms. Probiotics compete with disease-causing microorganisms in the gastrointestinal tract of humans and animals. When helpful bacteria such as acidophilus are reintroduced into the gastrointestinal tract, the result is balance. Probiotics are responsible for several activities in the gut, including manufacturing B vitamins, including biotin, niacin (vitamin B_3), folic acid, and pyridoxine (vitamin B_6); producing lactase; producing antibacterial substances that kill disease-causing bacteria; killing harmful bacteria by changing the acid/alkaline balance and by depriving the harmful bacteria of the nutrients they need; improving digestive tract function; and combating vaginal yeast infections.

ACIDOPHILUS is, technically, the *species* of naturally occurring live bacteria known as *Lactobacillus acidophilus*. However, products sold as acidophilus may also contain *L. bulgaricus* and other strains of lactic bacteria. Beneficial bacteria such as acidophilus are essential to the healthy functioning of the gastrointestinal system, where they play a role in the digestion of food and the production of B vitamins. Acidophilus is often recommended to replenish the population of friendly microorganisms that have been wiped out by a course of oral antibiotics. Supplementation helps prevent fungi like *Candida albicans* (a cause of yeast infections) from spreading. Acidophilus bacteria are also found in fermented milk products like yogurt and kefir, though most nutritionists agree such products are not high enough in acidophilus to replenish the intestinal flora. Acidophilus products must be kept refrigerated, unless specially formulated. Acidophilus is nontoxic.

BIFIDOBACTERIA (including *B. bifidum, B. infantis,* and *B. longum*) is a natural inhabitant of the human intestine. They are found in the stools of humans and help prevent colonization of the intestine by unfriendly bacteria, assist in the production of B vitamins, and increase acidity of the intestine, which is inhibitory to less desirable microorganisms. They also help infants retain nitrogen, which encourages weight gain. The Japanese scientific community now believes that bifidobacteria is the most important of all probiotics because it prevents reabsorption of toxins (such as amines and fennels) that, when allowed to reenter the system, place significant strain on the liver. Bifidobacteria also competes against *Candida albicans,* the bacteria that causes yeast infections. Bifidobacteria is the most common bacteria found in breast-fed human infants. Bottle-fed babies are low in bifidobacteria, however, as are most adults who have taken antibiotics or eaten pesticide-rich foods.

LACTOBACILLUS BULGARICUS is found in yogurt and cheese. When eaten or taken in a supplement form, these bacteria enhance digestion of the milk sugar, lactose, by producing the enzyme lactase. As with other lactic acid bacteria, these transient bacteria encourage a more acid environment, which inhibits less desirable microorganisms. *Bulgaricus* assists in the breakdown and absorption of proteins. It also boosts the immune system by stimulating the production of macrophages and immunoglobins, which are essential antibodies.

STREPTOCOCCUS THERMOPHILUS is found in yogurt and cheese, as well as heated and pasteurized milk. It is used along with *Lactobacillus bulgaricus* to form a culture that is used in the preparation of yogurt. When eaten or taken in a supplement, these bacteria enhance digestion of lactose by producing the enzyme lactase. *Thermophilus* also has unique growth-stimulating properties and combines with other probiotics to enhance the overall bacterial environment.

ENZYMES, CHARCOAL, CLAYS, FIBERS, AND HORMONES

Supplementing the body's natural catalysts, enzymes, are protein molecules that regulate the metabolism of proteins, carbohydrates (sugar and starch), and fats. They act as catalysts in starting chemical reactions in the body. Supplemental enzymes are usually taken when the body's natural enzymes have trouble doing their job. Most commonly, they are used to aid in digestion when the enzymes in the mouth, stomach, and small intestine are unable to break down food into components that can pass through the wall of the intestine. Undigested food components that pass through the intestinal wall have been linked to conditions such as rheumatoid arthritis and multiple sclerosis.

ACTIVATED CHARCOAL is pure carbon specially processed to make it highly absorbent of particles and gases in the body's digestive system. Activated charcoal slides through the intestines without being absorbed. It is taken internally to relieve gas pains, reduce flatulence, and absorb and excrete poisons and other toxins from the body. It may also lower blood cholesterol levels. It is best taken an hour before or after nutrient supplements to avoid eliminating them from the body as well. Activated charcoal can be applied externally (add water to the powder to make a paste) to alleviate pain and itching from bites and stings. It is safe and nontoxic. It is available in powder, tablet, capsule, and liquid forms.

BENTONITE is a powdered porous clay that gets its name from an area in Montana near Fort Benton. It is produced by the decomposition of volcanic ash. Bentonite is similar to cosmetic or green clay and can be mixed with water to make a paste that is applied to the skin for its drawing and drying powers against stings, poison ivy, and other conditions. Bentonite can also be taken internally to absorb toxins in the intestines if it is produced to meet special formulating standards. It comes in powder and liquid forms. (See clay.)

BROMELAIN is a naturally occurring enzyme derived from the pineapple plant. As a nutritional supplement, it is widely used to assist in the digestion of protein, to relieve painful menstruation, and to treat arthritis. It has also become a popular sports injury medicine, taken internally to reduce bruising, relieve pain and swelling, and promote wound healing. It can also be used externally, like papain, as a paste applied to stings to deactivate the protein molecules of insect venom. Reports have touted bromelain's immune-boosting properties as well. Typically it is taken with meals as a digestive aid, or thirty minutes before or ninety minutes after a meal to help treat sports injuries. It is available in tablets.

CITRIMAX is a trademarked derivative of the Asian fruit *Garcinia cambogia*. CitriMax is rich in the compound hydroxycitric acid (HCA). Chemically, HCA is similar to citric acid, but it has been shown to help curb appetite and inhibit the production of fats and cholesterol. It is intended for use in health and dietary supplements.

CLAY is the generic term for any finely grained, decomposed rock or volcanic ash with both external and internal medical applications. It can be mixed with water and applied as a paste to relieve insect bites, splinters, rashes, poison ivy, and other skin conditions. If classified as food grade, clay can be taken internally to cleanse the intestines after food or chemical poisoning. Some popular forms include cosmetic clay, green clay, and bentonite. It is sold as a powder or liquid. (See bentonite.)

COENZYME Q10 (CoQ10) is a vitamin-like compound, also known as ubiquinone, that occurs naturally in the body and is taken as a supplement to help activate the body's enzymes and, thereby, generate energy. It may help prevent or treat heart disease, hypertension, diabetes, Alzheimer's disease, and obesity. CoQ10 is an antioxidant, immunity booster, and may strengthen muscles and improve physical performance and endurance. It is taken to allow the body to adjust to higher altitudes and improve physical endurance. It has also demonstrated excellent results in clinical trials on periodontal disease by speeding up healing time, reducing gum pockets, and improving other factors associated with gum disease. It is available in capsules.

DIMETHYL SULFOXIDE (DMSO) is a liquid solvent that had only industrial uses until the 1960s, when it began to be widely sold in health food stores for its reported inflammation-reducing effects. Rubbed into the skin, it is easily absorbed, causing a distinctive odor on the skin and breath. It is claimed to help treat arthritis and sprains, stains, and bruises. Current federal law prohibits dispensing DMSO without a prescription, and its only federally approved use is for a type of cystitis, for which it is injected. Some states have approved other uses, but generally DMSO is no longer available in health food stores.

EPSOM SALTS are a white, crystalline product (purified magnesium sulfate) named for the town in England where the substance was first identified some 500 years ago. It has been a popular folk remedy ever since. Epsom salts are principally sprinkled in the bath for their relaxing effect. But they've also been used topically for stiff joints and aching muscles. (Make a pack by dissolving salts in hot water, soaking a hand towel, and applying.) They are also taken internally as a laxative. Epsom salts are a powder that is widely available in conventional pharmacies.

MELATONIN is a hormone produced by the tiny pineal gland in the center of the brain. It has been linked with changes in mood, performance, fatigue, sleep patterns, and biological rhythms. Levels in the body are affected by light and darkness, temperature, and other factors. Minute doses of 3 milligrams or so in pills are now being used to counter the effects of jet lag and to help jet lag sufferers to reset their biological clocks. Taken orally, melatonin is rapidly absorbed into the bloodstream, metabolized, and eliminated from the body. Side effects are negligible. It comes in tablets.

PAPAIN is a naturally occurring enzyme derived from unripe papayas. It is the ingredient in meat tenderizers that softens meat by breaking down muscle tissue. As a supplement, it is taken internally as a digestive aid. It is also applied topically, after water is added to crushed tablets, to make a paste to relieve bites and stings. It works by breaking down the large protein molecules of insect venom. Papain is available in tablets.

PECTIN is a water-soluble carbohydrate found in apples, oranges, and other ripe fruit. It is taken in supplement form for its rich fiber content. Like psyllium, it aids digestion and elimination and helps prevent constipation, diarrhea, and diseases of the colon, including cancer. As an additive, it is used by the food and cosmetics industries to thicken jellies, ice cream, and other products. It comes in powder and tablet forms. (See the description of psyllium.)

PSYLLIUM is the seeds or husks from the fleawort and other plantain (*Plantago ovata and P. psyllium*) plants. People take it in supplement form as a concentrated source of water-soluble dietary fiber. It promotes intestinal function and elimination and is often used in laxatives (Metamucil, for instance) to treat constipation, because it speeds transit time and eases bowel movements. Psyllium also adds bulk to stools and treats diarrhea. Since the mucilage in the seed husks absorbs water and forms a gel in the stomach, it gives a sense of fullness and decreases appetite, thus helping to treat obesity. Psyllium slows the digestion and absorption of carbohydrates, thus suppressing swings in blood sugar levels and helping to control diabetes. Finally, it may aid in lowering blood cholesterol levels. The whole seeds or husks should always be taken with liquids. It comes in dried and liquid forms. (See the description of pectin.)

PYCNOGENOL is a trademarked plant derivative that is a powerful antioxidant. It is derived from the bark of a pine tree (*Pinus maritima*) native to France, one of the few plants to yield significant amounts of certain bioflavonoids known as proanthocyanidins. Pycnogenol has been shown to strengthen blood vessels, prevent wrinkling of the skin, retard aging, improve vision, and possibly reduce the risk of cancer and heart disease. It is nontoxic and comes in capsules. (See the description of bioflavonoids in the section on vitamins and minerals.)

SHARK CARTILAGE is the semitough supporting and connective tissue that serves as a shark's skeleton, purified into a white powder and sold in supplement form. Shark cartilage contains a substance that slows the growth of blood vessels and thus may help inhibit tumors. It may also reduce the pain, inflammation, and joint stiffness of arthritis, alleviate inflammatory bowel disease, and reverse psoriasis. Pregnant women and people who suffer from vascular diseases should avoid shark cartilage. It comes in capsules.

TISSUE SALTS are twelve essential mineral compounds, including iron phosphate, calcium sulphate, and sodium chloride, that homeopaths call, respectively, ferrum phosphoricum, calcarea sulphurica, and natrum muriaticum. They are present in small amounts in healthy human cells. Practitioners prescribe tissue salt remedies, which are prepared similarly to homeopathic remedies, to treat various conditions (colds, headaches, and hay fever) that are said to result from imbalances or deficiencies in cell salts. The remedies are sometimes called Schuessler tissue salts after the nineteenth-century German chemist who pioneered the field. The salts come in tablets.

HERBOLOGY

Long before there was aspirin, there was the bark of the white willow tree, from which aspirin is derived. Long before there was digitalis, there was the foxglove plant, which provides today's pharmacologists with the raw materials to make the heart drug. Many plants have medicinal properties, and long before there was a pharmaceutical industry, there were traditional healers who understood how to use plants to help people overcome disease. That knowledge is the basis of herbal medicine.

Herbs are medicinal plants. Various parts of the plant—the leaves, stems, roots, and seeds—are used for their specific healing properties. Although scientists are discovering every day new therapeutic benefits of herbal medicines, pharmacologists tend to focus primarily on individual chemicals, rather than the synergistic effects of many compounds found in plants. Many herbs contain dozens of active constituents that combine to give the plant its therapeutic value. Consequently, herbalists believe that the plant itself, and even certain parts of plants, provide much more effective medicine than any single isolated constituent.

Herbs should be used with discrimination. Though they are generally much safer than prescription or over-the-counter drugs, some herbs can be toxic if taken in high doses. Read the descriptions below before using an herb, and use them as directed in Part II.

Below is a guide to herbs and healing foods that can be used to assist in the treatment of disease. Most of these herbs and foods are widely available in natural food stores and health food stores. Others are available through mail order sales.

At the very bottom of this list are formulas for preparing herbs. When terms such as infusion or decoction or teas turn up, refer to these instructions.

HERBAL PROPERTIES

The following terms are used to describe the properties of the herbs listed below.

- Alteratives are blood purifiers that are used to treat conditions arising from or causing toxicity. Over time, they will improve the condition of the blood, accelerate elimination, improve digestion, and increase the appetite.
- Analgesics are herbs that will relieve pain. Some relax muscles, others just reduce the pain signals to the brain.
- Antacids neutralize excess stomach and intestinal acids.

- Anticatarrhals are substances that eliminate or counteract the formation of mucus.
- Antipyretics are cooling herbs used to reduce or prevent fevers.
- Antiseptics are substances applied to the skin to prevent the growth of bacteria.
- Antispasmodics prevent or relax muscle tension.
- Astringents have a constricting or binding effect. They are used commonly to check hemorrhages and secretions.
- Carminatives are herbs taken to relieve gas and griping.
- Cholagogues are used to promote the flow and discharge of bile into the small intestine.
- Demulcents are soothing substances, usually mucilage, taken internally to protect injuries or inflamed tissues.
- Diaphoretics induce swelling.
- Diuretics increase the flow of urine.
- Emetics induce vomiting.
- Emmenagogues promote menstruation.
- Emollients soften, soothe, and protect the skin.
- Expectorants assist in expelling mucus from the lungs and throat.
- Galactogogues are substances that increase the secretion of milk.
- Hemostatics arrest hemorrhage. They are good for blood coagulation.
- Laxatives promote bowel movement.
- Lithotriptics help dissolve and eliminate urinary and biliary stones and gravel.
- Nervines calm nervous tension.
- Oxytocics stimulate uterine contractions.
- Rebefacients increase the flow of blood at the surface of the skin.
- Sedatives quiet the nervous system.
- Sialagogues promote the flow of saliva.
- Stimulants increase the energy of the body.
- Tonics promote the functions of the systems.
- Vulneraries encourage healing of wounds by promoting cell growth and repair.

HERBS

AGRIMONY *(Agrimonia eupatoria)*: Belonging to the Rose order of plants, agrimony was once drunk in springtime as a purifier of the blood. A mild astringent and tonic, it is useful in coughs and for diarrhea. Agrimony has had a reputation for curing jaundice and other liver complaints. It is also very useful in treating skin eruptions, such as pimples and blotches, and diseases of the blood. It is used by Native Americans to treat fever. It may be given either in infusion or decoction.

ALFALFA *(Medicago sativa)*: Alfalfa is an herb, a food, and the source of a nutritional green-food concentrate. Alfalfa is a perennial of the pea family, widely grown as a hay feed for livestock. The Arabs consider alfalfa so nutritious that they named it the father of all foods. In most forms it is rich in chlorophyll, beta-carotene, vitamins B_6, C, and E, and calcium. As an herbal preparation, it is traditionally used as a diuretic, an arthritis remedy, and an aid to gain weight. Studies indicate it lowers blood cholesterol levels and may help prevent heart disease and possibly some stroke. It is also used in sprouted form, but the leaves are more medicinal, and raw sprouts as well as seeds contain natural toxins that are potentially damaging to human health if eaten. Alfalfa's various forms include dried leaves, tablets, capsules, concentrated drops, tinctures, and extracts.

ALOE VERA *(Aloe vera* var. *officinalis)* juice or gel is a demulcent, emollient, laxative, vulnerary, and emmenagogue. It is used externally to treat skin problems, especially cuts, abrasions, wounds, and burns. It prevents scarring and encourages healing. The gel can be drawn directly from the pulpy aloe vera plant leaves. Apply the fresh juice or gel directly to the affected area. This herb has been in use since ancient Egypt. It is safe, highly effective, and increasingly turning up in products from skin lotions to shampoos.

ALUM ROOT *(Heuchera)*: The rhizomes of this plant were used by Nevada and Utah Indians to treat heart disease. It has a strong styptic taste. It is used internally and externally as an astringent. Due to its high tannin content, use it in small amounts, less than 5 to 10 grams of plant material. In high dosages, alum could cause kidney and liver failure.

AMARANTH *(Amaranthus hypochondriacus)* is more common in the tropics, especially in tropical America, but it recently has also been cultivated in cold countries. It has been known since ancient Greek times, when it was given its name, signifying *unwithering* or *immortal*. It is considered astringent and a decoction of the flowers has been administered for internal bleeding and menorrhagia. The fresh leaves of amaranth may be cooked and eaten to neutralize stomach acidity.

AMERICAN GINSENG ROOT *(Panax quinquefolium)* can best be described as an adaptogen, that is, it aids the body to adapt to various biological stresses. It contains panaxin, a stimulant for midbrain, heart, and blood vessels; panaquilin, a stimulant of internal secretions; panacen and sapogenin, volatile oils that stimulate the central nervous system; and gensinin, which has been shown to decrease blood sugar. Ginseng, in general, has a stimulant effect on the adrenal cortex and increases mental and physical effectiveness. It is variously recommended for anemia, atherosclerosis, depression, diabetes, edema, stress, and stomach ulcers. Typical dose is 1 to 4 grams.

ANGELICA *(Angelica atropurpurea)* is taken to alleviate respiratory complaints including colds and flu, as well as digestive problems. Studies confirm that it has chemical compounds that relax the windpipe and intestines and thus may be beneficial for bronchitis, asthma, indigestion, and heartburn. The roots are sold dried, since the fresh root is poisonous. It's also sold in capsules, concentrated drops, extracts, and tinctures. Diabetic patients should avoid angelica, as it lowers blood sugar. (See dong quai).

ANISE *(Pimpinella anisum)* was well-known to the ancient Greeks and has been used as a spice for centuries. Used as seed or as oil derived from the seed, anise has been used medicinally to aid digestion and decrease gas and abdominal pains. It has also been used as an ingredient in cough syrups and lozenges. Oil of anise is also used externally to kill lice.

APRICOT SEED *(Prunus armeniaca)* is the seed in the fruit of the apricot tree, originally from temperate regions of northern China. The oil extracted from apricot seed very closely resembles bitter almond oil. Medicinal uses: Apricot seeds contain the active ingredient amygdalin, from which Laetrile is produced. Some practitioners believe amygdalin cures cancer; the FDA strongly disagrees.

ARNICA *(Arnica montana* and *Arnica fulgens)* oil or gel is a popular external remedy indigenous to Central Europe. Recommended for sprains, bruises, and wounds, studies have shown arnica to have anti-inflammatory, analgesic, and even antibiotic activity. Externally, it is applied only to unbroken skin. Arnica is seldom used internally due to its toxic effect on the stomach. A homeopathic tincture, X6, has been used for epilepsy, as well as for seasickness.

ASTRAGALUS is derived from the root of a plant *(Astragalus membranaceus)* in the pea family. It is also known as milk vetch root (referring to astragalus species that grow in the Unites States) and as the Chinese herb, huang-qi. It is an adaptogen—that is, it has a balancing effect on bodily functions. Astragalus is used by practitioners of traditional Chinese medicine to strengthen or tonify the body's overall vitality, improve digestion, and support the spleen. Studies confirm it contains medicinally active compounds, including a polysaccharide that stimulates the immune system. Research has also shown that subjects with advanced cancer showed a two- to threefold increase in the strength of their immune response after being given astragalus. A second study showed that astragalus boosted immune response, even in animals that were treated with an immunosuppressive drug, cyclophosphamide. Astragalus is taken in China by cancer patients to boost immunity after drug or radiation treatment. It may protect body cells against heavy metals and chemical toxins. Astragalus is a good source of the essential trace mineral selenium. It is often combined in formulas with ginseng and other Chinese herbs. Herbal companies offer it fresh or dried and in capsules, concentrated drops, tinctures, and extracts.

BAMBOO leaves are diuretic. The root is astringent, styptic, and antipyretic. The epidermis or shavings of the young stems are sedative, antiemetic, antipyretic; they stop cough and clear the heart of invisible phlegm. The siliceous secretions are specifically anti-inflammatory and tonic for the lungs. Specifically, this part of the bamboo enters the heart, liver, and gallbladder.

BANCHA tea is made from the stems and leaves of mature Japanese tea bushes, also known as kukicha. Bancha aids digestion, contains calcium, has no chemical dyes, and contains only a minute amount of caffeine, which is generally unnoticeable. It is widely available in natural food stores. Pour two tablespoons of bancha or kukicha in four cups of water, boil, pour through a strainer, and drink hot. Add more tea if more water is used. Bancha or kukicha is very soothing and alkalizing to the spleen and liver.

BAPTISIA *(Baptisia tinctoria)* roots and leaves are powerful anti-inflammatories that have potent antibiotic and antiviral properties. It is used in extreme infections, blood poisoning, meningitis, and malignant sores. Baptisia is often combined with other anti-inflammatory herbs like echinacea and goldenseal. A decoction may be made by boiling a half ounce of the root in a pint of water for ten minutes. Drink one tablespoon every four hours.

BARBERRY *(Berberis vulgaris)* contains eight different alkaloids, the most important of which is berberine. Berberine produces vasodilatation, decreases heart rate, and, in higher doses, reduces bronchial restriction. The bark of the stem and roots is ground into a powder. It is used to treat liver problems including jaundice and hepatitis. It is also helpful in treating menstrual cramps and PMS. It is taken as a decoction or tincture.

BAYBERRY *(Myrica cerifera):* The dried bark of the bayberry root is astringent, stimulant, and in large doses, emetic. Bayberry bark has been used to stop excessive menstrual bleeding and in a douche to treat vaginal discharge. Folk remedies combined it with other herbs to treat colds and jaundice. It is also helpful to inflamed gums; apply the powder directly to the gums.

BEAR LICHEN is a new natural antibiotic. It is effective against most streptococcus and staphylococcus infections, and for trichomonas in women (for which it needs to be taken in tincture form every two hours for a week). It is also good applied full strength to infected cuts, fungus infections, impetigo, and for gastrointestinal tract, urinary tract, and streptococcus infections.

BILBERRY *(Vaccinium myrtillus),* also known as blueberry or huckleberry, is a folk remedy for better eyesight. Studies confirm a positive effect on vision due to the berry's flavonoid compounds, the anthocyanosides, that can cause biochemical reactions in the eye. It may also play a role in relieving menstrual problems; studies have found it helps to relax smooth muscles like those found in the uterine wall. Bilberry is nontoxic and comes in tablets, capsules, and extracts.

BISTORT *(Polygonurn bistorta)* root is one of the strongest vegetable astringents known and, as such, has been used to treat diarrhea, dysentery, cholera, and internal bleeding, including excessive menstrual flow. Applied as a poultice, it will stop a wound from bleeding. A paste made from equal parts bistort, alum, and pellitory and applied to a toothache will relieve pain and reduce infection of the tooth. Bistort is used as a powder or in a liquid extract.

BITTERROOT *(Apocynum androsaemifolium)*: The dried root of bitterroot contains elements closely related to digitalis, although it is more irritating to mucous membranes. It slows the pulse and increases the contractive strength of cardiac tissue. This is a toxic herb that should be used only under supervision.

BITTERS are herbal tonics whose pungent taste helps stimulate and revitalize the digestive system. Bitters assist in natural detoxification and cleanse the liver, intestines, and other organs. They work by promoting salivation and activating secretions and functions of the stomach, small intestine, and gallbladder. Bitters are typically made from herbs such as gentian, goldenseal, rue, rhubarb, yellow dock, or barberry steeped in alcohol or vinegar. They are usually taken by swallowing a teaspoon of the liquid tonic ten to twenty minutes before a meal. Though some proponents claim that bitters work best when the sense of taste is activated, they are available in capsules as well as the more common liquid form.

BLACKBERRY/RASPBERRY *(Rubus villosus)* is common around the world and specifically known in the United States as blackberry, dewberry, and a form with annual stems and no prickles, the raspberry (see the description of red raspberry). Leaves, roots, and bark contain up to 10 percent tannic acid. The root bark is used medicinally as an astringent tonic for diarrhea and dysentery. The leaves are helpful to treat fevers, colds, and sore throats. It is taken as decoction.

BLACK COHOSH preparations are derived from the dark root of a plant *(Cimicifuga racemosa)* also known as black snakeroot, which is native to North America. It is a popular Native American and folk remedy for female ailments and menstrual cramps, as well as for fatigue, anxiety, and respiratory conditions such as bronchitis. Black cohosh is also widely used in Germany for discomfort from menopause. It may have uses as a sedative and anti-inflammatory and can lower blood pressure and possibly help control diabetes. This herb promotes menstruation, so it should be avoided during pregnancy. It has other potential side effects as well and is often recommended to be used under the supervision of an herbalist. It comes in capsules, concentrated drops, and extracts.

BLACK PEPPERCORNS *(Piper nigrum)* are useful to control colds and mucous illnesses. It may also be used as a preventive. Take one-eighth teaspoon ground pepper mixed with honey daily.

BLACK WALNUT *(Juglans nigra)* leaves are used to make an extract that is used as an astringent. The leaves and bark were used by the early Greeks and Romans to treat fungal skin infections. In large doses, black walnut may irritate the stomach, due to its astringency.

BLAZING STAR *(Aletris farinosa),* also known as star grass, contains the sapogenin compound diosgenin, the substrate material used to chemically produce progesterone. Herbalists have used it to treat a variety of dysmenorrhea (painful menstruation) problems and to soothe sore breasts in nursing mothers. It is available as a powder and as a tincture.

BLESSED THISTLE *(Cnicus benedictus)* contains a bitter substance named cnicin, which reflexively stimulates gastric secretions. It is primarily used as a bitter to increase gastric function and to treat liver congestion.

BLOODROOT *(Sanguinaria canadensis),* an early and beautiful spring flower, is one of the best-known indigenous remedies in the United States. Its widespread use by physicians in the 1800s led to its reputation as a panacea, especially renowned as a cure for cancer. Studies have not borne out its antitumor properties. A considerable number of constituents have been isolated, the most useful being sanguinarine, which has diuretic and diaphoretic properties. Recent studies have shown bloodroot to be an effective rinse for counteracting dental plaque. If taken internally in large doses, bloodroot is extremely toxic.

BLUE COHOSH *(Caulophyllum thalictroides)*: The roots and berries of this plant are used as a menstrual aid and as an aid to childbirth. Studies have shown that blue cohosh has a stimulating effect on the uterine muscle but only when taken in large doses. The berries *must be heated* to detoxify them. Ingestion of unheated berries causes a variety of toxic reactions, including nausea, gastritis, and, in larger doses, cardiovascular collapse and convulsions.

BONESET *(Eupatorium perfolatium)* has a long history in herbal medicine as a bitter treatment for colds and fevers. Studies have confirmed its antiinflammatory properties due to a constituent named sesquiterpene. Other studies have suggested that boneset acts as a stimulant to the immune system. It acts as a relaxant to the stomach and liver. The bitter taste also has a strong appetite-stimulating effect.

BUCHU *(Barosma betulina)* is a weak diuretic and is used as an antiseptic to the urinary tract. It contains a volatile oil with a peppermint-like odor. Buchu is frequently given by herbalists as a treatment for kidney stones, inflammation of the bladder, and urethral irritation. Do not boil buchu; rather, make a cool-water infusion.

BUCKTHORN preparations are produced from the berries or bark of a shrub or small tree of Europe *(Rhamnus cathartica)* or North America *(R. ca-*

roliniana). The herb is renowned for its ability to loosen the bowels. In fact, because this laxative is so powerful, it can induce intestinal cramps. Most herbalists turn first to milder laxatives, like the related cascara sagrada. Buckthorn is an ingredient in some over-the-counter laxatives. The herb may have anticancer properties and is an ingredient in the controversial herbal Hoxsey Cancer Formula. In addition to cramps, its side effects may include vomiting and diarrhea, and it is not recommended for pregnant women or for long-term use. Herbal companies sell it as capsules and extracts. (See the description of cascara sagrada.)

BURDOCK *(Arctium lappa)* root is an alterative, diaphoretic, diuretic, and demulcent. It is used to promote the health and function of the kidneys, lungs, and liver, and also to treat chronic skin problems. Burdock root can be taken as a tea (boil 1 teaspoon of dried herb in 1 cup of water for 10 minutes; steep for 10 more minutes; drink twice a day for one week) or as a tincture (drops). Use 10 to 30 drops in water; twice a day, for one week. Do not take the herb longer than a week. Combine with dandelion and echinacea (see dandelion and echinacea herbs, below) for a strong immune-booster and antifungal treatment. Burdock can be found in most of our backyards. It's free for the taking and a wonderful promoter of health. It can be dried at home and chopped up to be used as an herbal tea. Use burdock for skin problems and as a tonifier and promoter of kidney function.

BUTTERCUP *(Crowfoot)* Apply buttercup directly to remove warts. The juice is topically applied to rheumatic and gouty joints to relieve these conditions. A tincture may be both externally applied and taken internally to treat shingles and sciatica.

CALAMUS ROOT *(Acorus calamus)* grows around ponds like cattails. Traditionally, it has been used to counteract an acidic stomach, as a carminative, and for treating coughs. Studies have shown that its volatile oil has a tonic and laxative effect. One constituent, beta-asarone, is reputed to be a hallucinogen, although the American variety often lacks this ingredient.

CALENDULA *(Callendula officinalis)* is astringent, vulnerary, antispasmodic, and diaphoretic. This plant is also known as marigold. It is used to treat skin problems, especially pimples and acne. It is antiseptic and anti-inflammatory, heals, and soothes. It is often found as part of an herbal salve. Apply it directly to the skin. Purchase calendula as a dried herb, boil, and use in a compress on the skin.

CALIFORNIA POPPY *(Eschscholzia californica)* is a flowering plant that produces a calming and quieting effect on the central nervous system. It is not as widely known as other herbal sedatives like valerian, but it is increasing in popularity. It is often taken about thirty minutes before bedtime to encourage restful sleep. It comes in concentrated drops and extracts.

CAPSICUM Red pepper is a commonly consumed spice worldwide. It lowers cholesterol and inhibits aggregation of platelets, thereby decreasing the tendency for the blood to clot and reducing the chances of suffering a coronary thrombosis, or a heart attack. Side effects can include heartburn, rectal burning, and sweating. It is best tolerated when taken before meals and it requires time to adapt to. Increase the dosage as tolerance increases. It's usually found in 500-milligram capsules, but you should adjust the dosage to avoid the unpleasant side effects. Capsicum has also been found to make the respiratory tract less sensitive, which reduces asthma attacks.

CARAWAY SEEDS *(Carum carvi)* contain 5 to 7 percent volatile oil. They are used as an aromatic, carminative, and as flavoring. The primary medical use is as an aid to digestion. Allow an ounce of the crushed seeds to steep in a pint of boiling water for twenty minutes. The normal dose is two tablespoons every two hours.

CARDAMOM SEEDS *(Elletaria cardamomum)* get their flavor and medicinal properties from their volatile oil. The mucous membrane–irritant properties make cardomom seeds a useful carminative and stimulant. Therapeutically, they are often combined with other purgatives.

CASCARA SAGRADA *(Rhamunus purshiana)* is a laxative, bitter tonic, nervine, and emetic. It is one of the most effective and powerful laxatives available. Use it as tincture (drops). Add 15 to 30 drops to a small amount of water, three times a day, once in the morning, once at midday, and once before bed. Use 10 to 15 drops for children. Do not use more than four days straight.

CASTOR OIL is a yellowish oil pressed from the toxic, beanlike seeds of the tropical castor oil plant *(Ricinus communis)*. Taken internally, the nontoxic but unpleasant-tasting oil has long been a widely recognized and effective laxative used after food poisoning or to relieve constipation. Applied topically, it readily penetrates the skin and is used to soften corns and skin tissue, prevent scarring, treat ringworm and abscesses, and promote the healing of bruises. It is often applied as a pack (an oil-dampened heated cloth).

CATNIP *(Nepeta cataria)* is diaphoretic, sedative, nervine, and carminative. Studies have found catnip to be a mild central nervous system stimulant and antispasmodic. It is well known as a sedative for nervous tension. Catnip is also used for insomnia and is a gentle cure for diarrhea. It is best taken as a tea.

CATTAIL *(Typha latifolia)* is an astringent root little used in modern herbology, but it is considered to be helpful to the kidneys and can also be chewed as a cough remedy.

CAYENNE, also known as red pepper, is both an herb and a spice obtained from the dried, ground fruit of various hot chili peppers *(Capsicum frutescens),* that contain the compound capsaicin, which reduces pain and inflammation, probably by blocking the activity in the body of substance P, a compound needed for transmitting pain impulses. Capsaicin is an ingredient in a prescription skin cream. Drops of cayenne concentrate are used to relieve toothache (though some will find it unpleasantly hot) and as a liniment to soothe sore muscles. Cayenne is also used topically to stop bleeding and is taken internally to stimulate circulation or induce sweating to break a fever. Some herbalists use it to treat colds and infectious diarrhea. In the Orient it is a popular crisis herb because of its heating and stimulating effects on the kidneys, lungs, stomach, and heart. It is widely used as a spicy seasoning. It is sold in the form of capsules, concentrated drops, and tinctures.

CEDAR BERRIES *(Juniperus communis)*: Of over sixty juniper species, the berries of *Juniperus communis* are best-known for their medicinal usage. Traditionally, they are used as an emmenagogue and externally as a remedy for skin disorders. (See also the description of juniper berries.)

CELANDINE *(Chelidonium majus)*: Renowned as a blood purifier, celandine is used to detoxify the liver in the treatment of jaundice, hepatitis, and certain skin ailments. It is used extensively by Chinese herbalists to heal bronchitis and whooping cough. Externally, the fresh juice may be mixed with milk and used directly to remove cataracts.

CELERY SEED *(Apium graveolens)* has a long reputation as a sedative as well as a treatment for dysmenorrhea and rheumatism. Modern studies have questioned its effectiveness.

CH'AI TEA is an Indian spice tea known for its warm, stimulating effect, especially recommended for uncontrollable shaking and cold chills. The tea is made by grating one ounce of ginger, adding seven peppercorns, a cinnamon stick, five cloves, and fifteen cardamom seeds. Simmer these in one pint of water for ten minutes. Add a half cup of milk and simmer ten more minutes. Combine a few drops of vanilla extract and a sprinkle of nutmeg with the tea, and drink one cup per day for warmth.

CHAMOMILE *(Anthemis floes; A. nobiles; Matricaria chamomilla; Compositae)* is a nervine, carminative, tonic, diaphoretic, sedative, antispasmodic, vulnerary, antiseptic, and emmenagogue. It is used to treat skin problems, soothes the skin, and makes it smooth. Chamomile is often an ingredient in herbal salves. The common herb tea speeds up a process called phagocytosis, or the proliferation of phagocyte cells, according to Dr. James Duke, a botanist and expert on herbs at the U.S. Department of Agriculture. The tea, which comes in tea bags and is commonly found in stores, also relaxes, makes sleep deeper and more restful, and helps relieve insomnia.

CHAPARRAL preparations are derived from the flowers, leaflets, and twigs of a woody, long-living shrub *(Larrea tridentata, L. divaricata)* of the American Southwest. Among its medically active compounds is a chemical with antibacterial action that can prevent infections when it is applied to wounds or can assist in clearing skin conditions. In the mouth, chaparral helps prevent tooth decay, mouth odor, and gum disease. Taken internally, it is a popular folk treatment for cancer; some studies confirm it may have antitumor effects. It also has potential anti-inflammatory and antioxidant properties, which may be useful in treating arthritis and helping retard aging. Chaparral was recently removed from the market by most herbal manufacturers after it was tied to five cases of acute toxic hepatitis, causing the FDA to issue a warning about it.

CHASTE BERRY *(Vitex agnus-castus)*. As its name implies, chaste berries were once thought to suppress sexual libido. While there is scant evidence that chaste berry decreases sexual desire, it is an effective tonic for the regulation of the female menstrual cycle. By stimulating the pituitary, this herb helps to create a balance between estrogen and progesterone production, thereby relieving much of the discomfort associated with PMS and menopause. Chaste berry is available as a powder and a tincture.

CHESTNUT LEAVES *(Castanea sativa)* are tonic, astringent, and antispasmodic. Regarded by some herbalists of the nineteenth century as a cure for coughs and chest inflammations, chestnut leaves are not widely used today, partly due to the blight that wiped out most chestnut trees.

CHICKWEED *(Stellaria media)* has antipyretic, demulcent, and alterative properties. It is used traditionally to treat fevers, inflammation, bronchitis, pleurisy, coughs, colds, and hoarseness. It can be applied externally as a poultice to treat skin diseases. As a tea, it is an effective way to curb cravings, assist digestion, and help lose weight.

CHRYSANTHEMUM *(Chrysanthemum morrifolium)*: The yellow flowers of the chrysanthemum are frequently used in China to combat inflammation, pneumonia, and fevers. It purifies the blood and calms the liver.

CINNAMON *(Cinnamomum verum; Lauraceae)* is a stimulant, astringent, diaphoretic, carminative, antiseptic, expectorant, and hemostatic. Research at the Human Nutrition Research Center at Tufts has found that cinnamon triples insulin's ability to metabolize glucose, or blood sugar. Because of this ability, cinnamon protects against diabetes and lowers hunger and sugar cravings, thus making it easier to control weight. At the U.S. Department of Agriculture, botanist and herb researcher Jim Duke, Ph.D., has found that cinnamon increases a type of immune cell, called a leukocyte, thus improving the body's ability to fight bacterial infections and viruses.

CITRUS SEED EXTRACT is a natural antibiotic that is very potent. It is derived primarily from the seeds of grapefruit and was developed after observing that citrus seeds do not readily decompose in nature from microbial action. This works in the body like most bitters and is good for drying damp conditions. This extract has been found to inhibit members of several classes of microbes and parasites, among them: protozoa, amoebas, bacteria, viruses, and at least thirty different types of fungi, including candida yeastlike fungi. Citrus seed extract is found in liquid extracts, capsules, sprays, ointments, and a variety of other forms for treating a host of maladies.

CLAY: Usually bought as French green clay, other clays are often just as good if French green clay cannot be found. To treat a boil or pimple, mix a tablespoon or more of the clay powder with just enough water to cause the powder to become a clay (usually it requires no more than a few tablespoons of water). Apply to the skin and let it dry. The clay can be applied in the morning and at night, until the boil or pimple has opened and drained. Then apply tea tree oil or herbal balm to promote healing. Clay, such as French green clay, can be purchased in most health and natural food stores.

CLEAVERS *(Galium aparine)* is alterative, astringent, and diuretic. Cleavers is used to help break a fever, treat inflammations of the kidneys and bladder, and to release suppressed urine. It is a strong diuretic and removes excess fluid from the body. Appalachian herbalists have long prescribed it for weight loss, due to its diuretic properties. It is also known as goosegrass.

CLOVE *(Caryophyllus aromaticus)* is antiseptic, aromatic, carminative, stimulant, anodyne, antiemetic, and aphrodisiac. A chemical extract of clove, *syzygium aromaticum*, has well-documented antitumor properties. According to Boston University Medical School immunologist Elinor Levy, Ph.D., immature cancer cells are the most dangerous because they tend to proliferate more rapidly than older, mature cancers. One of the active ingredients of clove, said Dr. Levy, has been shown to induce macrophages, a type of immune cell, to target and destroy these immature cells more rapidly. On the other hand, clove is particularly unhealthy when consumed as an extract or in clove cigarettes. It can cause toxic reactions in the lungs, which have resulted in death when taken in high doses.

COMFREY is a popular folk herb derived from the roots and leaves of a plant *(Symphytum officinale)* of the borage family. It is also known as boneset and knitbone. It has traditionally been taken internally as a digestive aid and, more frequently, applied externally to promote the healing of wounds and broken bones. Studies have found that comfrey contains compounds such as allantoin that promote cell regeneration and help relieve inflammation resulting from bruises, sprains, insect bites, and skin conditions. Allantoin is now widely used in body care products for its skin-soothing properties. Applied topically, comfrey is easily absorbed through the skin and reaches deep tissue. Oral ingestion of comfrey is now rare, due to concerns about potential liver toxicity. The American Herbal Products Association recently placed comfrey on its restricted use list, for external use only. Comfrey is frequently combined with calendula, witch hazel, Saint-John's-wort, arnica, and other herbs in salves and ointments. It is available fresh and dried, and in concentrated drops, tinctures, and extracts.

CONEFLOWER *(Echinacea angustifolia)* is reputed to be a natural antitoxin useful for internal and external infection, especially skin diseases. A study done in 1915 found no physiological active properties.

CORN SILK *(Zea mays)* is diuretic, lithotriptic (dissolves stones), and demulcent. The use of corn silk tea to treat kidney and bladder ailments was reported as early as the sixteenth century by an Inca writer, Garcilaso de la Vega. It is a traditional therapy for urinary tract complaints such as cystitis, urethritis, and prostatitis. Make a tea using one ounce of corn silk steeped in a pint of boiling water.

CORSICAN TEA is derived from Corsican seaweed, and is traditionally used for getting rid of intestinal worms. It is available at natural food stores and Oriental markets. Boil two to three tablespoons of seaweed in water. Drink when hungry. You can also drink it regularly instead of regular tea.

CRAMP BARK *(Viburnum opulus)* is an antispasmodic, sedative, nervine, and astringent. Cramp bark has a general tonic effect on the uterus and helps to regulate the menstrual cycle. It is often used in combination with its near relative, black haw, to treat PMS, menstrual cramps, and convulsions.

CRANESBILL ROOT *(Geranium maculatum)* is a pleasant astringent tonic used as a mouthwash or gargle. Taken internally, it is a remedy for diarrhea, colitis, and dysentery, especially when bleeding is present. Topically applied, it promotes healing of burns and can be used as a douche for vaginal discharge.

CULVER'S ROOT *(Leptandra virginica)* is a cholagogue, laxative, and diaphoretic. It is a markedly bitter, black root traditionally used to treat intestinal disorders as well as liver congestion with accompanying constipation.

CUMIN: Researchers from India have discovered that cumin *(Cuminum cyminum)*, a spice used commonly throughout the Middle East, inhibits platelet aggregation and lowers cholesterol in the blood. Israeli scientists have found that people who regularly add cumin to their food have lower rates of urinary tract cancers, including those of the bladder and prostate. Scientists in India confirmed these findings and discovered that cumin greatly increased the body's production of a detoxifying agent called GST, which is known to have strong cancer-inhibiting properties.

DANDELION *(Taraxacum officinale)* is a cholagogue, diuretic, hepatic, lithotriptic, stomachic, alterative, astringent, and galatogogue. It has been used traditionally to strengthen the liver, spleen, and heart. Dandelion promotes blood-cleansing functions of the liver, and lymph movement and drainage. It is also given to people suffering from hepatitis to promote the flow of bile from the liver. Dandelion greens are eaten as a vegetable, especially in springtime. The dried herb can be taken as tea (1 tablespoon of herb per 1 cup of water; boil for 10 minutes; steep for 10 minutes; drink daily for three days to a week). As a tincture, add 10 to 30 drops to a cup of water, and drink three to five times per week, for four weeks. The leaves of dandelion are common everywhere in North America. Harvest them before the plant flowers, however. After flowering, the plant becomes highly bitter and loses much of its vitality and healing effect.

DEVIL'S CLAW or WILD YAM *(Diascorea paniculata)* is traditionally used for gallstones and biliary colic. This herb was also used to treat rheumatic pains, though herbalists disagree over its effectiveness. For chronic liver problems, combine two parts wild yam, one part barberry root, and one-half part each of fennel seeds and ginger. Use as a tea or powder after meals.

DIOSCOREA (See the description of wild yam root, below.)

DONG QUAI (also dang-qui, danggui, tan kwe, and tang kui) is a favorite Chinese herb for women. It is derived from the root of Chinese angelica *(Angelica sinensis)*. It is used similarly to American and European angelica, and has long been prescribed by traditional Chinese and Indian herbalists to harmonize vital energy and nourish blood. Dong quai is widely taken in the West for gynecological problems and to regulate hormones, alleviate menstrual cramps, and end PMS distress. It has been extensively studied in China and found to nourish the reproductive system, enhance immunity, lower blood pressure, reduce pain, and improve circulation. Dong quai is often taken as a daily tonic by women entering menopause or before menstruation. It should be avoided during pregnancy. It comes dried and as tablets, capsules, concentrated drops, tinctures, and extracts. (See the description of angelica.)

EARTHWORM *(Pheretime aspergillum)* is an alterative, diuretic, and antispasmodic. It will open the bronchioles and the meridians of both the central nervous system and the circulatory system. Good for hypertension, lung inflammation that creates wheezing, arthritis, rheumatism, strokes, stiffness of the extremities, and high fever with convulsions and seizures.

ECHINACEA *(Echinacea angustifolia)* is an alterative, antibiotic, carminative, stimulant, and vulnerary. The organs affected are large intestine, lungs, stomach, and liver. Medicinal effects: Immune-boosting, antibiotic, antiinflammatory, and promotes digestion. Echinacea is one of the most powerful herbs against all types of infections. Dr. Jim Duke of the U.S. Department of Agriculture and herbalist Michael Tierra both say that echinacea stimulates phagocytosis (the process by which white blood cells consume bacteria, viruses, and cancer cells) and promotes the production of T cells (the immune cell that organizes the body's defenses against a disease-causing agent). Echinacea can be used in tincture (10 to 30 drops in water for adults; 10 to 15 drops in water or juice for children) or as a standard infusion. (See instructions, below.) Either as a tincture or infusion, echinacea is usually taken two or three times per day. Herbalists maintain, however, that it can be safely taken as many as five or six times a day with no ill effects. There are no contraindications. However, the author has noted that constipation occurs in some people when echinacea is taken in higher dosages for more than three days. Because of the herb's antibiotic qualities, fermented foods should be eaten consistently to maintain intestinal flora. Boiled grains, vegetables, and fruit should be eaten to maintain regularity.

ELECAMPANE *(Inula helenium)* is an expectorant, carminative, diuretic, and astringent. Elecampane root is specifically recommended for chronic mucus and coughs. It is also useful for asthma and bronchitis. It aids the digestive process, making mucus less likely to form.

EPHEDRA *(Ephedra vulgaris)* is an expectorant, astringent, diaphoretic, and stimulant. Ephedra is excellent for treating asthma, bronchitis, fever, headaches, low blood sugar, and respiratory conditions. It is especially powerful in the treatment of congestive sinus conditions. Ephedra increases blood pressure, and thus should not be used by people with hypertension. Weak or debilitated people should limit amounts and frequency of use. Ephedra has become increasingly controversial due to the tendency of some to use overdoses of the herb to create changes in brain chemistry and perception. Use only as directed. (See the related Chinese herb called ma huang, below.)

EUCALYPTUS is used as an inhalation against colds and flu to promote circulation in lungs, break up congestion, and improve breathing. It is often combined with pine needle, cloves, and thyme. Place the herbs in a vaporizer, along with water. Use leaves or oil of leaves. Hold a towel over the head to create a tent over the herbal steam and vaporizer. Inhale three times a day for ten minutes. This blend can also be added to a vaporizer left on in your room at night to help breathing. Herbs can be added to a pot of boiling water if a vaporizer is not available.

EYEBRIGHT preparations are derived from a northern plant *(Euphrasia officinalis)* with somewhat eye-shaped flowers. It has traditionally been used to make an eyewash for inflammations and other eye problems and is also taken internally for nasal congestion and coughs. Studies reveal that it contains compounds that are mildly astringent and anti-inflammatory. It is often combined with other herbs such as goldenseal, echinacea, and fennel seeds to relieve redness, swelling, and irritation of the eye. Eyebright is the source of the homeopathic remedy euphrasia. It comes in capsules, concentrated drops, tinctures, and extracts.

FALSE UNICORN ROOT *(Chamaelirium luteum)* is an emetic, diuretic, and vermifuge. False unicorn has been used traditionally to treat uterine disorders, especially painful and irregular menstruation. Studies have not been able to isolate its active ingredient or verify its effectiveness.

FENNEL preparations are produced from the seeds of a tall, stalky plant *(Foeniculum vulgare)* native to the Mediterranean. Fennel is primarily used as a digestive aid and to help expel gas. It is also used to treat diarrhea and infant colic. Women use it to stimulate milk flow, promote menstruation, and relieve menopausal ailments, although pregnant women should avoid it. As a tea it can be applied with an eyedropper to soothe the eyes. Aromatherapists use the essential oil medicinally, and the food industry uses it extensively as a flavoring. It is available dried and in capsules, concentrated drops, tinctures, extracts, and essential oils.

FENUGREEK *(Trigonella foengraecum)*: The seeds are tonic, astringent, demulcent, emollient, and expectorant. Fenugreek is one of the oldest recorded medicinal herbs. It is used to treat all mucous conditions and lung congestion. This seed is also helpful in treating inflamed conditions of the intestines.

FEVERFEW preparations are derived from the leaves and flowers of a bushy perennial *(Tanacetum parthenium),* and are used chiefly as a remedy for migraine headaches. Clinical trials in Britain indicate that a dosage of 50 to 100 milligrams daily of the dried leaves effectively prevents or significantly decreases the severity of migraine attacks for many people. Herbalists also use feverfew for its anti-inflammatory properties in the treatment of arthritis, as an antispasmodic to relieve menstrual cramps, and (as its name implies) a febrifuge to reduce fever. It is sold dried and in capsules, concentrated drops, tinctures, and extracts.

FLAXSEEDS *(Linum usitatissimum)* are a demulcent, emollient, and bulk-former. Traditionally, it is taken orally for coughs, due to its demulcent characteristics. Soaked flaxseeds are also prescribed for bowel irregularity.

FO-TI is one of the most widely used Chinese tonic herbs. It is derived from the root of a weedy, twining vine *(Polygonum multiforum)* in the buckwheat family. It is famous as a rejuvenating and longevity tonic in China, where it is taken to prevent premature aging, increase fertility, and maintain youthful strength and vigor. It is also used to treat dizziness, infertility, anemia, and constipation. There is evidence that it lowers blood cholesterol levels, and it is currently being studied for its ability to prevent heart disease and cancer. Fo-ti is sold dried and as powders, tablets, capsules, concentrated drops, tinctures, and extracts.

GARDENIA is called the happiness herb because it clears excess heat in the upper, middle, and lower parts of the body, which causes restlessness, irritability, anger, fever, hepatitis, jaundice, hypertension, ulcers, urinary tract infections, inflammation of burns, red eyes, mouth sores, bitter taste in the mouth, and insomnia. It is also used externally to reduce swellings from trauma. When partially charred, it stops blood in the vomit, stool, urine, or nose.

GARLIC *(Allium sativum)* is an alterative, antibiotic, antispasmodic, diaphoretic, expectorant, and stimulant. Garlic has antiviral, antibacterial, and antifungal activity. It promotes detoxification by the liver, specifically against carcinogens. Garlic has strong anticancer properties. It lowers both total cholesterol and LDL cholesterol, which causes atherosclerosis plaques. It also lowers triglycerides. Garlic raises HDL cholesterol, the cholesterol that protects against heart disease. It decreases platelet adhesiveness and inhibits blood clotting. Garlic also lowers blood pressure and improves blood flow by reducing the blood's viscosity. Various naturally occurring chemicals in onions and scallions have similar but less powerful effects.

GENTIAN *(Gentiana lutea)* is an intensely bitter root used as a stimulant to gastric secretions. One of the most popular bitters, it has been known since the time of the ancient Greeks. Gentian is useful to treat malaria but only in high doses.

GINGER *(Zingiberis officinalis)* is an aromatic, carminative, diaphoretic, stimulant, and diuretic. Ginger, commonly used as an herb in Oriental cuisine and a medicinal tea in Chinese medicine, has been shown to reduce the production of prostaglandins that cause inflammation, especially in people with arthritis. Such swelling, of course, is one of the factors that cause and exacerbate arthritis pain. Researchers have found that ginger also inhibits platelet aggregation, which means it prevents the blood from sludging, one of the factors that give rise to heart attacks and strokes. British researchers have found that ginger also prevents nausea, even in pregnant women. A study published in the *International Journal of Vitamin Nutrition Research* (61:364–369; 1991), showed that ginger also helped to reduce cholesterol in the blood of laboratory animals fed a high-fat diet. Thus, if you have any pain due to swelling, or nausea, or suffer from heart disease, a regular cup of ginger tea or a garnish of fresh grated ginger on your vegetables may be just what the doctor ordered.

GINKGO BILOBA (Chinese) preparations are derived from the fan-shaped leaves of one of the world's most ancient tree species *(Ginkgo biloba)*. It has been used by the Chinese for thousands of years to treat asthma, allergies, and coughs. Currently, it is gaining popularity for its reputed ability to improve brain function and boost memory and alertness. Researchers say that it stimulates circulation in the brain and ears and thus may help prevent dizziness, hearing loss, tinnitus, stroke, and depression. Ginkgo acts as an antioxidant. Studies indicate it has potential use in the treatment of impotence, varicose veins, and Alzheimer's disease. Extracts are often standardized to contain 24 percent ginkgo heterosides. It comes in tablets, capsules, concentrated drops, tinctures, and extracts.

GINSENG is a human-shaped root that is one of the most popular healing herbs of the East and West. It includes species from Asia *(Panax gin-*

seng, usually called Chinese or Korean ginseng) and North America *(P. quinquefolius,* called American ginseng). Siberian ginseng, or eleuthero, is also from the ginseng family and has similar effects and uses. Ginseng is commonly used as an adaptogen, meaning it normalizes physical functioning regardless of direction (for example, it will lower high blood pressure, but raise low blood pressure). It is also typically taken to lessen the effects of stress, improve performance, boost energy levels, enhance memory, and stimulate immunity. One study showed that two polysaccharides that could be isolated from ginseng stimulated the proliferation of CD4 cells in response to a disease-causing agent. Ginseng protects cells from damage caused by radiation and toxic substances. It is not as stimulating as herbs containing caffeine or ephedrine, but may be too strong for some people and should be used in moderation. It is sold as a whole root or powder, and in capsules, tablets, tea bags, tinctures, and extracts. (See also the description of Siberian ginseng.)

GOLDENSEAL *(Hydrastic canadensis; Ranunculaceae)* is an alterative, antiinflammatory, antiperiodic, astringent, diuretic, laxative, bitter tonic. Organs affected are colon, heart, liver, skin, and stomach. Goldenseal reduces inflammation, dries mucous membranes, regulates the menstrual cycle, cleanses the blood, promotes liver function, aids digestion, and treats bacterial infections. It reduces all forms of irritation from hemorrhoids (the herb is used in many medicinal salves). Goldenseal is also effective against yeast infections of all types, and the skin eruptions that normally accompany candidiasis. It treats the symptoms of flu, infections (including of the ears, eyes, and nose); it lowers fever, and relieves most digestive problems, including indigestion, gas, and heartburn. It can be applied externally for skin discharges and eruptions. Herbalist Michael Tierra says that when used over a ten-day period, it can be effective against dysentery *(Giardia).* Goldenseal, one of the most versatile and effective of all herbal plants known, should not be used for more than two weeks straight, say some herbalists. It is a strong stimulant that may irritate the urinary or digestive tract after two weeks or more.

GOTU KOLA is a principally Asian plant *(Hydrocotyle asiatica, Centella asiatica).* It should not be confused with kola, an unrelated, caffeinecontaining herb. For thousands of years, gotu kola has been a popular remedy in India and Pakistan, where it has a reputation for promoting longevity and is being investigated for use against leprosy and tuberculosis. In the West it is used mainly as a tonic to increase energy and endurance, improve memory and mental stamina, and alleviate depression and anxiety. It boosts circulation in the legs and is an effective remedy for varicose veins. Gotu kola also has important uses externally as a wound healer, burn remedy, and psoriasis treatment. Large doses taken internally may have a sedating effect. It is sold dried and in capsules, concentrated drops, tinctures, and extracts.

GRAPES (dark purple) are high in vitamins A, B, and C. They are good for blood deficiency and low energy, night sweats, excessive thirst, edema, dry cough, palpitations, and rheumatic and joint pains.

GRAVEL ROOT or QUEEN OF THE MEADOW *(Eupatorium purpureum)* is a diuretic, lithotriptic, nervine, tonic, and antirheumatic. Gravel root is a bitter root used for chronic urinary illnesses including stones, urinary gravel, hematuria, and frequent urination. It is also helpful for uric acid deposits in the joints and as a nerve tonic.

GREEN TEA, taken either in capsule form or as a beverage (both are available in natural food stores), provides numerous health benefits. Green tea contains chemical compounds called polyphenols (not present in the more common black teas), which act as powerful antioxidants. Studies show that people who drink approximately five cups of green tea a day (which contain about half the caffeine of coffee) or who take 500 milligrams a day of the caffeine-free capsules, have a lower risk of incurring cancer, suffering heart attacks and strokes, and contracting gum disease and cavities. Human population studies and animal research have shown a strong correlation between green tea consumption and reduced risk of certain cancers, especially esphageal cancer. The polyphenols in green tea also attack the bacteria that cause bad breath.

GRINDELIA *(Grindelia camporum)* is a stimulant, expectorant, mild sedative, and spasmolytic. Grindelia is used primarily as an expectorant and mild sedative. It is commonly used to treat asthma and bronchitis.

GUGULIPID is a plant extract that has been found to lower cholesterol as much as 21 percent and triglycerides by 25 percent in three to eight weeks, according to some studies. Typical doses are 500 milligrams, three times a day. Gugulipid causes no adverse effects on the liver or blood sugar. The only side effect reported is mild stomach upset, and that was seen in only one patient. At the same time, gugulipid was found to raise HDL cholesterol (the good cholesterol) by 36 percent. Gugulipid has also been shown to decrease platelet aggregation and increase fibrinolytic activity in patients, thus decreasing the tendency for the blood to clot and cause coronary thrombosis (*Indian Journal of Medical Research* 70:992, 1979).

Natural food and health food stores carry more concentrated preparations of gugulipid such as GuggulPlex; 25 milligrams, three times a day, is an effective dosage.

GUM PLANT (See the description of grindelia.)

HAWTHORN *(Crataegus oxyacantha)* is from a spiny tree, native to Europe. The berries, leaves, and blossoms contain biologically active flavonoids, which prevent constriction of blood vessels, thereby lowering blood pressure, according to the *Japanese Journal of Pharmacology* (43:242, 1987). Hawthorn may also strengthen the force of contraction of the heart muscle, which may assist those with heart failure, according to the

Fortschr medical journal (111; jr:20–21, 1993). Animal studies have shown that flavonoids lower cholesterol and reverse atherosclerosis. The British medical journal, *The Lancet* (342:1007, 1993), reported that hawthorn reduced the risk of death from heart disease and relieved chest pain (angina). Dosage varies depending upon the kind of preparation; 100 to 200 milligrams per day of the herb is a common dosage. Health food stores offer Solaray Hawthorn Extract of 100 milligrams, and tinctures, dried plant parts, and solid extracts. No adverse side effects have been encountered.

HONEYSUCKLE *(Lonicera periclymenum, Lonicera japonica)* is an alterative and an antipyretic. Although not well-known in American herbalism, honeysuckle is a basic ingredient in almost all Chinese detoxifying formulas. It is used to counteract inflammatory conditions such as acute flu and fever but, according to herbalist Michael Tierra, is not advisable for chronic conditions. Make an infusion by steeping an ounce of flowers in a pint of water. This infusion may also be applied externally for poison oak and other rashes.

HOPS is derived from the conelike fruits of a climbing plant *(Humulus lupulus)* best known for giving beer its bitter flavor. It is a digestive stimulant that is particularly effective for digestive complaints caused by anxiety. It is also a mild sedative and diuretic. It is sold dried and as concentrated drops, tinctures, and extracts. (See the description of bitters.)

HORSERADISH *(Armoracia radix)*: Best known as a condiment, horseradish is a stimulant to the digestive tract and is believed to inhibit intestinal worms. Traditional American herbalists applied it topically for rheumatism. Ingesting large doses of the raw root may cause vomiting.

HORSETAIL *(Equisetum arvense)* is an astringent, diuretic, lithotriptic, nutritive, and vulnerary. It is traditionally used as a diuretic for kidney ailments and, due to its high silica content, for skin and eye conditions. Humbart Santillo, author of *Natural Healing with Herbs,* specifically recommends it for internal bleeding and urine retention. Horsetail may have a toxic effect on the kidneys if it is used in high doses or for prolonged periods (more than a month).

HUCKLEBERRY *(Vaccinum myrtillus),* also known as blueberry or bilberry, is an astringent, diuretic, antiscorbutic, and a folk remedy for better eyesight. Studies confirm a positive effect on vision due to the berry's flavonoid compounds, the fifty-five anthocyanosides, which can cause biochemical reactions in the eye. Huckleberry may also play a role in relieving menstrual problems, as studies have found it helps to relax smooth muscles like those found in the uterine wall. Huckleberry is nontoxic and comes in tablets, capsules, and extracts.

HYDRASTIS (See the description of goldenseal.)

HYSSOP *(Hyssopus officinalis)* is a diaphoretic, expectorant, stimulant, and vulnerary. It is used to treat respiratory ailments, such as coughs, colds, asthma, and sinus problems. A fomentation of hyssop may be used externally for muscle pain and as a poultice to heal cuts.

IMPATIENS (See the description of jewelweed.)

IPECAC is prepared from the dried roots of a South American shrub *(Cephaelis ipecacuanha)*. The sweet-tasting syrup of ipecac is used to induce vomiting in poison victims. The syrup is widely available in conventional pharmacies and is safe even if not vomited. In other forms, the herb is sometimes used to bring up mucus from the lungs and relieve bronchitis. Formulations such as concentrated fluid extract of ipecac are much more toxic than the syrup preparations and need to be diluted before taking. Homeopaths use extremely dilute preparations to treat persistent and extreme nausea and some types of bleeding. Ipecac is sold as a syrup or concentrated fluid extract.

IRISH MOSS *(Chondrus crispus)* is an anticoagulant, demulcent, emollient, nutritive, and protectant. It is used to treat illnesses of the lung, upper respiratory tract and stomach. Irish moss is a seaweed used for the production of carrageenan, a thickening agent that is added to foods. It is soothing to those suffering from coughs or diarrhea. There are no apparent toxic properties.

JACK-IN-THE-PULPIT, also known as dragon root, grows in the damp localities of North and South America. The root is the only part that is used. It is an antispasmodic, carminative, diaphoretic, and expectorant. It opens up the meridians and treats disorders associated with blockage, such as spasms of hands and feet, lockjaw, seizures, strokes, facial paralysis, numbness, and dizziness. It's a drying herb and can be used to dry phlegm and to treat hoarseness, loss of voice, and discomfort in the throat, mouth, or tongue. It is good for asthma, whooping cough, stomatitis, chronic laryngitis, colic, and flatulence. A poultice or liniment can be made for sores, ulcers, swellings, and tumors.

JEWELWEED *(Impatiens nolitangere)* has been consistently used as an external treatment for skin rashes, especially poison ivy. The herb is not toxic if taken internally but has no clearly established therapeutic properties.

JUNIPER BERRIES *(Juniperus communis)* are antispasmodic, diuretic, astringent, carminative, and aromatic. They are traditionally used as an emmenagogue and externally as a remedy for skin disorders. Humbart Santillo, author of *Natural Healing with Herbs,* recommends juniper berries as an effective digestive tonic as well as a preventive for those who are nursing patients with serious airborne diseases.

KELP is a nutrient-dense, brown sea vegetable that is among the richest sources of the element iodine, which is needed by thyroid hormones to help regulate the body's growth and development. Iodine can also protect cells from damage by radioactive substances and heavy metals. As a food, kelp is usually eaten in small quantities; it is also used as a condiment and nutritional supplement. There are some potential adverse effects from long-term overuse. It is sold dried or as a liquid, powder, or tablets.

KUZU *(Pueraria thunbergiana)* is an antipyretic, diaphoretic, spasmolytic, and demulcent. A starch powder derived from the root of this fast-growing plant, kuzu powder is used by Asian healers to treat colds, flu, and intestinal ailments. It neutralizes stomach acidity and stops diarrhea.

LADY'S SLIPPER *(Cypripedium calceolus)* is a nervine, sedative, and antispasmodic used to treat nervous disorders such as insomnia, tremors, stress, and depression. Herbalist Michael Tierra reports that it is now an endangered species and should not be used until it has been reestablished.

LARKSPUR *(Consolida regalis)* is a parasiticide and insecticide. Larkspur is used externally to kill nits and lice. *Warning:* Do not take it internally; larkspur is a highly toxic poison. It is available in a tincture.

LEMON BALM preparations are derived from the aromatic leaves of a perennial mint plant *(Melissa officinalis)*. Also known as balm, bee balm, and sweet balm, it has traditionally been used to relieve nervousness and anxiety or to induce sweating. Studies confirm that it relaxes the nervous system and is an effective though mild herbal sedative. Herbalists recommend it to alleviate headaches, anxiety, and depression that are caused by nervous problems. It also improves digestion. Lemon balm is used topically as a wound healer. It has been found to have antibacterial, antiviral, and analgesic properties. Lemon balm is among the gentlest of the calming herbs, which include skullcap, valerian, hops, and passionflower. It is available dried and as concentrated drops, tinctures, and extracts.

LICORICE is an herb prepared from the roots of an Oriental and European perennial *(Glycyrrhiza glabra)* of the pea family. Licorice has long been used by traditional Chinese, Greek, and European herbalists as a general tonic and for respiratory problems such as asthma, coughs, and bronchitis. Studies have confirmed potential uses to relieve coughs, treat ulcers, alleviate arthritis, and control liver conditions such as hepatitis and cirrhosis. The herb's natural sweetness makes it a favorite flavor for herbal combination products as well as for candies and other foods. Overuse of extracts may cause adverse health effects related to salt and water retention. Retailers sell licorice in powders, capsules, concentrated drops, tinctures, and extracts.

LIFE ROOT *(Senecio aureus)* is an astringent. Part of the ragwort family and similar to ragweed, life root has been used to treat irregularities of menstruation. It contains more than forty pyrrolizidine alkaloids, many of which produce reactions toxic to the liver if taken in excess.

LIGUSTICUM is a Chinese herb prepared from the roots of a lovagelike plant *(Ligusticum chinensis, L. glaucesens)* and used similarly to dong quai as an herb for women's ailments. Ligusticum should not be confused with ligustrum or the Native American herb osha *(Ligusticum porteri)*. It comes in capsules. (See the description of osha.)

LIGUSTRUM is a Chinese herb *(nu-zhen-zi)* prepared from the dried and powdered fruits of an evergreen shrub *(Ligustrum lucidum)* also known in the United States as Chinese privet. It has traditionally been used as a general liver and kidney tonic. Recent studies in China and the United States indicate it may boost immunity and may be useful in the treatment of cancer by enhancing white blood cell counts after drug or radiation therapy. It is also a mild heart stimulant. Ligustrum is an ingredient in a number of herbal combination products sold in the United States. It is sold as a powder, extract, or concentrate.

LOBELIA *(Lobelia inflata)* is an expectorant, stimulant, antispasmodic, and emetic used to treat spasmodic lung and respiratory illnesses. Lobelia acts as a stimulant in small doses and as a sedative in larger doses. One of its active ingredients, lobeline, has a stimulating effect on the emetic medullary center. Lobeline acts in a similar way to nicotine and has been used as an aid in stopping smoking. Lobelia should be used carefully, since errors in dosage can produce opposite effects from those intended.

LOTUS ROOT TEA is made from the root of water lily, which is brown-skinned with a hollow, chambered, off-white inside. The tea is excellent for coughs and getting rid of excess mucus in the body. To make lotus root tea, grate ½ cup of fresh lotus root, squeeze the juice into a pot, and add a small amount of water. Cook for five to eight minutes, add a pinch of sea salt or tamari soy sauce, and drink it hot.

LUNGWORT is a tonic that is a relative of comfrey. It is an astringent, antitussive, demulcent, and expectorant and is used for dysentery, coughs, throat problems, and bleeding from the lungs. It can be made into a poultice and can be used for an enlarged thyroid gland, burns, tumor, and to reduce swelling and inflammation caused by injuries.

LYCII BERRIES *(Lycium chinensis)* are an alterative. Lycii is used primarily as a blood purifier, helping the body to assimilate nutrients.

MA HUANG is a Chinese herb derived from a primitive stemlike shrub *(Ephedra sinica)*. It is perhaps humanity's oldest medicine, traditionally used for millennia to relieve respiratory complaints such as bronchitis and asthma. Ma huang is a natural source of the powerful and long-acting stimulant compound ephedrine, which boosts heart rate, breathing, and metabolism and opens air passages, thus acting as a decongestant. The synthetically derived ephedrine relative, pseudoephedrine, is now widely used in conventional over-the-counter cold and allergy remedies such as Sudafed. (American species of ephedra have little or no ephedrine, a stronger stimulant than caffeine and one that could get you banned from participating in the Olympics.) High dosages and repeated use of ma huang may result in nervousness, restlessness, and increased blood pressure. It's sold as capsules, concentrated drops, and extracts. (See also the description of ephedra.)

MARIGOLD (See the description of calendula.)

MARSHMALLOW ROOT *(Althea officinalis)* is a demulcent, diuretic, emollient, and vulnerary. Marshmallow root is used internally to treat the intestines, kidney, and bladder. It is often combined with other diuretic herbs to help pass kidney stones.

MEADOWSWEET *(Filipendula ulmaria)* is an antispasmodic, analgesic, anti-rheumatic, diaphoretic, diuretic, and astringent. It is used for all kinds of urinary tract infections, fever, gout, arthritis, and rheumatism.

MILK THISTLE is a traditional liver remedy prepared from the seeds of a thorny, weedlike plant *(Silybum marianum)*. Milk thistle is often taken in the form of silymarin, a standardized extract of a complex compound found in the seeds. Studies show that silymarin helps liver cells regenerate and stabilizes liver cell membranes. It also boosts the organ's ability to filter blood and prevents liver damage from toxins including solvents, alcohol, drugs, most pesticides and herbicides, and bacterial compounds such as those associated with food poisoning. Milk thistle may help treat cirrhosis, hepatitis, and other liver diseases. It is often taken regularly as a preventive and after exposure to a toxin. It comes in capsules, concentrated herbal drops, and extracts.

MINT *(Menta piperita)* is an aromatic stimulant, stimulant, and carminative. Long used to calm the stomach, mint is used as a dried powder, volatile oil, or tincture. Dr. Jim Duke of the U.S. Department of Agriculture reports that mint increases the number of phagocyte cells, which are capable of destroying pathogens, bacteria, and cancer cells.

MISTLETOE (American) *(Viscum flavescens)* is an antispasmodic, nervine, diuretic, emetic, and tonic. American mistletoe is used to relieve tension and minor spasms. It is often given to women at the onset of labor because it stimulates contractions of the uterus and makes them more regular. Variable toxicity of plants call for caution in using this herb, especially with those prone to hypertension.

MOTHERWORT *(Leonuris cardiaca)* is an emmenagogue, nervine, diuretic, and cardiac tonic. It is used traditionally to treat slow menstruation and other female reproductive problems. Motherwort is also helpful as a cardiac tonic. It improves blood circulation and may be used to treat arteriosclerosis.

MUGWORT *(Artemisia vulgaris)* is a cholagogue, vermifuge, emmenagogue, hemostatic, antispasmodic, and diaphoretic. As a nervine, mugwort is good for treating nervousness, insomnia, and other nervous system ailments. It is also used as a bitter tonic for liver and stomach illnesses. Mugwort may also be used to bring on menstruation and may be combined with cramp bark to treat menstrual cramps.

MULBERRY *(Morus alba)*: Herbalist Michael Tierra reports that the properties of mulberry vary according to the part of the plant used. The fruit is a demulcent blood tonic used to treat anemia, dizziness, and nervousness.

Mulberry root bark is best known as a treatment for lung inflammation with expectorant properties. The leaf is diaphoretic with a cooling, calming effect on colds, sore throats, and feverish colds. The branch is antirheumatic and antispasmodic.

MULLEIN preparations are derived from the leaves, roots, or flowers of a tall, spikelike plant *(Verbascum thapsus)* used to make traditional respiratory remedies. Chemical analysis confirms that mullein contains mucilage, a substance that relieves coughs and soothes sore throats by absorbing water in the windpipe and becoming slippery. Mullein also acts as an expectorant by bringing up mucus. Herbalists use a mullein flower oil infusion (not the essential oil) as ear drops to relieve earaches. Mullein is sold dried or as concentrated drops, tinctures, extracts, oils, and essential oils.

MUSTARD SEED *(Brassica nigra)* is a stimulant, diuretic, alterative, and emetic. Mustard seed has been used for centuries in a plaster as a counterirritant, that is, by irritating the skin, it was felt that deeper-lying infections would be counteracted. It is still frequently used to stimulate circulation in cases of sprains, aches, and colds. Care should be exercised not to leave the plaster on for long after it begins to produce a burning sensation. It may also be taken internally: a teaspoonful for a mild laxative and a tablespoonful for an emetic.

MYRRH *(Commiphora myrrha)* is an antiseptic, emmenagogue, stimulant, astringent, and expectorant. Myrrh is a well-known and powerful antiseptic. It may be combined with goldenseal to treat wounds and skin diseases, especially when pus is present. As a tincture, it is diluted with water and used as a mouthwash for spongy gums, pyorrhea, and sore throats. Internally, myrrh stops putrification in the intestines and helps in the treatment of ulcers. It is also given for arthritis, rheumatic, and bronchial complaints. Due to its high resin content, avoid continuous use unless combined with other demulcent herbs.

NETTLES *(Urtica urens)* are an alterative, nutritive, antiseptic, expectorant, and hemostatic. Nettles have been used traditionally to treat asthma, baldness, calcium deficiency, goiter, night sweats, stomach disorders, urinary tract disorders, and externally for baldness. It has antihistamine and anti-inflammatory properties.

NIGHT-BLOOMING CEREUS *(Selenicereus grandiflorus)* is a diuretic, sedative, and cardiac tonic. Primarily used for heart problems, night-blooming cereus may be combined in equal parts with hawthorn berry and motherwort. Suggested dosage is ten drops three times daily; higher dosages may cause irritation.

OATS, like nettle, are a kind of healing herb and nutritional supplement. It is prepared from the whole plant and seeds of a hardy, widely cultivated cereal grass *(Avena sativa)*. The edible grain is a popular breakfast cereal. The herb is traditionally used as an aphrodisiac and as a remedy for exhaustion and depression. Studies confirm that oats contain an alkaloid that stimulates the central nervous system. Oats provide a range of therapeutic and nutritional substances that feed a debilitated nervous system. As a nutritional supplement, it is high in calcium and other nutrients and acts as an excellent nerve tonic, gently stimulating the system and providing nourishment. It is also now used to help break addictions. In high concentrations, oats can make people (and horses) excitable. It is sold dried and as capsules, concentrated drops, tinctures, and extracts.

OAT STRAW *(Avena sativa)* is a tonic and nutritive. Tea made from oat straw is useful for chest and kidney ailments. Body retention of calcium is increased, making it a good treatment for bone disease and lactation difficulty. It is also a good tonic for stomach problems and a helpful treatment for bed-wetting. Put a gallon of the warm tea in a bath for gout and rheumatic pain.

OREGON GRAPE ROOT *(Berberis aquifolium)* is a cholagogue, antiseptic, alterative, and laxative. It is a blood purifier used for all liver ailments, especially hepatitis, jaundice, and gallstones. It works by stimulating the flow of bile through the liver and gallbladder, which helps to eliminate constipation, and it also stimulates the thyroid. It is also highly recommended for skin diseases.

OSHA is prepared from the dried roots of a North American plant *(Ligusticum porteri)* that Native Americans have traditionally used to treat sore throats, colds, and flu. Recent research indicates potential antiviral and immune-boosting properties. Osha may have applications in the treatment of bronchitis, herpes, and flu. It is often sold in combination with other herbs. It is available in capsules, extracts, and concentrated drops. (See also the description of ligusticum.)

OYSTER or CLAM SHELL: Crushed or whole oyster shell *(Ostrea gigas*; in Mandarin, it is called *mu lin)* and clam shell *(Meritricix meritrix*; in Mandarin called *hai ge ke)* can be purchased in Chinese herb stores or collected at the ocean beach. They need to be crushed and then decocted into a tea. Oyster-shell calcium supplements can also be taken.

PARSLEY *(Petroselinum sativum)* is a lithotryptic, diuretic, nutritive, antiseptic, and expectorant. Parsley has been used traditionally to treat urinary infections, and especially for expelling stones. A tea made from the root and leaf is also useful as a mineral supplement.

PASSIONFLOWER preparations are made from the leaves of a climbing vine *(Passiflora incarnata)*. Passionflower has traditionally been used as a sedative and analgesic. It can help induce a contemplative state or mild euphoria, and it can relieve headaches or muscle spasms from nervous tension. Passionflower is gentle enough for children who are overly nervous and for the elderly suffering from insomnia. It is also an antispasmodic sometimes recommended as a digestive aid and menstrual reliever. It is not an aphrodisiac, despite its name, which derives from the plant's supposed resemblance to the crown of thorns in the biblical Passion. It should be avoided by pregnant women and should not be taken in large amounts. It is sold dried and in concentrated drops, tinctures, and extracts.

PAU D'ARCO preparations derive from the inner bark of a tall, flowering tree *(Tabebuia avellanedae, T. impetiginosa)* native to Brazil. The herb, also known as lapacho and taheebo, has been used for centuries in South America to heal wounds and treat snakebites. Its popularity is spreading among herbalists in the United States and Europe due to its broad clinical applications, including antibacterial, antiviral, and anti-inflammatory properties. The tea and extract can be taken orally or applied topically for bites and stings, infections, and inflammations. It comes as dried, shredded bark or as capsules and liquid extracts (often standardized for lapachol content).

PEACH SEED *(Amygdalus persica)* is a sedative, laxative, stomachic, and demulcent. The kernel of the peach contains hydrocyanic acid. It has been used traditionally as a sedative. It is a bitter seed similar to apricot.

PEONY ROOT *(Paeonia lactiflora)* is an alterative, liver tonic, and antispasmodic used to treat liver ailments and as a blood purifier.

PEPPERMINT *(Menta piperita)* is an aromatic stimulant, diaphoretic, stimulant, and carminative. Long used to calm the stomach, peppermint is also used for insomnia and headaches. Due to its high tannin content, it should not be taken on a daily basis for periods longer than a month.

PIPSISSEWA *(Chimaphila umbellata),* also known as pyrola, is a diuretic, astringent, alterative, and bitter tonic. It is excellent as a disinfectant for the urinary tract. Pipsissewa has also been used extensively to treat arthritis and rheumatism. It is a bitter, astringent herb similar to uva ursi but containing less tannin.

PLAINTAIN *(Plantago major)* is a diuretic, alterative, anti-inflammatory, and astringent that is widely used both internally and externally. Taken internally, it is best known for treating urinary infections. It contains acubin, which helps to regulate the secretion of uric acid from the kidneys. Plaintain tincture is also useful for all inflammations, including jaundice, bronchitis, hepatitis, and dysentery. Externally, it is used for insect bites, skin rashes, or poison ivy.

PLEURISY ROOT TEA *(Asclepias tuberosa)* is a diaphoretic, expectorant, antispasmodic, diuretic, and tonic. As its name implies, it is useful for pleurisy and pneumonia. Pleurisy root will bring on a sweat and has been used to treat colds, fevers, and flu.

POMEGRANATE *(Punica granatum)* is an astringent and anthelmintic. The rinds and bark of pomegranate have been used as an astringent tonic. The root had frequent use historically as a treatment for worms but is very toxic in large doses, in some cases having caused complete paralysis.

PRICKLY ASH BARK *(Zanthoxylum americanum)* is a stimulant, antirheumatic, alterative, diaphoretic, and emmenagogue. The bark, leaves, and fruit of prickly ash have all been used, but the bark is considered most healing. It stimulates blood and lymph circulation, making it helpful in treating arthritis and rheumatism. Prickly ash is also useful for stomach ailments as a gastric stimulant. Powdered bark may be applied to the gums for pyorrhea and receding gums.

PSYLLIUM *(Plantago psyllium)* is a laxative and demulcent. The seeds are used to relieve constipation. Herbalist Michael Tierra recommends a mix of two parts psyllium soaked in water with equal parts flax and chia seeds.

PULSATILLA *(Pulsatilla vulgaris)* is an anodyne, alterative, sedative, and bactericidal. It is historically used to treat syphilis. Recent use is as a sedative in nervous disorders. Pulsatilla is also recommended for amenorrhea and dysmenorrhea.

PYROLA *(Pyrola maculata)* (See the description of pipsissewa.)

RED CLOVER *(Trifolium pratense)* is an alterative, antispasmodic, and expectorant sedative. It is a good blood purifier with blood-thinning properties. Red clover is used for the treatment of cancerous tumors. For treatment of cancer, it is often combined with other herbs, especially yellow dock, echinacea, dandelion, and sassafras. Red clover is also used for mucous congestion and as a salve for skin problems.

RED RASPBERRY is prepared from the leaves and berries of a prickly bush *(Rubus idaeus)*. It has traditionally been used as a woman's herb to control morning sickness during pregnancy and to ease the pain of menstruation and childbirth. It has also long been used as a remedy for childhood diarrhea. Studies confirm that it helps relax the uterus and contains astringent compounds that can treat diarrhea. It is sold dried and in capsules, concentrated drops, tinctures, and extracts.

REHMANNIA *(Rehmannia glutinosa)* is a diuretic, alterative, and tonic. It is an important heart tonic and kidney treatment in Chinese herbal medicine. It is available as the raw root, which is best for treating the kidneys, and as a powder, which is used for anemia and heart disease. Rehmannia helps the body to recover from illness and combats anemia.

RHUBARB *(Rheum palmatum)* is a purgative, astringent, aparient (in small doses), alterative, and antibiotic. Rhubarb root has combined properties; it is both laxative and astringent, making it useful for constipation and, in smaller doses, for diarrhea and dysentery. When taken for diarrhea, it is best combined with ginger to reduce griping pains.

ROSE HIPS are the small, cherrylike, ripe fruit of various roses *(Rosa carolina* and other species). They are an excellent source of vitamin C and bioflavonoids. Vitamin companies frequently use rose hips in natural vitamin C supplements (although vitamin C from synthetic sources makes up the bulk of the tablet). Hips are gathered in autumn or winter, split open to remove the seeds, dried, and then finely ground into a fragrant powder used in supplements. The seeds of one species *(Rosa mosqueta)* yield an oil that is high in essential fatty acids.

ROSEMARY is a strong-smelling herb and essential oil made from the thin leaves of a small evergreen shrub *(Rosmarinus officinalis)*. It has long been a popular cooking herb and an ingredient in a stimulating tonic wine said to have a positive effect on the nervous and circulatory systems. Rosemary is used to treat chronic circulatory weakness, including low blood pressure. It is also an appetite stimulator, digestive aid, and antioxidant. It is applied topically to soothe sprains and bruises and heal wounds. A few drops of the essential oil put in the bath act as a relaxant. Taken internally, the essential oil may induce menses and thus should be avoided by pregnant women. Rosemary comes dried and in tinctures, concentrated drops, and essential oils.

SAFFRON *(Crocus sativus)*: A study published in the *Developments in Biological Standardization* (77:191, 1992) indicated that saffron has been shown to inhibit the growth of tumors in mice. It also stimulates T cells—perhaps the most important of immune cells—to multiply. Saffron also acts as an antioxidant.

SAINT-JOHN'S-WORT *(Hypericum perforatum)* is a sedative, astringent, alterative, and antidepressant. It is used for nervous system disorders, including neuralgia. It is also helpful with boils, uterine problems, dysentery, and jaundice. To treat depression, herbalist Michael Tierra recommends a mixture of equal parts of powdered Saint-John's-wort, red rose petal, and lemon balm.

SANTICLE *(Sanicula canadensis)* is a vulnerary, nervine, and antitumor. It is used as a blood purifier and a specific remedy for rheumatism. Santicle is mentioned by Humbart Santillo, author of *Natural Healing with Herbs,* as an ingredient in an antitumor herbal combination.

SARSAPARILLA *(Smilax medica)* is an alterative, anti-inflammatory, antipruitic, and tonic widely used historically in herbal preparations for skin eruptions including psoriasis and eczema. In addition to skin ailments, it is useful in treating venereal diseases and liver ailments.

SASSAFRAS *(Sassafras albidum)* is an alterative, diaphoretic, diuretic, and antirheumatic. An Appalachian folk favorite, sassafras is prescribed for skin ailments, including acne. It is a blood purifier that is also used to cleanse the liver and treat rheumatism. There is controversy over the presence of *safrole,* a constituent of sassafras, which, according to herbalist Michael Tierra, has been shown to cause tumors in rats. Tierra points out that studies on humans have not shown this result.

SAW PALMETTO is derived from the dark berries of a small southeastern palm tree *(Serenoa repens, S. serrulata)* with swordlike leaves that grow in a fan shape. It has traditionally been used as an aphrodisiac and to tonify the male reproductive system. Studies confirm an effect on male sex hormones, and an extract has exhibited positive clinical results in treating enlargement of the prostate. It is also an expectorant used to treat respiratory complaints like colds, coughs, and bronchitis. Saw palmetto contains polysaccharides with potential immune-boosting effects. It is sold as tablets, concentrated drops, extracts, and tinctures.

SCHISANDRA (also spelled schizandra) is a common Chinese herb derived from the dried, berrylike fruit of a hardy vine *(Schizandra chinensis)* of the magnolia family, native to East Asia. The Chinese refer to it as *wu-wei-zi*. Schisandra is a major tonic herb in Chinese medicine, long prized by emperors for its ability to prolong youth, increase stamina, and prevent fatigue. It is an adaptogen, balancing bodily functions. It nourishes the liver and kidneys and improves the body's response to stress. It is sometimes used as a mild sedative to treat insomnia and as a respiratory stimulant for coughs and asthma. Schisandra may be beneficial in the treatment of prolonged diarrhea. Herbal companies frequently combine it with Siberian ginseng and other Chinese herbs in adaptogen formulas. It comes as a powder and in capsules, concentrated drops, tinctures, and extracts.

SCORPION *(Buthus martensi)* is used to balance the body's overall energy and promote pain relief.

SKULLCAP *(Sculletaria lateriflora)* is an antispasmodic, nervine, and antipyretic used for nervous system ailments, including insomnia and hysteria. Skullcap works on the cerebrospinal centers, calming excessive excitement.

SENNA is derived from the leaflets and seed pods of a small shrub *(Cassia angustifolia)* grown in India. An ingredient in conventional laxatives, it is taken for its powerful effects on constipation. Herbalists often combine it with ginger or other herbs to reduce its side effects, which may include sudden, sharp bowel pains. Most herbalists recommend trying milder laxatives like cascara sagrada first. Senna should be avoided by pregnant women and should not be taken over an extended time. It comes in capsules, tinctures, and extracts.

SHEPHERD'S PURSE preparations are derived from the flowering tops of a common North American weed *(Capsella bursapastoris)* of the mustard family. Its name comes from its distinctive purse-shaped seed pods. Shepherd's purse has been used since ancient times to stop bleeding, both internal (menstrual bleeding, for instance) and external (cuts, scrapes, and nosebleeds). Chemical analysis confirms that it contains tyramines and other chemicals that promote blood coagulation and constrict blood vessels. It also has compounds (choline and acetylcholine) that reduce blood pressure. Shepherd's purse may trigger labor during pregnancy. It is available dried and in capsules, concentrated drops, tinctures, and extracts.

SHIITAKE MUSHROOMS *(Genus lentinula)* are wide flat-capped mushrooms traditionally grown in the Orient and now widely available in the United

States and Europe. Studies at the U.S. National Cancer Institute and the Japanese National Cancer Institute have established the shiitake mushroom as an immune-booster, a cancer fighter, and a powerful cholesterol-lowering herb. Shiitake has antiviral and antibacterial properties; it also causes the immune system to mount a stronger attack against an invading antigen or a tumor. Both animal and human studies have shown that shiitake mushrooms substantially lower blood cholesterol; some research suggests that the cholesterol-lowering effect of shiitake extract—the concentrated form of the herb—may be as much as 25 percent when used over a couple of weeks.

SIBERIAN GINSENG (also widely known as eleuthero) is a popular Oriental herb derived from the root or leaves of a northern shrub *(Eleuthero coccus senticosus)* from the Far East. It is from the same plant family as other ginsengs and like those has long been used by the Chinese to increase longevity and improve overall health. Like other ginsengs, it is an adaptogen, a substance that normalizes and regulates all of the body's systems. It supports the working of the adrenal glands and prevents the worst effects of nervous tension, increases energy, extends endurance, and fights off fatigue. Siberian ginseng may play a role in the treatment of heart disease, kidney infection, and psychological ailments. It is safer for daily consumption than most energy-boosting herbs. Herbal producers often combine it with other adaptogenic herbs such as schisandra. It is usually less expensive than other ginsengs. It is available dried and in capsules, tinctures, and extracts. (See also the description of ginseng.)

SKUNK CABBAGE is an antispasmodic, and is used as a cure for hiccups. Either prepare a tea or use the tincture. It is also useful for hoarseness, muscular cramps, and convulsions.

SLIPPERY ELM preparations are derived from the ground inner bark of a tree *(Ulmus rubra, U. fulva)* recently ravaged in the United States by Dutch elm disease. It has been a popular folk medicine, healing food, and digestive tonic for thousands of years. Today, it is most widely used in lozenges for symptomatic relief of sore throats, coughs, and colds. As a paste, it can be used externally to soothe and heal minor skin injuries, rashes, and irritations. Even the FDA calls it an excellent demulcent, or soothing agent. Slippery elm can be mixed with water or milk to make a food that, because it is nutritious and easily assimilated, is often recommended for those recovering from illness. It is sold in powders, lozenges, tablets, and extracts.

SOYBEANS: Soybean products, such as tofu, tamari, shoyu, and miso, contain a compound known as genistein that, according to recent research, blocks blood vessels from attaching themselves to tumors. Cancer cells and tumors, like all other cells and tissues in the body, need oxygen and nutrition to survive. By blocking blood flow to tumors, genistein prevents needed nutrients and oxygen from getting to both benign and malignant growths.

SPEARMINT *(Mentha viridus)* is an aromatic, carminative, stimulant, and diaphoretic. Spearmint is a mild, soothing stomach tonic. It is also a mild diuretic useful for treating colds and flu. It will help to stop vomiting.

STINGING NETTLE *(Cirsium altissimum)* is an alterative, nutritive, expectorant, and hemostatic. Nettle tea is good for diarrhea, dysentery, and hemorrhoids. It is a nutritious vegetable high in iron, silica, and potassium. For this reason, it is useful as a tea for anemia in children.

STONEROOT *(Collinsonia canadensis)* is an astringent, diuretic, hepatic, emmenagogue, and alterative. Used primarily as a treatment for hemorrhoids, stoneroot is a specific tonic to strengthen the portal vein of the rectum and varicose veins in general. It is good to take after rectal surgery. It is also strengthening to the heart.

SUMA *(Pfaffia paniculata)* is an adaptogen, energy tonic, and demulcent. Suma is equal to Siberian ginseng as an energy booster. Herbalist Michael Tierra reports studies showing five constituents of suma that inhibit tumor cell melanomas. It has a mild flavor, similar to vanilla. It is very helpful in treating chronic fatigue syndrome.

TEA (GREEN AND BLACK) contains antioxidants, flavonoids, tannins, and indoles, all of which are being demonstrated to have anticancer effects on the body. Human population studies and animal research have shown a strong correlation between tea consumption and reduced risk of certain cancers, especially esophageal cancer. These teas, in regular or decaffeinated form, were also found to reduce the development of skin cancer in animal studies.

Green tea has been touted throughout the popular media as a protective agent against cancer, especially after it was learned that it is rich in antioxidants and that Japanese who drink green tea have lower rates of cancer. *The Lancet* reported recently that black tea contains just as many antioxidants as green tea, which means that it may well provide the same protection.

TEA TREE OIL is a broad-spectrum fungicide and antiseptic and is highly effective against a wide variety of skin problems, including acne. The oil is derived from the leaves of *Melaleuca alternifolia,* a tree that grows in New South Wales, Australia. It is also used to treat bruises and on wounds to prevent infection. For children or those with sensitive skin, tea tree oil can be diluted with water or vegetable oil.

THYME *(Thymus vulgaris)* is an antiseptic, parasiticide, diuretic, antispasmodic, and expectorant. Taken as a tea, thyme is good for expelling intestinal worms and as a general stomach tonic. It is also recommended for bronchial and throat ailments from bronchitis to whooping cough. Limit intake to one ounce of tea daily. Externally, the tincture is a good antiseptic for ringworm and athlete's foot. In combination with myrrh and goldenseal, it makes a good salve for herpes and other skin problems.

TURMERIC, derived from *Curcuma longa,* has been shown to reduce inflammation and inhibit platelet aggregation, thus protecting against heart attacks and strokes. Research has shown that curcumim, a compound found in turmeric, is even more effective than beta-carotene in preventing the development of cancer in animals that have been fed a powerful carcinogen. "Turmeric inhibits cancer by disrupting certain chemical processes that would otherwise lead to malignancy," said Michael Wargovich, M.D., professor of medicine at the University of Texas's M. D. Anderson Cancer Center in Houston. Turmeric may also have a therapeutic role in the treatment of HIV and AIDS. Dr. Elinor Levy, professor of immunology at Boston University, says that turmeric inhibits the spread of HIV in laboratory animals and is now being tested in human trials.

USNEA is derived from two species of tree lichens *(Usnea barbata, U. longissima)* that are widely used in Europe for their antibiotic and antifungal properties. It is also known as old man's beard. Unique plantlike organisms formed by the marriage of a fungus and an alga, lichens grow abundantly around the world. Usnea is used externally (applied topically to stop bacterial skin infections and alleviate athlete's foot and ringworm) and internally (to treat urinary tract and respiratory tract infections). Studies of lichens have identified over two hundred potentially therapeutic compounds in their tissues, including antibiotic acids and immune-boosting polysaccharides. Usnea may help counter colds and flu. It comes in tinctures, concentrated drops, and extracts.

UVA URSI *(Arctostaphylos uva-ursi),* also known as bearberry, is a diuretic, urinary antiseptic, and astringent. It is used specifically in the treatment of urinary tract infections including nephritis, cystitis, urethritis, and kidney stones. Humbart Santillo, author of *Natural Healing with Herbs,* advises always combining uva ursi with marshmallow root or some other mucilaginous diuretic. For hemorrhoids and skin infections, put one cup of leaves in a sock and add to a hot bath.

VALERIAN *(Valeriana officinalis)* is a nervine, hypnotic, antispasmodic, and stimulant. A powerful nerve tonic and sedative, valerian is used to treat insomnia and the symptoms of emotional stress. It is also good for gas, spasms, menstrual cramps, and general pain relief. Valerian acts first as a stimulant until the body breaks it down to valeramic acid, which brings on a calming effect. Proper dosage is one half to one teaspoon. Large dosages may cause depression.

VIOLET LEAVES *(Viola odorata)* are demulcent, expectorant, alterative, antipyretic, and antiseptic. They are good for treating the lungs and upper respiratory tract; chronic dry cough, asthma with a dry cough, and sore throat are all alleviated by the syrup made from violet leaves. Humbart

Santillo, author of *Natural Healing with Herbs,* also recommends it for tumors and cancerous growths.

VITEX, well known in Europe as the women's herb, is derived from the berries of a Mediterranean plant *(Vitex agnus-castus)*. The herb is also known as chaste tree, chasteberry, and agnus castus. In the Middle Ages, vitex was thought to have an antiaphrodisiac effect. Today, it is used principally to treat women's conditions such as PMS, menopausal discomfort, fibroids, and excessive menstrual bleeding. It works to balance hormones by strengthening the sexual organs and glands. Vitex also stimulates the flow of breast milk and may clear acne during puberty. It is safe for use over an extended period of time. It comes in tablets, capsules, concentrated drops, tinctures, and extracts.

WAHOO *(Euonymus atropurpureus)* is a purgative, blood cleanser, emetic, and tonic. It is used as a laxative, often in combination with other herbs such as psyllium and flaxseeds. Wahoo bark is also used to treat the liver.

WATERMELON *(Citrillus lanatus)* is cooling and diuretic. The fruit of the watermelon works as a diuretic, helping the kidney to function. The seeds have been used to treat cystitis and also, in children, to relieve pain in passing urine.

WHEAT GERM OIL is an emollient and a blood cleanser. It is used externally to treat skin ailments. It can be used as a treatment for burns, especially in combination with comfrey, slippery elm, and lobelia. It is also used in stimulation of the scalp to reduce dandruff and hair loss. Wheat germ oil may be taken internally, two teaspoons daily for two weeks, to stimulate the heart and treat heart disease.

WHITE BRYONY *(Bryonia alba)* treats connective tissue pain anywhere in the body and rheumatic pains in the chest caused by fluid accumulation and chronic cough. It is very widely used in homeopathic medicine where its specific conditions are symptoms aggravated by motion. White bryony can be toxic and irritating to the skin, although a plaster of the crushed roots may be used in place of a mustard plaster.

WHITE PEPPER *(Piper glabrispicum)* is a stomachic, stimulant, and carminative. White pepper is made by removing the pungent resin, chavicine, from black pepper. It is used as a tonic for stomach ailments.

WHITE WILLOW preparations are made from the bark of a tree *(Salix alba)* and are used to relieve pain and reduce fever. Like the herb meadowsweet *(Filipendula ulmaria),* white willow bark is a natural source of salicin, a chemical relative of the synthetic salicylic acid used to make aspirin (acetylsalicylic acid). Some willow-based aspirin substitutes are standardized for the salicin content. Because of the risk of Reye's syndrome, white willow preparations shouldn't be given to children who have a fever that may be due to certain viral illnesses. The herb comes fresh and dried and in tablets, concentrated drops, tinctures, and extracts.

WILD CARROT *(Daucus carota)* is a stimulant, diuretic, and nutritive used to treat kidney problems and obesity. An infusion of the roots and leaves is also recommended for diabetes. As a vegetable, it is high in vitamin A.

WILD CHERRY BARK *(Prunus serotina)* is an antitussive, sedative, astringent, and carminative. Historically, one of our most popular indigenous remedies, wild cherry treats the respiratory system, especially coughs and asthma. It is available as a syrup, usually in combination with other herbs. It is also used in treating digestive disorders such as colitis, gastritis, and dysentery.

WILD YAM ROOT *(Diascorea villosa)* is an antispasmodic, anti-inflammatory, cholagogue, expectorant, and diaphoretic. It contains a steroid from which progesterone and cortisone have been made. Wild yam root aids in the removal of accumulated waste products, which makes it useful in curing rheumatism. It is best known as the traditional herbal treatment for biliary colic, gallstones, and abdominal cramps.

WITCH HAZEL is a widely used medicinal herb derived from the leaves and bark of a North American shrub or small tree *(Hamamelis virginiana)*. It is used as a liniment even by medical doctors and is available in conventional pharmacies. It has well-established astringent properties that reduce the pain and swelling of hemorrhoids, varicose veins, insect bites, and bruises. It is also an effective styptic that can stop the bleeding from small cuts such as shaving nicks. Witch hazel is a component in some cosmetics. Herbalists generally recommend concentrated drops and tinctures, which are more potent than the distilled commercial witch hazel solutions sold in conventional pharmacies. Witch hazel is mild enough to be applied directly to the skin and is a popular ingredient in herbal skin salves. It comes in concentrated drops, tinctures, and extracts.

WOOD BETONY *(Stachys betonica)* is a nervine, sedative, astringent, and bitter tonic. It is a good remedy for chronic headaches and other problems of the head, nervousness, and anxiety, and it is often combined with equal parts of feverfew, rosemary, and skullcap for migraines.

WORMSEED, also known as American wormseed, Jerusalem oak, chenopodium, and Mexican tea, is a common name given to various plants of the genus *Chenopodium* and their derivatives. The plant grows two to four feet high and has yellowish green flowers. The black seeds ripen in the autumn and should be collected then. The smell is not very pleasant. The medicinal parts are the seeds and the top. They are used to expel intestinal worms, promote menstruation, and to overcome uterine colic and hysteria.

WORMWOOD *(Artemisia absinthium)* is an antiseptic, anthelminic, diaphoretic, and tonic. It is a very bitter tonic used to break fevers and relieve hot stomach pains. Wormwood is good for all liver-related ailments. Herbalist Michael Tierra reports that studies have found a compound in some varieties of wormwood that attacks and destroys the membranes of parasites, especially malaria. Wormwood will also expel pinworms and intestinal parasites.

YARROW *(Achillea millefolium),* also known as milfoil, is an astringent, diaphoretic, hemostatic, and stimulant. It is used to treat all types of skin problems, including pimples, acne, infections, itching, rashes, and other skin irritations. Yarrow heals and acts as a styptic, a substance that reduces blood flow and inflammation to the area. It is usually found as part of an herbal salve that includes other medicinal herbs, such as goldenseal, chamomile, and sage.

YELLOW DOCK *(Rumex crispus)* is an alterative, astringent, cholagogue, laxative, and nutritive. It is used traditionally to promote liver cleansing and the health of the colon. It is also excellent for treating hemorrhoids. Yellow dock is a mild laxative. It is used primarily to help support and restore liver function and improve iron metabolism of blood, so it is often used for people suffering from anemia. Take ten to thirty drops in a tincture, three to five days per week, for two weeks.

YERBA MANSA is used for diarrhea, dysentery, malaria fevers, pulmonary infections, gonorrhea, catarrhal conditions, indigestion, cough, and digestive weakness. Externally, it may be used as a tincture or ointment for infections, especially fungal infections.

YERBA SANTA *(Eriodictyon californicum)* is an expectorant, alterative, and carminative. Primarily used as a treatment for upper respiratory ailments, coughs and colds, it is also often combined with other bitter herbs as it contains a resin that absorbs and masks their bitter taste. Native Americans used it as an expectorant for hay fever and also to treat hemorrhoids. Externally, it is sometimes combined with grindelia and applied to the skin for the relief of poison oak and poison ivy.

YOHIMBINE is an aphrodisiac derived from the bark of the yohimbé tree *(Corynanthe yohimbe),* an evergreen indigenous to West Africa. Studies demonstrate its aphrodisiac effects on men. Yohimbine can cause erectile stimulation of the penis and help in the treatment of male impotence. The compound yohimbine hydrochloride is the active ingredient in some prescription drugs (Actibine, Aphrodyne, Yohimex) for certain types of male impotence. The herb may also elevate mood and may be a weight loss aid. According to FDA regulations, it cannot be promoted in herbal form as an aphrodisiac. It is a potent herb with potential for abuse. Yohimbine is sold dried and in tablets, capsules, concentrated drops, and extracts.

FORMULAS FOR MAKING HERBS

Congee

Congee is eaten throughout China as a breakfast food and is often called rice water. The way to make congee is to simmer a handful of brown rice in five to six times as much water as rice. Cook in a covered pot for four to six hours on warm or use the lowest flame possible. It is not possible to cook congee for too long because the longer it cooks, the stronger it becomes.

This rice soup is very easy to digest and has a cooling, demulcent, and tonifying effect. It is also useful for increasing the milk supply of nursing mothers. The liquid can be strained from the porridge to drink as a supplement for those with weak digestion and assimilation. Other things that have therapeutic properties may be added to the congee and they will be easily assimilated because of the strengthening effect of the rice on digestion.

Herbal Preparations

When making herbal preparations, use stainless steel, earthenware, or ceramic pots.

INFUSION

An infusion is used to extract the volatile oils from herbal plants, their flowers, or their leaves. Infusions are used hot or cold (strain them and let them sit). Many times they are made into a sun tea, which is made by putting the contents into a jar with the cover on and setting it in the sun for two to four hours. The heat from the sun will do the extraction.

To prepare an infusion, use one ounce of herb to one pint of water. Bring the water to a boil and pour it over the herb. Cover with a tightly fitting lid so steam does not escape. Let it stand for twenty minutes, strain, and drink.

Tinctures are concentrated herbal extracts that can be preserved over long periods of time. They can be carried around easily and taken in a little water or under the tongue. If they are bitter, they can be added to a little bit of juice.

DECOCTION

To extract the deeper healing qualities of stems, roots, and barks, herbs must be simmered for about fifteen to forty-five minutes. Many times the pot is left uncovered during simmering to evaporate some of the water. Decoctions and infusions must be used before they sour or growth starts (usually within twenty-four to seventy-two hours).

DECOCTION AND INFUSION COMBINED

Roots and barks are made into a decoction by simmering for a period of time. Leaves and aromatic herbs are more sensitive to heat and are only steeped so as not to lose the volatile oils. To combine the two, you would first make your decoction, then pour it over your leafy herb and let it steep for twenty minutes. Therefore, use one more cup of water while making the decoction. Another way is to make the decoction and infusion separately and then combine them. Make sure you use stainless steel, earthenware, or ceramic pots.

FOMENTATION

To make a fomentation: Soak a cotton towel in a large pot of herbal tea (in this case, either agrimony or lobelia). Make the herbal tea as hot as can be tolerated. Wring the towel to get rid of the excess water and place over the affected area. Place another thick towel over the wet towel to contain the heat. When cool, soak the towel again in the pot of herbal tea and reapply.

HERBAL POULTICE

To make a poultice: A poultice is a mass of herbs that have been pulverized or powdered and then moistened with water. The poultice is then applied wet to the affected area of the skin. Wrap a cloth around the poultice to keep it in place. Poultices heal bruises; draw out pus, toxins, and particles; break up congestion; restore circulation; reduce inflammation; and soothe the injured area.

THERAPEUTIC MASSAGE TECHNIQUES

"The issues are in the tissues," says the old axiom, and to a practitioner of therapeutic massage, or bodywork, the aphorism is both an insight into human nature and a gateway to healing. As simple as a shoulder rub and as intricate and far-reaching as acupressure, bodywork has emerged over the past twenty years as one of the most important preventive and therapeutic tools in natural healing.

While there are many forms of bodywork today, the practices all have several things in common, the most fundamental of which is the recognition of the unity of body and mind. Your every thought and emotion changes the condition of your muscular, circulatory, nervous, and endocrine systems. Thoughts and emotions affect the health of your heart, the flow of blood and oxygen to cells, and the function of your immune system. Many thoughts and emotions create feelings of calm and well-being. They relax muscles, enhance circulation, and promote hormonal balance. Others excite: they activate the nervous system and awaken the senses. Still others weaken us physiologically. They create tension, promote the production of stress hormones, impair the function of the heart and circulatory system, and depress the immune response.

In certain areas of the body there are mounds and knots of tension that may be years old; in other places, there is flaccid tissue, weakness, and a perceptible lack of vitality. Parts of the body are cold from lack of circulation; others are warm from a recent injury. Look at people carefully as they walk down the street. See their postures as outward expressions of their inner worlds: their attitudes, self-esteem, and emotional condition. Look at the imbalances that make up the human form, how one shoulder is higher than the other, how one leg and one arm stride boldly forward, while their counterparts passively, almost meekly, follow suit. By the time we reach adulthood, each of us seems like a cacophony of distortions, each one the symptom of our own history: a never-fully-healed injury here, accumulated emotional and physical tension there, an unresolved conflict made manifest over here. The notion that the mind and body are separate seems ludicrous even to the superficial observer.

To a trained bodywork practitioner, these alternating conditions of stress and relaxation, joy and sadness, fear and strength exist in the tissues like a three-dimensional map of the psyche. Each practice has its own approach to the bumps, valleys, strengths, and weaknesses. However, practitioners agree that outward imbalances are a reflection of the inner world, and that with a careful and healing hand, both the outer imbalances and the inner wounds can be healed.

Below is a summary of some of the most popular and most widely available practices throughout the United States and around the world.

ACUPRESSURE

Based on the principles of acupuncture, acupressure uses the fingers and hands instead of needles to stimulate acupuncture points. (See the section on Chinese medicine in Part III.) The body is traversed by fourteen energy patterns, or meridians, along which life energy, or qi, flows. On these meridians exist more than a thousand acupuncture points, or generators of qi energy. An acupressurist stimulates these points to stimulate qi along specific meridians and to specific organs to bring about healing.

ALEXANDER TECHNIQUE

Created by the actor F. Matthias Alexander, the technique focuses on improving overall posture, which practitioners say is responsible for a whole range of disorders, including tension and pain, as well as respiratory, muscular, and hormonal imbalances. Practitioners teach and use gentle, hands-on methods to correct distortions in posture and create coordinated, graceful, and balanced movement.

DANCE-MOVEMENT THERAPIES

Practitioners use movement and dance to help people experience and express inner feelings, resolve conflicts, and heal body, mind, and spirit. The practice is especially popular among those with addictions, disabilities, histories of sexual abuse, eating disorders, and long-standing emotional wounds.

FELDENKRAIS METHOD

Also referred to as "awareness through movement," Feldenkrais uses movement training, gentle methods of healing touch, awareness, and psychological dialogue to release the body of old, restrictive patterns and the psychological states that reinforce those patterns. Feldenkrais uses two approaches to bodywork: a hands-on approach, using massage techniques to work with breathing and body alignment; and classes designed to create new, balanced, and harmonious movement.

HELLERWORK

Developed by Jospeh Heller, former aerospace engineer, Hellerwork uses deep-tissue massage to release tension and "stuck" muscle and connective tissue. The person is also made aware of imbalances in his or her movements, and the body is reeducated to move with greater balance, coordination, and freedom. The underlying psychological issues that influence movement are also dealt with in sessions with a Hellerwork therapist.

JIN SHIN JYUTSU

This technique was developed by Jiro Murai, a twentieth-century Japanese sage who cured himself of life-threatening illness by developing a system of healing touch that focuses life energy into twenty-six "safety energy locks." These twenty-six safety energy locks, which close when imbalances manifest in the body, are found at precise locations on the body. Symptoms arise whenever a safety energy lock is closed. The practitioner gently touches a part of the body where one of the safety energy locks is located, infusing it with life energy. Unlike acupressure, no real pressure is applied; rather, the body is held gently at the safety energy lock. When the safety energy lock is opened, life energy flows to a related organ or part of the body, restoring health. The leading practitioner in the United States is Mary Burmeister, who maintains an office in Scottsdale, Arizona.

KINESIOLOGY

This is a diagnostic and therapeutic system based upon muscular reactions to specific questions, situations, or objects held within the client's hand. The client's posture, gait, and lifestyle are analyzed. Muscles and joints are manipulated; nutritional advice is given. Practitioners of kinesiology include chiropractors, nutritionists, dentists, and medical doctors.

NEUROMUSCULAR THERAPY

Neuromuscular therapy illuminates the role muscles play in applying pressure on nerves and the creation of pain. Therapists attempt to relieve muscle tension, congestion, and lack of flexibility to release tension on nerves and restore nerve supply.

OHASHIATSU

Developed by Waturo Ohashi, Ohashiatsu combines shiatsu massage, exercise, meditation, and ancient diagnostic techniques to relieve tension, restore life energy to meridians and organs, boost vitality, and create inner harmony. Ohashiatsu uses the hara, or the vital center located in the area of the navel, as a diagnostic tool to assess the person's condition. The practitioner then applies Ohashiatsu to strengthen the client's meridians, organs, and hara.

PHYSICAL AND OCCUPATIONAL THERAPIES

Therapists use massage, exercise, electrical stimulation, ultrasound, and other modern methods to relieve pain, release tension and stress, and restore strength to injured parts of the body. Occupational therapists help injured or disabled people return to the workforce and resume active, productive lives.

POLARITY

Polarity therapists maintain that energy fields exist throughout nature and within the human body, where they sustain both health and life. Therapists use massage techniques and laying on of hands to restore balance to these fields, open blocked pathways, and restore energy that is currently deprived of life force. Polarity therapists also use diet, lifestyle counseling, and exercise to promote the flow of energy within a person's body and overall life.

REFLEXOLOGY

Reflexology is an ancient practice that stimulates specific points on the feet and hands to promote the flow of life energy to specific organs and parts of the body. The practitioner massages these points to relieve stress, promote healing, and restore balance to parts of the body that are currently blocked or deprived of life energy.

REIKI

Reiki is a Tibetan form of laying on of hands or palm healing. Reiki therapists gently place hands over specific parts of the body to channel energy to the client's body. Reiki practitioners attempt to boost the life force of the client so that he or she can experience greater health, emotional and psychological harmony, and the realization of the true inner self.

ROLFING

Rolfing is a form of deep-tissue massage designed to restore the body's correct alignment and posture. The practice was developed by Ida P. Rolf, who maintained that emotional, psychological, and physical trauma impacted directly on the body and made its connective tissue, or fascia, become shorter and more rigid. Practitioners use each session to correct a specific part of the body's alignment, ultimately integrating and restoring the body's correct, upright stature.

THE RUBENFELD SYNERGY

The Rubenfeld method, developed by Ilana Rubenfeld, applies gentle touch, guided and spontaneous movement, and dialogues between the client and the practitioner to elicit a deeper understanding of the emotional and psychological issues that are manifesting in the body. The method, which is more than thirty years old, combines gestalt therapy, Alexander technique, Feldenkrais method, and hypnotherapy to gain insight into long-standing mental, emotional, and physical issues. Practitioners complete a three-year course for certification.

SHIATSU

The Japanese form of acupressure, shiatsu is more than a thousand years old. As with acupressure, shiatsu uses finger pressure to stimulate life energy at specific acupuncture points and along meridian lines to restore health and vitality to organs and tissues.

SWEDISH MASSAGE

Swedish massage combines therapeutic massage, Oriental techniques, and the principles of anatomy and physiology to release tension, restore circulation, and relieve pain. Therapists apply deep-tissue massage techniques, along with gentle touch, manipulation, and rubbing to treat back pain, sleep disorders, and stress-related disturbances. Swedish massage is among the most widely practiced massage therapies in the United States and around the world.

THERAPEUTIC TOUCH

Therapeutic touch is a form of laying on of hands, one of the oldest forms of healing. It has been developed and studied scientifically by Dolores Kreiger, a nursing professor and practitioner, who demonstrated its efficacy in the treatment of a wide variety of disorders, including pain relief, the healing of injuries, and stress-related disorders. It has been shown to boost immune response, as well. Therapeutic touch practitioners evaluate a person's energy field and attempt to restore harmony and balance to weakened or injured parts of the field.

TRAGER

Tragerwork uses gentle rocking, cradling, massage, and movement to relieve physical tension and discover the mental and emotional sources of physical imbalances. Tragerwork is designed to promote greater flexibility, a wider range of motion, and mental clarity. The person is shown where tension resides in his or her body, and is assisted in reeducating the body to move in less-restricted patterns. Tragerwork is used by many athletes to enhance performance and by people with back pain and muscular and skeletal disorders.

HOMEOPATHY

Homeopathy was created by German physician Samuel Hahnemann, who lived from 1755 to 1843. Hahnemann created the practice because he had become discouraged by the practices of bloodletting, blistering, and the use of toxic substances, such as mercury, to treat the sick. He found that these methods were not only ineffective, but made the patient sicker and often caused death.

After much experimentation, Hahnemann discovered that "a substance that produces a certain set of symptoms in a healthy person has the power to cure a sick person manifesting those same symptoms." With that, he had articulated the first of several principles of what would be his new medicine, a principle he called the Law of Similars. In essence, the principle states that like cures like.

Hahnemann called his new medicine homeopathy, which joined the Greek words, *homoios,* which means *like,* and *pathos,* meaning *pathology* or *sickness.* The Law of Similars revealed to Hahnemann how the body reacts to disease. He maintained that the presence of an illness stimulates the body's defense system to eliminate the illness. That defensive reaction produces symptoms, which are part of the body's effort at eliminating the underlying disease. The symptoms are not the illness, said Hahnemann, but part of the curative process. Hahnemann maintained that the effective medicines actually produce a condition similar to the illness itself, but effectively arouse the body's defense system against the underlying disease. In effect, the medicine makes it easy for the body to recognize the underlying disease and mobilize its defenses against the illness. The outward manifestation of this effort are symptoms. A cough, for example, is the body's attempt at expectorating the pathogen; fever is hostile to the underlying pathogen; mucus attempts to isolate it and allow it to be driven from the body as a runny nose, sneezing, and watery eyes.

This was, of course, an ancient understanding of symptoms, as was Hahnemann's belief that the body was animated by an underlying life force, which he called the vital force. Strictly speaking, the Law of Similars was not by itself a new principle, either. It was known among Ayurvedic physicians two thousand years earlier, and was central to the medical approaches of Hippocrates (400 B.C.) and Paracelsus (the sixteenth-century philosopher, alchemist, and physician). Still, it was a direct opposite to the prevailing medical approach, which Hahnemann termed *allopathy,* which used drugs to create the opposite effect on symptoms. Allopaths treat swelling, for example, by administering drugs that will directly reduce swelling, rather than stimulate the body's defense system against the swelling, and thereby cure it. However, the suppression of symptoms forces the disease to go deeper into the body, said Hahnemann, causing a more serious condition, and one that is harder to cure.

Hahnemann wanted to reduce the severity of the symptoms caused by medicine, and thus he decided to reduce the size of the dosage. Remarkably, he found that the smaller dose was even more effective against the underlying illness. Further experimentation led Hahnemann to his next principle, which he called The Law of Potentization, or the Law of Infinitesimals. Hahnemann stated that the smaller the dose of medicine, the greater its potency, or its effect on the body's vital force. A microdose of the medication actually strengthened the vital force against the illness. He developed a method to dilute medicines down to infinitesimal doses by diluting the quantities and then shaking (what is called *succusion* by homeopaths). This process is done successively until only molecular amounts of the original medicine remains.

Homeopaths draw these molecular quantities of substances primarily from plants, such as chamomile, but also from animal products like snake and bee venom, and from minerals. Homeopathic remedies come in either single or combination form (two or more single remedies combined to make a cold and flu formula remedy, for instance). The use of combination remedies is almost as old as the classical form of homeopathic practice, which uses only single remedies. Most homeopathic manufacturers make both types of remedies. Single and combination remedies look the same, coming in small tablets or pellets. Remedies are also combined to make ointments, lotions, and tinctures for external application. From the natural food retailer's viewpoint, homeopathic remedies have some notable advantages over other natural remedies. Homeopathic remedies are considered over-the-counter drugs by the FDA and thus can make certain health claims on their labels. The labels help simplify customers' purchase decisions, and they protect the retailer from charges of practicing medicine. Also, the store owner need not refer the customer back to a practitioner, since homeopathic remedies are basically self-care treatments for minor, self-limiting problems. Homeopathic remedies' protected status as over-the-counter drugs also makes them safer to position point-of-purchase materials and literature, which help educate consumers about homeopathy.

ACONITE is prepared from the poisonous aconite *(Aconitum napellus)*, or monkshood plant. It is used to relieve states of acute emotional upset, especially those that come on suddenly from extreme anxiety, intense fear or pain, and shocking or violent situations. It is also used after surgery, during the early stages of inflammation or fever, and for certain types of colds, headaches, and insomnia. Aconite may be helpful for a person who is fearful and restless and who may experience sudden nausea and vomiting. Aconite is a common ingredient in combination remedies for colds and flu, earache, fever, and headache. It comes in tablets and pellets.

Apis is prepared from whole honey bees or bee venom and used to relieve bee sting–type symptoms, such as a burning sensation with rapid, red swelling. Apis is recommended to treat certain types of insect stings and bites, sunburn and other minor burns, skin irritations, hives, the early stages of boils, and frostbite. It may also help relieve joint pain, eye inflammations, and fevers. Apis is effective against pain that is typically improved by cold and made worse by pressure. Apis is a common ingredient in combination remedies for allergies and hay fever, bites and stings, burns, and sore throat. It comes in pellets, tablets, and ointments.

Arnica is the premier homeopathic contusion remedy. Derived from the whole fresh arnica plant (especially *Arnica montana*), it is often the first medicine given after an injury or a fall to counter bruising, swelling, and local tenderness. It is also recommended for aching muscles, sprains, and other sports injuries. Unlike herbal preparations of arnica, homeopathically diluted arnica tablets are safe for internal consumption. Arnica is taken orally to relieve contusions, calm someone who is in a dazed or shocked state, and dispel the distress that usually accompanies accidents and injuries. It is also used before and after surgery and childbirth to prevent bruising and speed recovery. Externally, it is applied only to unbroken skin. Arnica is a common ingredient in combination remedies for back pain, bruises, fatigue, and hemorrhoids. It comes in pellets, tablets, creams, ointments, and sprays.

Arsenicum is a homeopathic remedy prepared from arsenic trioxide, a compound of the poisonous chemical element arsenic. In microdilute homeopathic dosages, arsenicum is used to treat certain skin rashes, anxiety-induced asthma, vomiting, diarrhea, or stomach upsets from food poisoning. It is also taken for exhaustion, fevers, and headaches. Arsenicum is typically recommended for people who are anxious, restless, pale, and fearful. Arsenicum is a common ingredient in combination remedies for colds, diarrhea, fatigue, headache, and insomnia. It is sold in pellet and tablet form.

Belladonna is a homeopathic remedy derived from the extremely poisonous deadly nightshade plant *(Atropa belladonna)* of Europe. In dilutions it is used to treat sudden-onset conditions characterized by redness, throbbing pain, and heat, including certain types of cold, high fever, earache, sore throat, and sunstroke. Belladonna may be recommended for a person who has a flushed face, hot and dry skin, and dilated pupils. Belladonna is a common ingredient in combination remedies for teething, colds and flu, earache, fever, headache, menstrual problems, sinusitis, and sore throat. It comes in pellets and tablets.

Bryonia is a homeopathic remedy prepared from the poisonous root of wild hops *(Bryonia alba)*, a European climbing perennial. In dilutions it is used to treat certain types of flu, fevers, and coughs and colds, especially those that come on slowly. It also relieves some headaches, digestive problems, and muscle aches and pains. Bryonia may be helpful for a person who is typically irritable and aggravated by motion. Bryonia is a popular ingredient in combination remedies for colds and flu, constipation, fever, and headache. It comes in pellets and tablets.

CALENDULA is derived from the whole calendula plant and is used to promote the healing of minor cuts and scrapes, cool sunburns, and relieve skin irritations. Homeopathic calendula is principally a topical remedy but is available in pellet and tablet form for the same symptoms. Calendula is a common ingredient in combination remedies for burns, skin conditions, and yeast infections. It comes in ointments (usually 1X strength; a 10 percent calendula extract), tinctures, oils, and calendulated soap bars.

CHAMOMILLA is derived from the whole, fresh chamomile plant *(Matricaria recutita* or *Anthemis nobilis)*. Recent research has shown that chamomile tea is an effective immune-booster. Chamomile is used to treat restlessness and insomnia, toothaches and childhood teething pains, colic, earaches, fever, and joint pain. Chamomile is generally recommended for people who are frequently irascible, stubborn, and inconsolable. Chamomilla is a common ingredient in combination remedies for teething, diarrhea, earache, insomnia, and menstrual problems. It comes in pellets, tablets, and ointments.

EUPHRASIA is a homeopathic remedy made from dilutions of the juice of the eyebright plant *(Euphrasia officinalis)*. It is most frequently used as an external and internal treatment for various injuries to the eyes, especially when there is profuse watering, burning pain, and swelling and redness of the eyelids. It is also taken for some coughs and colds. Euphrasia is a common ingredient in combination remedies for allergies and hay fever, colds, and flu. It comes in pellets and tablets.

FERRUM PHOSPHATE is a homeopathic remedy derived from iron phosphate. It is used primarily for the early stages of inflammatory and feverish conditions that develop gradually rather than having rapid onset, including colds, flus, and viral illnesses. It is also widely used as a first aid treatment for sprained and bruised muscles, and as a childhood remedy for ailments like headaches, earaches, and nosebleeds. Ferrum phosphate is a common ingredient in combination remedies for fever. It comes in pellets and tablets.

GELSEMIUM is derived from the flowering yellow jasmine plant *(Gelsemium sempervirens)* native to the southeastern United States. It is used principally to relieve dull, heavy aches and pains associated with colds, flu, tension headache, jet lag, and fatigue. It is also recommended to help relieve bed-wetting among nervous children, middle ear infections, and blurred vision. Gelsemium is a common ingredient in combination remedies for fever, headache, and menstrual problems. It comes in pellets and tablets.

HYPERICUM is prepared from the Saint-John's-wort plant *(Hypericum perfo-ratum)*. It is used topically and internally to relieve pain and trauma related to nerves and the central nervous system. Hypericum is best for an injury that causes the type of shooting pain that seems to ascend the length of a nerve and for wounds to an area of many nerve endings, such as the ends of the fingers and toes. It also speeds the healing of jagged cuts and relieves the pain from dental surgery, toothaches, injuries to the tailbone, and some burns. Hypericum is a common ingredient in combination remedies for bites and stings, bruises, and burns. It is manufactured as pellets, tablets, tinctures, lotions, and sprays.

LEDUM is prepared from the leaves and twigs of wild rosemary *(Ledum palustre),* a small evergreen shrub. The plant is toxic and thus not widely used by herbalists. Homeopaths use dilutions to treat puncture wounds from various sharp objects, including nails and needles, and bites by insects (especially mosquitoes) and small animals. It is also used to relieve stiff joints, sprained ankles, black eyes, and severe or persisting bruises. Ledum is more appropriate than apis if the site of the injury is cold and numb or if it is swollen and relieved by cold rather than heat. Ledum is a common ingredient in combination remedies for bites, stings, and bruises. It comes in pellets, tablets, and ointments.

NUX VOMICA is derived from the toxic, strychnine-containing seeds of the poison nut evergreen tree *(Strychnos nux-vomica)*. Homeopathically diluted, it is used principally to treat nausea and vomiting, especially from ailments due to overeating or drinking. The remedy may be beneficial for flatulence, constipation, or indigestion. It is also used to treat motion sickness and some types of colic, coughs, backaches, fevers, headaches, and insomnia. Nux vomica is frequently combined with other ingredients in combination cold and flu remedies and in combination remedies for back pain, constipation, fatigue, flatulence, headache, hemorrhoids, indigestion, and insomnia. It comes in pellets and tablets.

PULSATILLA is derived from the poisonous pasqueflower *(Anemone patens)*. In homeopathic dilutions, people take it internally for colds characterized by a profusely running nose and coughing. Homeopaths also recommend it for certain eye and ear ailments, skin eruptions, allergies, insomnia, fainting episodes, and gastric upsets, particularly when the patient is sensitive and prone to crying. Pulsatilla is a common ingredient in combination remedies for colds and flu, earache, fever, indigestion, insomnia, menstrual problems, and sinusitis. It comes in pellets and tablets.

RHUS TOXICODENDRON is prepared from leaves of the poison ivy plant *(Rhus tox-icodendron)*. Dilutions are taken to alleviate poison ivy and other skin conditions that are red and swollen, like rashes, hives, and burns, as well as joint stiffness. Rhus toxicodendron is also a prominent sports medicine used for pain and swelling that affects muscles, ligaments, and tendons, such as from sprains and overexertion. It is known as the rusty gate remedy: It works best for the person who feels stiff and sore at first but better after movement. Rhus toxicodendron is a common ingredient in combination remedies for back pain, strains and sprains, and skin conditions. It comes in pellets and tablets.

RUTA is prepared from the flowering rue *(Ruta graveolens)*. It is used to treat injuries to the periosteum, the tough connective tissue that covers the shin and other bones. Homeopaths also recommend it for bruised kneecaps and elbows, sprained wrists and ankles, torn tendons, stretched ligaments, and tennis elbow. Ruta is a common ingredient in combination remedies for bruises. It comes in pellets, tablets, and ointments.

SULPHUR is derived from the naturally occurring yellowish chemical element sulfur. It is commonly taken for certain chronic (as opposed to acute) conditions and skin problems, and during the early stages of the flu. Depending on the symptoms, it may also be used to treat sore throats, allergies, and earaches. Sulphur is a common ingredient in combination remedies for back pain, constipation, diarrhea, hemorrhoids, and skin conditions. It comes in pellets and tablets.

SYMPHYTUM is prepared from the roots of the comfrey plant *(Symphytum officinale)*. It is primarily used to treat bruises (especially black eyes), bone injuries, and sprains. Symphytum is a common ingredient in combination remedies for strains and sprains. It comes in pellets, tablets, lotions, and ointments.

URTICA is a first aid remedy prepared from fresh, flowering stinging nettles *(Urtica urens)*. It may be taken internally or applied topically to treat skin conditions characterized by red, raised, rashlike welts, including bites, stings, burns, hives, and prickly heat. Urtica is a common ingredient in combination remedies for bites, stings, and burns. It comes in pellets, tablets, and ointments.

Hydrotherapy and Physiotherapy

The following plasters, compresses, and poultices have been recommended in the remedies sections of Part II of this book. Below are instructions for making these poultices, as well as advice on the conditions for which they are best suited.

CASTOR OIL PACKS

Castor oil packs gently break up stagnation and shrink masses within the body. They restore circulation. Apply the packs to the lower abdomen nightly for forty-five minutes to one and a half hours. Use three or four thicknesses of undyed wool saturated with castor oil and then wrung out lightly. This is then heated in a special pot used for this purpose only. You may reuse the same cloth twenty to forty times. Just store it in the pot and add more castor oil as needed with each use. This cloth is applied as hot as the body can bear to the area from the lower right rib cage border over the entire right side of the abdomen, down to just above the pubic bone. The pack is then covered with an oiled cloth or plastic and kept warm with a heating pad. If necessary, the bed may also be protected by plastic. After the application, wash the area with a weak solution of bicarbonate (one teaspoon to one quart of warm water).

GINGER COMPRESS

A ginger compress stimulates blood and body fluid circulation and helps loosen and dissolve stagnated toxic matter. Boil a four-quart pot of water. Grate (on the small side of a grater) about a half cup of gingerroot. Place ginger in cheesecloth and tie it up. Turn off the boiling water and squeeze the grated ginger into the water. Throw the cheesecloth packet of gingerroot into the water. Now apply compresses of hot ginger water to the area of the body indicated. Take the compress as hot as you can tolerate it. Leave the compress on for a few minutes or until it loses its heat. Another towel can be placed on top of that towel to retain the heat. At that point, reapply the compress and keep on reapplying until the pot of water is no longer hot. This same water can be used for two days.

TARO ROOT PLASTER

A taro root plaster is often used after a ginger compress to draw toxins from the body. It often will draw out toxins by breaking the skin and allowing accumulated waste products to drain. Peel off taro potato skin and grate the white interior. Mix with 5 to 10 percent grated fresh ginger. Spread this mixture in a two-thirds- to one-inch-thick layer onto a fresh cotton linen and apply the taro side directly to the skin. Change every four hours. Try to use the smaller taro potatoes, if possible. They can be purchased in a natural food store or an Oriental market.

COMFREY ROOT POULTICE

This poultice is used to treat poison ivy. Mix the following herbs in equal portions into the gel of aloe vera pulp and apply over the affected area:

1 part comfrey root
1 part marshmallow root
1 part slippery elm
aloe vera, as moist base
1 part witch hazel
1 part plantain
1 part mugwort

CHICKWEED POULTICE

Use this poultice to draw out toxins and shrink oils, skin eruptions, and inflammations. Boil one ounce of chickweed in one and one half pints of water till water is down to a pint; apply it over the surface of the skin; leave it on for ten minutes.

BROWN RICE PLASTER

A brown rice plaster will help to reduce the fever around an infected area. Grind up in a suribachi (which is a mortarlike bowl with a rough interior): 70 percent cooked brown rice, 30 percent raw leafy vegetables, and a few crushed sheets of raw nori. Add water if the mixture is a little sticky. Grind as much as possible. Apply to the affected area. If there is burning, remove it with warm water, because that is when it is no longer effective.

DRIED DAIKON LEAVES

Apply dried daikon leaves as a compress or use them in a hip bath. Dried daikon leaves are used to treat the skin and female sex organs. They warm the body and draw out odors and excessive oils.

To prepare the compress, dry fresh daikon leaves in the shade until they turn brown and brittle. Use turnip greens if daikon is not available. Boil four to five bunches of the leaves in four to five quarts of water and cook until the water turns brown. Add a handful of sea salt. Dip cotton linen into the water and wring it out. Put it against the affected area until the skin turns red.

A sitz bath is used for problems related to sex organs, especially for women. Boil the leaves and add salt as in the instructions for making a compress. Pour the liquid into hot bathwater. Sit in the hot bath. The water should come to the waist and the upper part of the body should be covered with a towel. Sit until sweating begins. This can be repeated up to ten days. Following this bath, douche with warm bancha tea, a half teaspoon of sea salt, and the juice of half a lemon or brown rice vinegar.

MUSTARD PLASTER

Mustard plasters stimulate blood and body fluid circulation. They are good for conditions where there is stagnation. Add hot water to dry mustard powder, stir well, and spread it onto a paper towel and sandwich it between two thick, cotton towels. Apply the plaster to the skin and leave it on until the skin becomes red and hot. After removing, use a towel to wipe the remaining plaster off.

SALT PACK

A salt pack is used to treat pain, especially on a bone or the back of the head. It is also good for providing deep warmth to an injured or painful part of the body, such as the low back. Roast salt in dry pan until it is hot, wrap it in thick cotton linen, and tie it up. Apply the salt pack to the troubled area, and remove it when area feels cool.

TOFU PLASTER

This is a good way to draw out a fever. Squeeze out the water from tofu. Mash tofu up well and mix in 10 to 20 percent pastry flour and 5 to 10 percent grated ginger. Put the mass into cheesecloth and apply it to the affected area. Allow it to sit for up to two to three hours, or change the plaster when it feels hot.

FAITH AND HEALING

What is the nature of healing? What does it take to heal?

Ask any traditional healer—and, indeed, most medical doctors—to define the nature of healing, and they will include some nonmaterial, nonquantifiable element in their perspective. Some will speak of a person's attitudes and beliefs. Others will use the word faith—not only the faith of the patient, but of the healer, as well.

"In my view there are four essential qualities of a healer: trust, faith, love and humility," wrote Elisabeth Kübler-Ross, M.D., in her essay "The Four Pillars of Healing." These qualities, Kübler-Ross says, affect the patient in a positive way, causing his or her own faith and trust to arise.

Why is the patient's faith so important to healing? Why is this intangible element so vital to the healing process? After all, if we take a strictly materialistic view of life and of healing, drugs alone should be sufficient to bring about the desired results. But this is not the case, as we all know. In order for anyone to be healed, he or she must have faith and trust that healing is possible, and that the medicine being offered will bring about such a healing. "Drugs are not always necessary," Norman Cousins wrote in *Anatomy of an Illness.* "Belief in recovery always is."

There are a great many intangibles involved in healing, just as there is in the process by which we become ill. Something mysterious and powerful in each of us plays a pivotal role in determining our state of health and even our longevity. For example, when comparing men in similar age groups, those who suffer the loss of their spouse die in far greater numbers than men who do not experience such a loss. After examining this phenomenon in the laboratory, Mount Sinai's Stephen Schliefer, M.D., found that a crucial part of the immune system, a group of immune cells called lymphocytes, were not "turning on" in the face of a pathogen. The body's lymphocyte cells didn't attack the pathogen but remained inert when confronted with a disease. Consequently, the illness proliferated. Scientists are finding that, each year, thousands of people die because their immune systems collapse in the face of bereavement, which is to say, they die of broken hearts.

Bereavement is only one emotional condition that can cut short a person's life. In fact, scientists have found that simply believing that one will suffer a premature death can sometimes be enough to bring it about. The British medical journal, *The Lancet,* in November 1993, reported that people who, early in life, believed that they were predisposed to an earlier-than-normal death actually died prematurely. Researchers followed Chinese-Americans who were born during certain years that were believed to be predisposed to lethal diseases. These Chinese-Americans actually died four years sooner, on average, than Chinese-Americans born during other years, and at least four years sooner than Anglo-Americans who, in fact, had the same diseases as the Chinese-Americans but had healthier beliefs about the outcomes of those illnesses. "Our findings and those of others suggest that mental attitude is associated with health," said the study leader, David P. Phillips, Ph.D., professor of sociology at the University of California at San Diego.

Just as negative beliefs can have an altogether weakening effect on health and longevity, positive beliefs are capable of restoring health. Volumes of research have been published on the healing power of placebos. Scientists have found that a placebo, a pill or potion with no therapeutic value, can have the painkilling power of morphine and the healing effectiveness of science's best drugs—as long as the patient believes in the power of the placebo to bring about the desired results.

Such a belief is translated into optimism or faith, which in turn sparks some inner power to heal. Recently, researchers from the University of Pittsburgh Medical School, Yale University, and Pittsburgh Cancer Institute combined to conduct a study of cancer patients who took relaxation and cognitive therapy designed to boost optimism and overcome self-defeating beliefs. The patients, thirty in all, suffered from a type of cancer that had an extremely high likelihood of recurrence. "The course was designed to make them more optimistic about events in their lives; it didn't focus on cancer," said Martin Seligman, a psychologist at the University of Pennsylvania, one of the scientists who participated in the study.

Remarkably, the training did, indeed, make the participants more optimistic, which in turn showed a marked improvement in immune function. The scientists discovered that the patients who took the course had more natural killer cells than the control group, which was made up of patients who only received the standard medical treatment. Natural killer cells are one of the most important immune constituents in the body's fight against cancer because they target and destroy tumors and cancer cells.

Craig A. Anderson, a psychologist at Rice University in Houston, says that optimists tend to feel more in control of their circumstances than pessimists. If events go badly for an optimist, an optimist usually creates a new approach or strategy, believing that if he persists, the events will turn in his direction. The pessimist, says Anderson, feels cursed by fate. He perceives things as hopeless and therefore gives up sooner.

As a practical matter, optimists have a better chance at success, since repeated effort raises the odds in their favor. Behavior based upon optimism is obviously more self-empowering, since there is an implicit belief that one's efforts will eventually pay off.

After studying women with advanced breast cancer, Dr. Sandra Levy, of the Pittsburgh Cancer Institute, found that women who were generally optimistic experienced longer disease-free periods, the best predictor of survival. On the other hand, the disease recurred sooner among the pessimists.

Dr. Christopher Peterson, of the University of Michigan, has found that pessimists tend to have poorer health habits, are more likely to indulge in high-fat foods, are more likely to drink excessively, and do not exercise as much as optimists. As this book points out in our section on the immune system, such behavior can have a depressing effect on the body's defenses.

Optimism or pessimism alone have dramatically different effects on immune response and one's quality of life, as the pioneer of stress research, Hans Selye, M.D., has demonstrated. In his book *The Stress of Life* (1956), Dr. Selye states that the two most significant attitudes in our lives are gratitude and revenge. Indeed, Selye maintains that these two emotional conditions determine whether or not a person experiences deep and abiding stress or is healthy and capable of enjoying life. As he put it, "It seems to me that, among all the emotions, there is one which, more than any other, accounts for the absence or presence of stress in human relations: that is the feeling of gratitude—with its negative counterpart, the need for revenge. . . . I think in the final analysis that gratitude and revenge are the most important factors governing our actions in everyday life."

Gratitude and revenge, optimism and hostility—each of these opposite poles create, in their own way, the internal conditions that give rise to health or illness. All of this points to the paradoxical nature of reality. Both optimists and pessimists have plenty of evidence to support their opposing views of life. The evidence for both sides is everywhere. But that's the trouble with reality: It tends to be so rich, so complex, and so thoroughly paradoxical that you can find just about anything you want to find in any given day. In the end, it is the individual who determines the nature of reality. No one has an objective view of life.

In fact, objectivity doesn't even occur in the laboratory, as quantum physics has proven. Heisenberg's Uncertainty Principle teaches us that the observer of an event actually shapes the outcome of that event by his expectations and beliefs. In the end, both the pessimist and the optimist see those facts or circumstances that support his or her worldview, which—as subjective as that worldview may be—nevertheless can make a difference between health and illness.

This is why healers maintain that before any medicines are applied, a patient must examine himself and his way of thinking, so that the therapy can have the best chance of succeeding.

Two of the most important factors involved in healing, writes Native American Healer Sun Bear, are "overcoming negative blocks, and developing positive, life affirming attitudes. . . . From the spiritual standpoint, the most common blocks are the negative attitudes and emotions that a lot of people carry around all the time. These blocks must be overcome for healing to occur. . . . Although such factors start within the mind, they quickly manifest in the body."

Sun Bear uses a variety of tools to help people rid themselves of negative beliefs, among which is the exercise of digging a large pit in the earth and yelling every negative thought, feeling, or belief into that pit. "If they feel up-tight about something concerning their mate or someone else, if they have had rage bottled up for a long time, if they have unexpected grief or dread, all of this gets dumped into the hole. Thus they give their negativity to the earth."

At Southern Methodist University, Professor of Psychology James W. Penne-baker, Ph.D., discovered that writing down one's most painful and intimate se-crets, especially those involving past traumas, has the remarkable effect of relieving depression and boosting immune function.

Pennebaker discovered the healing power of writing when he himself became depressed. He spent a year writing about his life, personal struggles, disappointments, and losses, after which he realized he was no longer de-pressed. In fact, he felt that he had undergone a kind of rebirth. Astounded by the healing effect writing had on him, he decided to study the phenome-non in the laboratory. He sought the help of two immunologists, Janice Kecolt-Glaser and Ronald Glaser, whom he enlisted to measure the immune systems of student-volunteers before and after they wrote about their most traumatic experiences. The scientists found that the participants who wrote about such events experienced a marked improvement in their immune func-tion.

Pennebaker designed the study so that each participant conformed to a specific writing regimen. The volunteers had to write about a specific trau-matic event in their lives, one that they had never talked about with other peo-ple, or that contained details they had never divulged before. Rather than write in general terms about the traumatic event, each participant was to re-port in detail any negative feelings that the event had engendered in him or her, including sadness, grief, anger, remorse, or guilt. They were to do this writing four days in a row, and each session was to last at least twenty min-utes.

The researchers measured specific immune responses before and after the writing exercise and found that the number of T cells (also referred to as CD4 cells), which are the governing cells of the immune system, were more nu-merous and responded more aggressively to an immune-stimulating chemical than those who did not participate in the writing exercise (otherwise known as a control group).

Pennebaker found that those students who did the writing exercise also ex-perienced fewer visits to the health clinic than the study's control group. Re-markably, the immune responses were the greatest among those volunteers who confessed feelings that they had never considered or addressed before they started writing. Termed "high disclosers" by Pennebaker, these volunteers had the most remarkable improvement in T cell response than all other par-ticipants.

Pennebaker explains the improvement in immune response by saying that such confessional writing releases a long-standing psychological inhibition, which he describes as the mechanism by which we keep things secret, especially from ourselves. This inhibiting response requires a certain degree of psychic and physical energy, which, he says, is a demanding form of physical and mental work. Pennebaker noted that physical symptoms of disease, such as elevations in blood pressure, heart rate, breathing, skin temperature, and perspiration levels, frequently occur as a result of such inhibition. Once the secrets are disclosed, even to a journal, the painful events are made conscious and the inhibition is released. The energy that had gone toward maintaining that inhibition is now circulating through the body and mind in new ways.

Pennebaker repeated this experiment numerous times with similar results and wrote a book about his discoveries, entitled *Opening Up: The Healing Power of Confiding in Others.* Pennebaker's work, which has come to be known as the Pennebaker method, has been duplicated with similar results by researchers at the State University of New York at Stonybrook, the University of Miami, and the University of Nebraska.

THE PENNEBAKER METHOD

To get the most out of the Pennebaker method, or confessional writing, use the following guidelines.

1. Write for twenty minutes each day, for four consecutive days.
2. Write continuously about the most upsetting experience or trauma of your entire life.
3. Don't worry about grammar, spelling, or structure of the piece.
4. Write your deepest thoughts and emotions regarding the experience. Include all the details you remember and insights into the events.

Researchers have found that those who perform this exercise experience similar changes during the four days of writing. During the first two days of the exercise, people experience negative emotions, such as anger, sadness, anxiety, and grief. On the third or fourth day, they experience feelings of relief, insight, and resolution, suggesting that they have released the inhibiting energy and integrated the traumatic events into their consciousness.

Pennebaker points out that one does not necessarily have to write the event. Confessing it to someone else will have the same effect.

All of the research now points to a healing power that exists in all of us that can be called forth, inhibited, or repressed. Such repression has a depressing effect on immune response. Conversely, our efforts to become more intimate with our inner selves, to know ourselves more deeply—even when it means confronting painful memories or old wounds—clearly boosts immune response and supports healing.

Clearly, some power exists within us to restore health, even when we confront serious illness or have suffered traumatic experiences.

Waturo Ohashi, author of *Healing the Body* and the creator of a therapeutic massage method called Ohashiatsu, likes to say that no one is purely sick, no matter what the state of their health may be. "The state in which sickness has achieved complete victory is called death. As long as we're alive, health and sickness exist side by side. In order to heal, we must promote the health that already exists so that sickness has a smaller influence on our lives."

"The conditions for healing involve faith in the possibility that healing can occur, and resonance with the deeper and wiser parts of the self where healing is," wrote spiritual teacher, author, and healer Ram Dass.

The power of healing flows from a place "where healing is," as Ram Dass put it, or where health already exists in each of us. The belief that a higher power, or divine aspect, exists within all of us, of course, is the basis for virtually every major religion. Many healers believe that this power can be encouraged within us to support the recovery of health.

Traditionally, people have called upon that healing power within themselves during times of crisis through prayer and meditation. Now science is showing that prayer and meditation can stimulate this inner power to bring about healing.

Randolph Byrd, M.D., a cardiologist and medical doctor, had a computer randomly select 393 patients who were admitted to the coronary care unit at San Francisco Hospital and divide them into two groups. One group (192 patients) was prayed for by home prayer groups; another group (201 patients) were not prayed for. Not only was the study randomized, but it was also double-blind, meaning neither the patients nor the scientists and doctors knew who was being prayed for and who wasn't. The prayer group was given the first names of the patients and a brief description of their illnesses. Each patient had five to seven people praying for him or her. The prayer group prayed for the patients every day, but were not told how to pray. The study was conducted over a ten-month period.

The differences between the two groups were remarkable. The group that was not prayed for was five times more likely to need antibiotics than those who were prayed for; the not-prayed-for group was three times more likely to develop pulmonary edema (a very common illness among cardiac patients) than the prayed-for group. None of the prayed-for group required endotracheal intubation (another common procedure for cardiac patients), while twelve of the not-prayed-for group needed the treatment. Finally, fewer of the prayed-for patients died.

The power of prayer and meditation to heal has been studied extensively on everything from human health to its effect on blood cells, plants, and even fungi, and the results have demonstrated that prayer frequently causes measurable improvement in health.

At the University of Miami Medical School, researchers have found that daily meditation or relaxation exercises caused CD4 cells to increase in men with HIV. CD4 cells normally decline when HIV is contracted. One year after this initial study was done, Gail Ironson, M.D., a psychiatrist and researcher at the University of Miami Medical School, followed up on the same group of men and discovered that those who had continued to meditate were less likely to suffer from AIDS symptoms than those who did not continue meditating.

Other research has shown that meditation or relaxation exercises have increased immune cell activity in the face of an antigen. One study showed an increase in natural killer cells and greater proliferation of lymphocytes in medical school students who practiced a daily relaxation regime.

"There are many forms of relaxation or meditation exercises," said Dr. Ironson. "They can be as simple as muscle relaxation, or meditating on a beautiful place in nature, or repeating a single word (like a mantra) over and over again in your head. We don't have enough data to distinguish the effects of each of these practices on the immune system, but the research so far suggests that all of them—if practiced regularly—seem to have a positive effect."

Research at Harvard University has found that Transcendental Meditation (TM)—a technique in which a mantra, or a specific word or words, is repeated over and over again—creates deep states of relaxation and may be associated with increased longevity. Researchers found that a group of nursing home residents who practiced TM lived longer than matched controls who didn't meditate.

Herbert Benson, M.D., associate professor of medicine at Harvard Medical School, has extensively studied the effects of prayer and meditation on health and found that such methods create what Benson calls the "relaxation response." Ten to twenty minutes of meditation per day, Benson says, lowers blood pressure, slows heart rate, relaxes muscles, and creates a more balanced hormonal condition, all of which can contribute to a stronger immune response.

Psychotherapist and mind-body expert Jon Kabat-Zinn told television reporter Bill Moyers, "Emotions are not bad—they're just what you're feeling. The point is to get out of the same emotional ruts. Meditation can wake you up to the fact that in the present moment there may be new options, and new ways of relating to old situations. We've found that people who were very dissatisfied in their relationships with their bosses or their spouses or children, were able to encounter these people in a totally different way. Even if a lot of negativity is coming at them, they can learn to breathe with it and find a new kind of response that completely changes the ground on which everybody's standing."

Meditation and prayer open us up to the larger possibilities associated with the healing power that lies within. That healing power is frequently experienced as optimism, gratitude, and faith. And with such psychological conditions frequently come physical changes, including the improvement of health and psychological rebirth.

Below are suggestions for meditations and guided imagery exercises. These can be used as they are described or modified in whatever way you desire to bring about a greater sense of faith, security, and optimism. They also can be helpful in promoting immune response. Find one or two that particularly appeal to you and, if possible, do it daily.

READING SPIRITUAL AND RELIGIOUS LITERATURE

Many people find that dramatic changes in beliefs and outlook occur with consistent reading of spiritual or religious literature. Among the most powerful and popular forms of this practice are the daily reading of the Bible, the Old or New Testaments, or both; the Koran; the Bhagavad Gita; the Vedas; the Upanishads; the Sutras of the Buddha; and the Tao Te Ching.

Many short passages in spiritual literature, such as the Psalms in the Bible, or poetry and music, can be used as a meditation or chanting exercise. If one stays with you, it probably is because it touches some deep chord and may be exactly what you need to focus on in order to stimulate something in your psyche.

RELIGIOUS PRAYERS

In times of crisis, many people turn to the powerful and evocative prayers taught to them in their youth, especially by their religious teachers. Hence, the Rosary is recited by many Roman Catholics; the Lord's Prayer by both Catholics and Protestants; the Sh'ma by Jews; and the Sutras by Buddhists, the Heart Sutra being one of the most popular.

CONCENTRATE ON A WORD OR SHORT PASSAGE

Chanting a word or phrase has been the basis for religious and spiritual devotion in both the East and West. Such words, or mantras, are repeated over and over again in a slow, rhythmic fashion until other thoughts are gradually eliminated from the mind. A sense of deep relaxation and well-being will begin to fill up your inner being. These good feelings will strengthen you and promote health by restoring your energy and sense of balance.

Chanting is easier for some people than just thinking of the word, and the inner vibration that is created from the sound will promote an integration of your feelings and emotional balance. Common words or phrases used are *amen, father, abba, Mary, mother, shalom* (the Hebrew word for peace), *om* or *aum* (used in Oriental traditions to signify the universal sound), *nam myo ho renge kyo* (a popular Buddhist chant thought to be very empowering), and also the names of common spiritual and religious figures. Both Alfred Lord Tennyson and Walt Whitman chanted their own names. This practice has been known to awaken parts of one's identity that were previously unknown or misunderstood.

CONCENTRATE ON A SINGLE IMAGE

A single image can be used to enter into deep relaxation and instill security and strength. The image must be seen in as much detail as possible. There are also qualities associated with the image that should be felt as much as possible. Focus as long as you can before coming out of this meditation. Common images are a mountain, which is the picture of stillness, tranquillity, and strength; a pool of water, which can represent stillness, but also an embrace; the ocean—the picture of primal power, the primordial mother of all of life on the planet—combines strength with serenity, patience, and longevity; a tree suggests peaceful yet relentless growth and beauty; and the grace and buoyancy of a single white cloud.

FOCUS ON YOUR BREATH

Both Eastern and Western traditions have encouraged this type of meditation for centuries. Begin by concentrating on inhaling and exhaling your breath. Picture life, health, and love fill up your body as you inhale and all undesirable emotions, sickness, and difficulties leave you on the exhalation. With every breath you become more aligned with the movements of the universe, the very basic expansion and contraction that takes place in the cosmos as well as on the level of subatomic particles.

The most important thing is to achieve a very deep state of relaxation, which will encourage as many positive emotions to well up inside of you as possible.

GUIDED IMAGERY

The Relaxation Exercise

- Go to a softly lighted room and sit in a straight-backed, comfortable chair. Take off your shoes and sit back.
- Notice your breathing. Slow down so that your breath is drawn deep into your stomach, and then release it in a very gradual and relaxed manner. Continue to breathe deeply and slowly.
- Focus on the muscles in your face. Make a tense prune face and then relax. Allow the tension to melt away.
- Turn your attention to the muscles of your neck and shoulders. Lift your shoulders to your ears and then relax. Feel the tension fall away from your neck and shoulders.
- Let your arms rest in your lap or on the arms of the chair, and feel the tension and energy drain from them.
- Focus on your stomach and chest. Your breathing should be slow, calm, and deep. Relax your stomach and chest and picture the tension falling away.

- Concentrate now on your legs and feet. Tense them first, then feel the tension dissipate, as if it were draining down your legs and out the bottoms of your feet.
- Feel warm, relaxed, and healthy.
- Picture a natural setting with which your being resonates. See it as clearly and in as much detail as you can. Feel the sun and gentle wind against your skin. Feel the peace and joy that this place creates for you.
- Concentrate as long as you can and then gradually come out of this meditation.

It's not necessary always to concentrate on the same place in these meditations, but it will be most effective if you add as much detail as possible and also experience it with as many of your senses as your imagination allows.

The Light Meditation

- Perform the relaxation exercise.
- Imagine a small beam of light emanating from your heart.
- Notice that this light is tiny but powerful.
- Watch the spark of light gradually become larger, until it fills your entire chest area, then spreads to every part of your body, emanating from your every pore.
- Imagine that the cells of your body are radiant with light. This light is all-powerful and has an entirely energizing and transforming effect on your being, filling you with joy, love, and limitless energy. Hold this state for as long as you can.

Exercise for Those in Poor Health

- Notice that every cell within you that is ill cannot absorb the light; these cells are therefore dark and weak.
- Picture your white blood cells, which are clothed in light, bearing down on the dark, weak, diseased cells. The light cells are infinitely more powerful, numerous, and organized than the dark cells.
- Picture the light cells routing the diseased cells and forcing them into your digestive tract, where they will be eliminated from your body.
- Picture a large but distinct source of light just above you. This source of light is infinitely radiant and has limitless power.
- Imagine this source of light sending energy into your body, making you all the more radiant and filled with vitality.
- Bathe in the warmth of this energy. It is love.
- Continue the meditation for as long as you wish.

PART IV

DISEASE PREVENTION AND HEALTH MAINTENANCE OF INDIVIDUAL ORGANS

INTRODUCTION

An old Oriental aphorism about health goes something like this: "A man who lives according to his weaknesses will have great vitality and good health his whole life long, but a man who lives by his strengths will suffer endless misery." The wisdom of this statement is clear to anyone who has a weak stomach, yet still insists on eating those hot chili peppers. The tongue and the intestines may be able to tolerate the heat, but the conflagration in the stomach causes him misery all day (and night) long.

An old sage from any tradition might counsel our weak-stomached friend to heed the advice of his own stomach and avoid those foods that give it pain. Such behavior will not only please his stomach, but will place less stress on his palate and intestinal tract. This, of course, is the easy solution to chronic misery. By living according to the dictates of our weaker organs, we place less stress on the entire body. This, say the Chinese, is the basis for good health and long life.

Many of us are aware of some chronic weakness in our health but do not have the same kind of clear and ready answer for our weak intestines, congested lungs, stressed kidneys, or chronically distressed sex organs, for example. While such discomforts usually do not cause serious illness, they nevertheless diminish the quality of our lives, and, at the very least, distract us from the things we'd rather be doing.

This part of the book offers guidance for strengthening the organs. For example, it will outline easy methods for supporting and strengthening the health of the heart, kidneys, sex organs, and lungs. Advice about diet, exercise, and herbs is offered to make the large intestine function better on a daily basis, or help the skin radiate a healthy glow.

Although specific illnesses and disorders are dealt with in Part II of this book, this section emphasizes *prevention* of disease, rather than the cure. It focuses on making the weaker aspects of the body stronger and more resistant to illness. Thus, this is a guide to treating the body—or more specifically, the organs—well.

THE BLADDER

A muscular, spherical sac located in the lower abdomen, the bladder holds urine, the body's liquid waste, which is produced by the kidneys as they filter the blood. It is located within the pelvis, directly behind the pubic bone. The bladder's walls are three layers thick. The first layer is composed of longitudinal muscles; the second with circular; and the third, again, with longitudinal. This patterning of muscles provides the bladder with tremendous control, as well as the ability to expand and contract.

The bladder of an adult can hold as much as one pint of liquid, which flows from the kidneys via two tubes, or ureters. Another tube, called the urethra, passes from the bladder to the penis in men or to an opening in the muscles of the pelvic floor, right next to the vagina, in women. The muscles of the pelvis also control the anus, and, in women, the vagina. They also support the developing fetus during pregnancy.

As the kidneys cleanse the blood of waste, urine flows into the bladder, which causes the walls to expand. This expansion causes nerve signals to be sent to the brain via the spinal cord, making one aware of the need to urinate. When one decides to urinate, nerve impulses from the brain order a series of muscular reactions. First, the muscles that surround the urethra expand, thus allowing urine to flow through the tube. Second, two sets of sphincter muscles—one that exists internally, within the bladder, at the opening of the urethra, and another that exists externally, or just on the other side of the bladder around the urethra—open to allow the urine to flow out of the body. At the same time, the brain orders the bladder walls to contract, and continue contracting, until all the urine has been expelled.

COMMON ILLNESSES AFFECTING THE BLADDER

Urinary tract infections, incontinence, and stones (also called calculi) are among the most common illnesses affecting the bladder (see the specific sections on these conditions). Men can suffer a variety of disorders of the prostate, which can prevent the bladder from fully eliminating urine (see the section on the prostate).

Women tend to suffer urinary tract infections far more frequently than men because their urethras are shorter than men's and they are located closer to the anus, from which bacteria can easily pass. There are numerous other causes of urinary tract infections. In general, anything that prevents full elimination of urine from the bladder and urethra will increase the likelihood of bacteria build-up and infection. Common causes include injury to the urethra or bladder, causing inflammation, which can impair full elimination of urine; swelling of the urethra from sexual intercourse, most common in women; kidney or urethra stones; pregnancy; irritants present in bubble baths, douches, feminine hygiene sprays, and diaphragms; vaginitis; congenital abnormalities of the urethra or some other

The Bladder

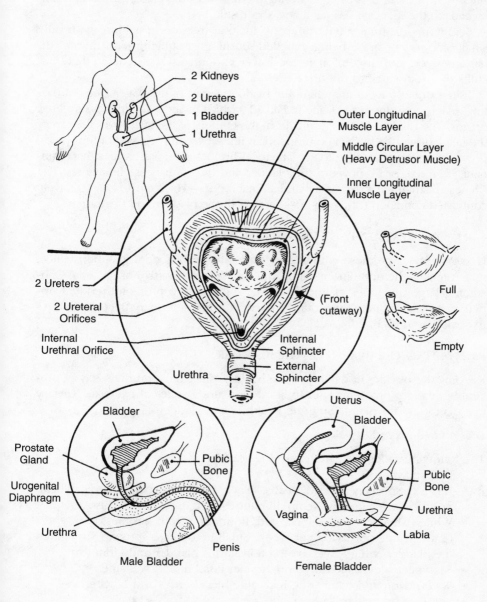

2 Kidneys
2 Ureters
1 Bladder
1 Urethra

Outer Longitudinal Muscle Layer

Middle Circular Layer (Heavy Detrusor Muscle)

Inner Longitudinal Muscle Layer

2 Ureters

2 Ureteral Orifices

Internal Urethral Orifice

(Front cutaway)

Internal Sphincter

External Sphincter

Urethra

Full

Empty

Bladder

Prostate Gland

Urogenital Diaphragm

Urethra

Pubic Bone

Penis

Male Bladder

Uterus

Bladder

Pubic Bone

Urethra

Labia

Vagina

Female Bladder

part of the urinary tract; prostate enlargement or inflammation; psychological stress; and the use of a catheter during medical tests or surgery. If the infection spreads to the kidneys, serious illness can result.

Symptoms of urinary tract infection include frequent urination, with only small amounts of urine being expelled; burning or stinging pain during urination; fever; and discomfort in the lower abdomen. Occasionally, there are chills or a foul smell to the urine.

In the Chinese medical system, the bladder is part of the Water Element (see the section on Chinese medicine in Part III), which includes the kidneys and sex organs. The bladder meridian runs from the corners of the eyes, over the top of the head, down the back (in four meridian lines, two on each side of the spine), down the backs of the legs, to the little toe. This long meridian assures that abundant life force, or qi, flows to the bladder and thus enhances elimination. The Chinese maintain that excess salt and animal foods—which create an excessively contracted condition (or over yin)—harm both the bladder and the kidneys.

COMMON TREATMENTS OF URINARY PROBLEMS

Doctors encourage those with urinary tract infections to drink cranberry juice, which makes the urine more acidic and thus less supportive of bacteria. Consuming large quantities of liquids also is suggested to promote frequent urination, which will help flush out the bacteria from the urinary tract. Antibiotics may also be prescribed.

PROTECTING THE HEALTH OF THE BLADDER

Keeping the bladder fit while you are healthy is the most prudent way of preventing bladder problems later in life. Below are a series of exercises, dietary tips, and ideas for maintaining the health of the bladder.

Diet and Foods to Eat

The following foods will strengthen the bladder:

- Beans, especially adzuki beans, black beans, soybeans and soybean products, such as tofu, tempeh, natto, shoyu, tamari, and miso
- White fish, such as haddock, cod, flounder, scrod, sardines, and others (Eat fish once or twice per week. Small amounts of protein strengthen the bladder, while excessive protein harms bladder and kidneys.)
- Sea vegetables, especially nori, arame, kombu, and wakame
- Watermelon and other fruit, including blackberries and blueberries
- Spirulina and chlorella
- Black sesame seeds

Herbs

- Marshmallow root
- Prepared rehmannia root
- Asparagus root

Foods to Reduce or Avoid

The following foods have been shown to irritate the bladder and make one more vulnerable to incontinence and other bladder problems, according to the Public Citizen Health Research Group *Health Letter.*

- Salt (The body needs about one-fourth of a teaspoon of salt per day to maintain healthy blood pressure and nerve and muscle function. The National Academy of Sciences recommends that people add no more than one and a half teaspoons of salt from all sources, including at the table; in cooking; and from processed foods. When using salt in cooking, add no more than a pinch to grains or vegetables. Excess salt harms both bladder and kidneys, but small amounts strengthen these organs. High-quality sea salt is slightly richer in minerals than regular table salt.)
- Caffeine
- Alcohol
- Sugar
- Acidic juices and foods
- Spicy foods
- Milk products (Dairy foods have been shown to make some women incontinent.)

Other foods that have been shown to irritate the bladder in sensitive people include:

- Caffeine-containing foods
- Carbonated beverages
- Vinegars
- Cranberry and guava juices
- Citrus fruits (along with apples, cantaloupe, grapes, peaches, pineapples, plums, strawberries, and tomatoes)

Stop Smoking

Approximately one-third of women who suffer bladder problems, particularly incontinence, are or have been smokers, according to research at the Medical College of Virginia at Richmond. Smokers have twice the risk of bladder problems and incontinence than nonsmokers.

Exercise

KEGEL EXERCISES AS A ROUTINE WORKOUT FOR THE BLADDER

Dr. Arnold Kegel, a professor of obstetrics and gynecology at the University of California at Los Angeles, created a set of exercises for preventing and treating incontinence. Those exercises are as follows:

1. Practice controlling the bladder by slowing urine flow, and then stopping it. When you are able to stop the flow, hold it one or two seconds. Do this six or eight times as you urinate. You may have to do this exercise numerous times before you are able to stop the flow entirely, but eventually you will be able to control the flow without leakage. Practice relaxing and contracting the pelvic floor muscles, as well.
2. Practice relaxing and contracting the same muscles used in the first exercise throughout the day. Hold the contraction for several seconds and then relax. Do this exercise anywhere from 50 to 100 times per day, and repeat the first exercise when urinating.
3. Contract the pelvic floor during lovemaking.

All exercises that strengthen the abdomen will help to restore strength and control to the pelvic floor, as well. A complete guide to prenatal and postnatal exercises are included in the book, *Essential Exercises for the Child-Bearing Year,* by Elizabeth Nobel.

Exercises to Reduce or Avoid

High-impact aerobics may increase a woman's likelihood of losing control of the bladder later in life, according to research done by John Delancey, M.D., at the University of Michigan. He studied 326 women ranging in age from seventeen to sixty-eight and found that more than a third of the women who run or do high-impact aerobics experience lost bladder control during their workouts. Dr. Delancey's advice is to empty the bladder before exercise, do Kegel exercises daily, and if the problem persists, switch to a more bladder-friendly regimen, such as bicycle riding.

LOSE WEIGHT

Excessive weight places additional strain on the bladder and may weaken it sufficiently to cause incontinence and other urologic problems, according to a study published in the *Journal of Urology* in November 1991. "A link between body mass and incontinence supports the concept that weight gain may increase susceptibility to incontinence, and suggests that weight loss may decrease incontinence," concluded researchers Kathryn L. Burgio and her colleagues.

Drink Clean, Pure Water

Drinking clean, pure water is essential to a healthy urinary tract because it eliminates unfriendly bacteria from the bladder. The standard recommendation of 6 to 8 glasses of water per day may be inappropriate, based on the individual's size and weight.

THE EAR

For people living in the United States and much of the Western world, hearing gradually deteriorates with age, though this is not the case among those living on more traditional diets and lifestyles in Asia and some European countries.

The primary dietary factor affecting hearing is dietary fat, which causes atherosclerosis in the tiny arteries and passageways within the hearing mechanism of the inner ear. One study compared the hearing of citizens living in Wisconsin with that of the African tribespeople, called the Mabaans. Researchers found that not one Mabaan—even at the age of seventy—suffered the hearing loss that the average Wisconsinite had suffered by the age of thirty-five. Other research compared the hearing of Finnish people with Yugoslavians. The Finns, whose diet is high in fat, have the highest per capita blood cholesterol level (290 mg/dL) of anyone in the world, and consequently the highest rates of heart disease in the world. The average cholesterol level among Yugoslavians is 180 mg/dL. Researchers found that Finnish children begin to suffer hearing loss at age ten. By the age of nineteen, they have distinct hearing impairment, especially at the higher range of 16,000 to 18,000 cycles per second. No such hearing loss was found among Yugoslavians.

The most important way to protect yourself from loss of hearing is to eat a diet that is low in fat and cholesterol. Such a diet will promote optimal circulation, especially within the inner ear. Any injury to the ear will heal faster and more thoroughly when circulation is good, and waste products will not be able to accumulate within the ear mechanism.

Of course, loud noises should also be avoided. Noise can be extremely harmful to hearing. Once the ear is injured, you should eat a diet that will boost immune function and assist in healing.

The Chinese maintain that the ear is nourished with life force by the kidneys. Consequently, taking good care of your kidneys is also a way to support the health of your ears and hearing.

The following recommendations will help to prevent hearing loss and ear problems, including earache and ear infection.

Diet and Foods to Eat

- Collard greens, broccoli, brussels sprouts, squash, carrots, and other foods rich in beta-carotene
- Broccoli (one of the richest sources of vitamin C), tangerines, leafy greens, and other foods rich in vitamin C
- Whole grains, green vegetables, pumpkin seeds and other seeds, vegetable oils, salmon and other fish and seafood are all rich in vitamin E.

- Food rich in zinc, including whole grains, shrimp, and pumpkin seeds
- Garlic is antifungal and antibacterial.

Herbs

Use the following herbs, especially when ears are congested or infected.

- Mullein is an antibacterial; four drops in each ear, four times per day.
- Chamomile is especially beneficial for children, as a tea. It will promote perspiration and elimination of accumulated toxins. Take 2 to 3 times per day.

Foods to Reduce or Avoid

- Dairy foods, especially those that are combined with sugar, promote congestion within the ear and ear infections.
- Foods high in fat
- Sugar
- Refined flour products, especially white bread, white rolls, and white pastry foods
- Fried foods

Parents of children who are prone to ear infections and other ear problems should be conscious of the possibility of food sensitivities in their children. Foods to which children may be sensitive include:

- Wheat products
- Dairy foods
- Excessive fruit and fruit juice (Small amounts of fruit may not be a problem, but there may be a point at which fruit and fruit sugars cannot be tolerated.)
- Nightshades, such as tomatoes, potatoes, and eggplant
- Sugar (Children are often able to tolerate a certain amount of sugar, but they can react negatively once their tolerance is exceeded.)
- Artificial ingredients, such as synthetic flavors and colors, preservatives, pesticides, and herbicides

See also the sections on earache and ear infections in Part II of this book.

THE EYE

The eye's ability to see is made possible, in part, by the facility of the crystalline lens to change shape in order to focus on an object. This is called *accommodation*, meaning the ability of the lens to adjust, or accommodate, to the distance of the object being focused on. Typically, the lens becomes less elastic and flexible with age, requiring eyeglasses for most older people. This loss of accommodation is more common in the West than it is among traditional peoples.

The ciliary body, a muscular ring that surrounds the lens, makes it possible for the lens to change shape and focus on objects. The ciliary body contracts and allows the eye to focus on objects that are near; it relaxes and expands to allow the eye to focus on objects that are relatively far away. Focusing the eye is an involuntary action.

Since the muscles of the ciliary body focus the eye, many leading eye therapists maintain that visual acuity is largely a function of eye-muscle fitness. Indeed, numerous exercise programs have been developed that can successfully restore visual acuity to those suffering from a wide variety of eye disorders. (See below.) The Chinese, on the other hand, have traditionally maintained that the health or fitness of these muscles, as well as the health of the eye overall, depends on the qi, or life force, sent to it by the liver. Therefore, from the perspective of Chinese medicine, all eye problems stem, in part, from an imbalance within the liver, preventing the organ from sending the eyes adequate qi. A Chinese healer would not only treat the eyes themselves, but would offer herbs, acupuncture, and other therapeutic measures to strengthen the liver. (See the section on the liver for more information.)

Around the cornea is a drainage ditch called the canal of Schlemm, that allows waste from inside the eye to drain from the eye and into the capillaries below. Before the waste reaches the canal of Schlemm, it passes through a filter-meshwork that exists where the cornea and iris meet. This filter-meshwork can become clogged with waste (urea, cholesterol, or other waste products), causing pressure to build within the eye, and thus give rise to a disease called glaucoma. (See below.)

Nathan Pritikin, the pioneer diet and health advocate, maintained that both high-fat and high-protein diets causing fat, cholesterol, and protein by-products (such as uric acid crystals) to infiltrate the eye, block the filter-meshwork and canal of Schlemm, thus preventing optimal elimination of waste products from the eye. As the filter-meshwork and canal of Schlemm become less efficient, aqueous fluid is prevented from flowing out of the eye and thus causes interocular pressure to build, resulting in glaucoma. Waste accumulation causes other eye-related problems, as well, including the appearance of floaters in the visual field. Waste prevents the optimal functioning of the eye and prevents true accommodations. Thus, it plays a role in the eye's ability to focus.

Pritikin encouraged people to use the Bates Method exercises to restore vision and to eat a low-fat, low-cholesterol diet to restore maximum circulation and waste removal within the eye.

Diet and Foods to Eat

See also related sections on vision in Part II and on the liver in Part IV.

- Barley and whole wheat strengthen the liver, which supports the eyes with life force.
- Asparagus, broccoli, brussels sprouts, cabbage, carrots, cauliflower, green beans, leafy greens, lettuce, mushrooms, okra, parsley, peas, sprouts, and zucchini are all rich in beta-carotene, the vegetable source of vitamin A, which supports the health of the optic nerve.
- Apples, grapes, oranges, pears, prunes, and raisins all help heal the liver.

Foods to Reduce or Avoid

- Fatty foods prevent maximum circulation to the eyes.
- Avoid excesses of alcohol and excessive exposure to chemicals that impair liver function.

Exercise

The work of behavioral optometrists has its roots in the theories of pioneer vision therapist, Dr. William Bates. Bates developed exercises to improve vision that were used throughout this century to help restore eyesight. The Bates Method was used successfully by many young men who wanted to be fighter pilots during World War II, but who were unable to pass the eye exam at the first try. Among the most common practices Bates encouraged was to lie on a bed and trace the outline of the room, where the walls meet the ceiling, at a steady but rapid pace. As the eyes rotate, the muscles that focus the eyes are exercised. Bates also encouraged reading for short periods—ten to twenty minutes— without the use of glasses. When the eyes tire, rest them, and then read again for as long as possible until they tire again. This time, stop. Bates encouraged people to do as much as possible without the use of eyeglasses, which tend to weaken the eyes by making them dependent upon the corrective lenses.

A simple exercise for the eyes is to hold your finger up before your face, at the level of your nose, about one foot away from your face. Focus your sight on your finger. Hold it ten seconds. Now shift your focus to a detailed object, such as a painting, about ten feet away. That is considered one round. Do ten repetitions of this single round, and then relax. Do several sets of these exercises throughout the day. This will exercise the ciliary body and strengthen those muscles that focus the eye.

THE GALLBLADDER

About three inches long, shaped like a pear, and found in the back of the liver, the gallbladder serves as a reservoir for bile, a liquid emulsifier produced by the liver and used to break down fats in the stomach and small intestine. Bile is the body's liquid detergent, you might say. When food is moved from the stomach to the small intestine, hormones signal the gallbladder to release bile, which breaks up the fat into smaller particles, which are then absorbed by the small intestine.

Bile is composed of both bile acids (also known as bile salts) and cholesterol. The cholesterol buffers the acids in the bile, preventing them from eating holes in the gallbladder, stomach, and small intestine.

The most common disorder affecting the gallbladder, of course, is gallstones, which are highly preventable. About sixteen million Americans suffer from gallstones, twelve million of whom are women. Scientists believe the disparity is due to the drop off of estrogen levels that women experience after menopause. Some 500,000 gallbladders are removed each year due to gallstones.

Gallstones, which are composed almost entirely of cholesterol, appear when the delicate balance between bile acids and cholesterol gets thrown off due to a high-fat diet. Cholesterol buffers the bile acids; the bile acids, meanwhile, keep the cholesterol in solution, preventing them from forming stones. Problems arise when too much cholesterol and fat are consumed, causing the cholesterol level within the gallbladder to rise. According to the late Nathan Pritikin, the pioneer nutritionist who used diet and exercise to restore health to tens of thousands of people with serious illness, a healthy cholesterol level within the gallbladder is approximately 350 milligrams. Most Americans, by contrast, have cholesterol levels within their gallbladders of 650 milligrams. Once the cholesterol becomes excessive, the acid within the gallbladder can no longer keep the cholesterol in a liquid state. Gradually, the cholesterol congeals and forms crystals, which become the nuclei for stones.

Pritikin maintained that if people simply lowered their cholesterol levels, the bile acids within the gallbladder would dissolve the stones, and in the process prevent many unnecessary gallbladder operations.

Other forms of traditional medicine, such as naturopathy, argue that the liver and gallbladder become congested through excessive consumption of fat, cholesterol, artificial ingredients, sugar, and alcohol. When forced to overwork due to a diet that is essentially toxic, the liver can overproduce bile and cholesterol, thus flooding the gallbladder, causing stagnation within the organ, and eventually creating stones.

Naturopaths often recommend a variety of herbs and a diet rich in antioxidants to treat both the liver and gallbladder, because free radicals are usually the underlying cause of most liver and gallbladder disease.

The Gallbladder

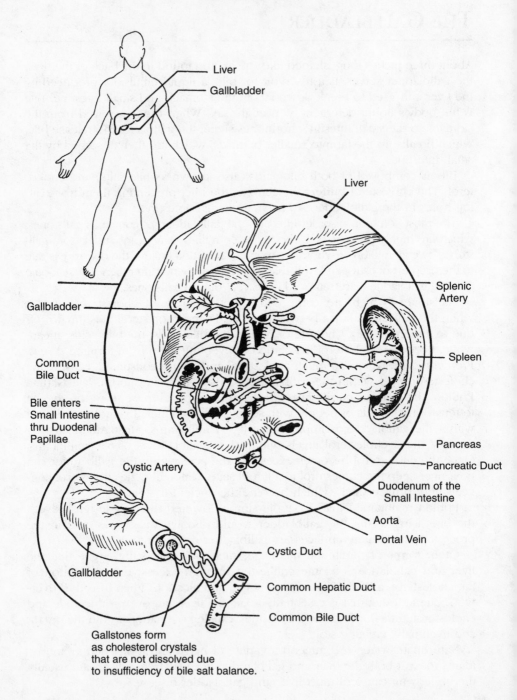

Liver

Gallbladder

Liver

Gallbladder

Splenic Artery

Common Bile Duct

Spleen

Bile enters Small Intestine thru Duodenal Papillae

Pancreas

Pancreatic Duct

Duodenum of the Small Intestine

Cystic Artery

Aorta

Portal Vein

Gallbladder

Cystic Duct

Common Hepatic Duct

Common Bile Duct

Gallstones form as cholesterol crystals that are not dissolved due to insufficiency of bile salt balance.

According to the Chinese, the gallbladder is responsible for sound decision making, or, as *The Yellow Emperor's Classic of Internal Medicine* puts it: "The gallbladder occupies the position of an important and upright official who excels through his decisions and judgment." The Chinese maintain that every organ is associated with an emotion and specific psychological function. (See the section on Chinese medicine in Part III for more information on the five element theory and the emotional and psychological associations of the gallbladder.) The gallbladder is associated with anger (as is the liver) and has the role of maintaining emotional equilibrium. When the emotions are balanced, the mind is clear and decisions are sound, say the Chinese. But when the gallbladder is disturbed, anger and frustration dominate the psyche, and decision making becomes clouded by emotional imbalances.

The Chinese also maintain that whole wheat, wheat products, a wide variety of leafy green vegetables, carrots, and carrot juice will assist in the healing of the gallbladder. In addition, sour taste stimulates the cleansing of the liver and gallbladder, say the Chinese.

The following recommendations will help to prevent gallbladder disease and assist in the restoration of the organ.

Foods to Eat

- Whole wheat and whole wheat products, such as wheat berries, bulgur, and noodles
- Broccoli, cabbage, collard greens, kale, and dark leaf lettuce
- Lemon as a condiment
- Carrot juice
- Grapefruit juice
- Apple juice
- Beet root tops, beet juice
- Figs
- Pears
- Radish; eat one or two between meals for three weeks
- Prunes
- Dandelion greens
- Chicory
- Olive oil
- Grated apples
- Small amounts of olive oil used on salad or greens twice a week cleanses the gallbladder.
- Sesame seeds
- Oranges
- Celery
- Garlic
- Onions
- Tomatoes

- Dates
- Melons
- Pineapple

Foods to Avoid

- Meat
- Eggs
- Refined carbohydrates
- Dairy
- Hydrogenated fats
- Nuts and nut butters
- Sugar
- Alcohol

Herbs to Treat

- Chamomile tea, to dissolve stones
- Dandelion tea and greens clear obstruction

Chinese Medicine

- Treat liver stagnation with the foods and herbs listed above.
- Acupuncture or acupressure, especially treating liver and gallbladder meridians

Supplements

- Beta-carotene: 15–30 mg per day
- Thiamine: 1.5 mg per day
- Riboflavin: 1.8 mg per day
- Vitamin B_6: 2–10 mg per day
- Vitamin B_{12}: 2–10 mg per day
- Niacin: 20 mg per day
- Vitamin C: 100 mg one time per day
- Vitamin E: 100–200 IU one time per day

The Heart

In the average person, the heart beats between 60 and 80 times per minute, 100,000 times per day, and 2.5 billion times in the average life span. The entire blood supply flows through the heart every sixty seconds. About the size of a man's fist, the heart is not one pump, but two. The right side of the heart, composed of two chambers—an upper chamber called the atrium, and the lower called the ventricle—pumps blood to the lungs, where it receives oxygen and gives up its carbon dioxide load. The left side, also composed of upper and lower chambers by the same names, pumps blood to the general circulation. The two jobs require vastly different amounts of effort. There is a great deal more resistance in the seemingly endless network of blood vessels, arteries, and tiny capillaries than there is within the lungs. Consequently, pumping blood to the general circulation is much harder. This makes the left side of the heart stronger and more muscular. Yet, the two sides must beat in perfect union and harmony if the heart is to function properly.

For most Westerners, the greatest threat to the heart is a diet rich in fat and cholesterol and low in fiber, coupled with a sedentary lifestyle.

More than sixty million Americans suffer from illnesses of the heart and arteries, and nearly one million die each year of such diseases. The standard American diet is a formula for cardiovascular illness. Meanwhile, our lifestyles promote stress, with which we have not yet learned to cope. The three most important factors that can prevent heart disease are a diet low in fat and cholesterol and high in fiber and antioxidants, a regimen of stress reduction, and the development of faith. (See the section on faith.)

CHECK YOUR CHOLESTEROL LEVEL

The most critical gauge as to whether or not your diet is low enough in fat and rich enough in fiber and antioxidants is your cholesterol level. Ideally, your cholesterol level should be 100, plus your age, never to exceed 160 mg/dL. Scientists find a significant drop in the rate of heart attacks and diseases of the heart among those with cholesterol levels below 180 mg/dL, and heart disease is rare among those with cholesterol levels of 160.

DIET AND FOODS TO EAT

For more detail on the most effective diet for preventing illnesses of the heart, see the section on nutrition. A diet rich in cholesterol-lowering fiber, abundant in heart-healthy antioxidants, and low in fat and cholesterol is the best way to promote heart health.

The Heart

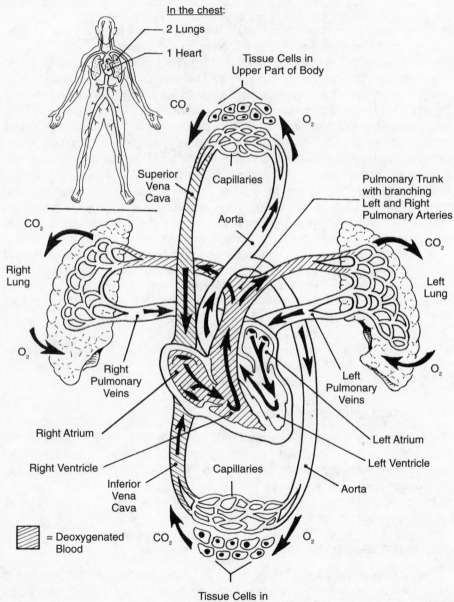

In the chest:
- 2 Lungs
- 1 Heart

Tissue Cells in
Upper Part of Body

CO_2

O_2

Superior
Vena
Cava

Capillaries

Aorta

Pulmonary Trunk
with branching
Left and Right
Pulmonary Arteries

CO_2

Right
Lung

Left
Lung

CO_2

O_2

O_2

Right
Pulmonary
Veins

Left
Pulmonary
Veins

Right Atrium

Left Atrium

Right Ventricle

Left Ventricle

Inferior
Vena
Cava

Capillaries

Aorta

⬦ = Deoxygenated
Blood

CO_2

O_2

Tissue Cells in
Lower Part of Body

- Make whole grains, such as brown rice, barley, millet, corn, and oats, the central part of most meals.
- Include at least one green and one orange or yellow vegetable at dinner every evening to be sure you are getting an abundance of antioxidants (as well as cancer-preventing vegetables).
- Eat two servings per day of green vegetables, such as collard greens, kale, mustard greens, broccoli, brussels sprouts, cabbage, lettuce, or some other green vegetable.
- Include regular amounts of cholesterol-lowering foods, such as shiitake mushrooms, garlic, and soybean products, such as tofu and tempeh. All of these foods lower cholesterol, boost immune function, and protect against other diseases, including cancer.
- Eat beans and legumes, including adzuki beans, black beans, garbanzo beans, lentils, mung beans, navy beans, pinto beans, split peas, green beans, and soybeans.
- Corn and glutinous millet are both considered herbs for the heart in Chinese medicine.

According to the Chinese, each taste has a healing property. Slightly burnt foods, such as toast or roasted seeds, have a healing effect on the heart.

Foods to Reduce or Avoid

- Avoid red meat. If you are currently eating meat on a regular basis, increase the number of meatless meals gradually (see the nutrition section).
- Substitute skim milk and low-fat and nonfat cheeses for whole milk and whole-milk products.
- Oils that are filled with saturated fats, such as palm kernel, coconut, and peanut oils should be avoided or eliminated.
- Limit alcohol consumption to two drinks per day.
- Caffeine stimulates the heart excessively and weakens the kidneys and bladder. According to Chinese medicine, kidneys control the heart. Weak kidneys weaken the heart.
- Excess salt weakens the kidneys and arteries and causes high blood pressure.

DEAL EFFECTIVELY WITH STRESS

- Begin each day with a conversation with your own higher self or the divine, however you conceive of It, Him, or Her. Carry on this conversation throughout the day.
- Do the progressive relaxation exercises described in Part IV of this book.
- Exercise daily.

- Enjoy diversions from work or problems. Read, or see films (especially those that uplift your spirit or make you laugh).
- Join a social club. Get out into the world. Avoid isolation.

Exercise

- Before you begin any exercise training program, have a thorough cardiovascular medical examination by your doctor. This is particularly important if you are over forty and have any of the risk factors for heart disease, including a history of cigarette smoking, a previous heart attack, if you currently have a high cholesterol level, high blood pressure, diabetes, disorders of the lungs, claudication, or if you have a family history that includes heart disease, heart attack, or stroke.
- Twenty to thirty minutes of aerobic exercise, three to five times per week is recommended.

See the sections on heart disease in Part II and exercise in Part III of this book.

THE IMMUNE SYSTEM

"A new form of medicine" is what scientists at M. D. Anderson Cancer Center, Louisiana State University, and other leading research centers are calling the immune-boosting and cancer-fighting effects of certain foods, herbs, and stress-reduction activities. These and other health-promoting methods are being given that singular designation because they treat the very causes of disease rather than its symptoms.

The majority of today's medicines address only the outer manifestations of illness: Medications for headaches or the common cold, for example, don't address the cause of pain or the cold virus; they simply alleviate the symptoms. In the same way, drugs that treat angina pectoris, or chest pain, only address the pain itself and not the clogged arteries that caused the angina and that could eventually lead to a heart attack.

The medicines that nature provides—namely, certain foods, herbs, nutrients, and immune-boosting behaviors—work on the molecular and cellular levels, restoring health where illness originates. And they do it with little or no side effects.

NEW INSIGHTS INTO THE ORIGINS OF DISEASE

The use of diet, herbs, and immune-boosting activities as medicine is emerging from a larger understanding of how we become ill and age. Scientists today are finding that more than sixty major disorders and even aging itself all have the same cause. That cause, referred to as *free radical formation,* is a kind of decay that occurs when highly reactive oxygen molecules interact with atoms within our own tissues. These oxygen molecules cause atoms to lose electrons, triggering a chain reaction that results in the breakdown of cells and tissues. That breakdown of cells and tissues is the underlying aging process, but it can lead to a wide variety of disease states, including heart disease, cancer, arthritis, cataracts, Alzheimer's disease, and Parkinson's disease.

Remarkably, certain nutrients in foods and herbs reverse the free radical process. These nutrients, called *antioxidants,* donate electrons to atoms, and thus halt the breakdown of cells and tissues. They establish order and health on the cellular level.

There are many antioxidants, but the three most commonly known are vitamins C and E and beta-carotene, the vegetable source of vitamin A. In addition to these are selenium, a mineral, and glutathione, a chemical found in whole grains, whole grain breads, fruit, and vegetables. Antioxidants, however, are only one of the immune-boosting and cancer-fighting tools now emerging. Other nutrients stimulate the production of enzymes and proteins within the body that directly fight cancer cells and tumors. These foods inhibit the growth of cancer. According to Michael Wargovich, M.D., a professor of medicine at M. D. Anderson Cancer Center in Houston, some cancer-fighting foods not only prevent malignancy, but actually attack tumors that have already developed.

Yet, diet is only one of at least six major immune-boosting and cancer-fighting tools that are both easy to adopt and accessible to virtually everyone. These six health promoters are: diet, culinary herbs, exercise, stress-reduction techniques, social support, and intimacy.

IMMUNE BOOSTER #1: DIET

Within diet, there are four areas on which scientists are now focusing: The first is the antioxidants; the second, nonantioxidant vitamins; third, minerals that promote immunity and cancer-fighting mechanisms of the body; and fourth, an overall low-fat diet. Scientists have found that when these nutrients are at their optimal levels within the blood, immune reaction is significantly enhanced.

The Antioxidants

The antioxidants include vitamins C, beta-carotene, vitamin E, glutathione, and selenium. They are all free radical scavengers, and thus act in similar ways to prevent disease. At the same time, each boosts immune function or stimulates a specific response within the body to fight cancer.

VITAMIN C

Some researchers believe that vitamin C is the strongest antioxidant available in the food supply. That's the conclusion of researchers Balz Frei, Laura England, and Bruce N. Ames, who reported their findings in the *Proceedings of the National Academy of Sciences* in August 1989. Other research has confirmed that vitamin C is particularly protective against heart disease because it prevents macrophage cells and blood cholesterol from combining to form atherosclerotic plaques, according to a study published in 1990 in *Atherosclerosis*. When the researchers compared the anti-atherosclerosis effects of vitamin C and E, the researchers concluded that C was the most protective nutrient.

Vitamin C also stimulates production of interferon, which prevents viruses from taking hold in the system. Researchers believe that this is one of the ways the vitamin prevents colds and flu. It also helps maintain the health and vitality of macrophages, which produce chemicals that kill bacteria. In addition, vitamin C plays a role in the body's ability to destroy tumors.

Cornell University's T. Colin Campbell, who studied the health and dietary patterns of 6,500 Chinese living in China, found that Chinese with optimal blood levels of vitamin C had the lowest rates of all forms of cancer, including those of the breast, colon, rectum, and prostate. The Chinese got those optimal levels exclusively from their daily food supply.

Good sources of vitamin C include broccoli, cabbage, strawberries, oranges, grapefruit, cantaloupe, leafy greens, sauerkraut, squash, and red and green peppers. Rose hip and hibiscus teas are especially rich sources of vitamin C.

Recommended Amounts

The scientists at the Human Nutrition Research Center on Aging at Tufts University suggest that the daily optimal amount of vitamin C is 60 mg a day for both men and women. Some studies suggest as much as 100 mg a day as an optimal amount.

Research published in the *Journal of Age and Aging* in May 1991 revealed that 100 mg was sufficient to bring blood levels back to normal and, when combined with vitamin E and beta-carotene, positively affected all aspects of the immune system (as we will see shortly). You can easily get these amounts from diet alone. One spear of broccoli contains 134 mg of vitamin C.

"The use of megadoses of any nutrient is unwise," says pioneer immunologist R. K. Chandra, Ph.D., of the Health Sciences Center at St. John's, Newfoundland, Canada.

Dr. Chandra, whose research is frequently cited by scientists working on nutrition and immune response, says that "when it comes to any nutrient, it's important to meet the RDA, but not to exceed it. Studies have shown that taking too much of a nutrient will actually depress immune response, even if that nutrient boosts immunity in smaller quantities."

BETA-CAROTENE

Beta-carotene stops the breakdown of cells and tissues caused by free radical formation. It also increases the overall number of several types of immune cells, and makes them more potent against disease, including cancer, according to Ronald Ross Watson, Ph.D., an immunologist at the University of Arizona Medical School.

Beta-carotene has been shown to strengthen the immune system's effort against *Candida albicans,* the bacterium that causes yeast infections. Remarkably, beta-carotene is only one of hundreds of chemicals known as carotenoids, all of which may have immune-boosting potential. Carotenoids are the color-producing nutrients in many green, orange, red, and yellow vegetables. Beta-carotene may not even be the most effective immune booster, say some researchers.

Heart Disease and Beta-carotene

The underlying cause of heart disease is the formation of atherosclerotic plaques, which occur when blood cholesterol reaches unhealthy levels and then oxidizes, forming free radicals within the blood. When the body recognizes that these decaying cholesterol particles are becoming too numerous in the blood, it calls out a group of immune cells called macrophages. These cells consume and destroy cancer cells, viruses, bacteria, and other threats to health. The macrophages gobble up the decaying cholesterol particles. As they do, these macrophages become engorged and sink into the walls of arteries, becoming embedded in the artery wall and forming what are called foam cells. This is the first stage of heart disease. As more and more macrophages consume decaying cholesterol particles, they also become engorged and embedded in the artery wall, causing those initial foam cells to become a larger injury to the artery wall, called a fatty streak. As more and more macrophages become bloated with decaying cholesterol particles, that fatty streak can become a full-blown cholesterol plaque.

As the plaques get bigger, they block optimal blood flow to the heart or brain. This condition, called ischemia, can eventually shut off blood to the heart or brain, resulting in the suffocation and death of part of the heart, called a heart attack, or the suffocation or death of part of the brain, which is a stroke.

Antioxidants prevent heart attacks and strokes by preventing cholesterol from oxidizing, or forming free radicals. This, in turn, prevents macrophages from having to consume the decaying cholesterol particles, and thus reduces the risk of forming a cholesterol plaque in the first place.

Studies show that daily intake of beta-carotene–rich foods offers significant protection against major illness. A study of 90,000 female nurses over eight years revealed that those nurses who ate regular amounts of fruits and vegetables rich in beta-carotene had a 40 percent reduction in their incidence of stroke and a 22 percent reduction in their risk of heart attack when compared to control populations. Some studies have shown that a single carrot a day is sufficient to lower your risk of illness.

Cancer and Beta-carotene

Beta-carotene stimulates the macrophages against cancer cells and tumors. A macrophage is capable of producing chemicals that can destroy cancer cells and tumors, said Dr. Watson. Dr. Campbell's study of the Chinese revealed that consumption of foods rich in beta-carotene was "found to have a protective effect . . . particularly for stomach cancer." A study published in the *New England Journal of Medicine* showed that when smokers took supplements of beta-carotene, they had higher rates of cancer than those who took no supplements or whose daily intake of beta-carotene came only from food. Scientists are not sure why supplements may bring about a higher-than-average rate of cancer, while food sources of the same nutrient actually lower the risk of disease. One theory suggests that supplementation may overburden and weaken the liver, which must target and eliminate toxins in the blood, including carcinogens.

Sources of Beta-carotene

Foods that are rich in beta-carotene are squash, collard greens, carrots, broccoli, kale, mustard greens, sweet potatoes, and cantaloupe.

Recommended Amounts

There is no RDA for beta-carotene, though 6 mg is frequently cited because it provides 100 percent of the RDA for vitamin A. Six milligrams is easily achieved through dietary sources alone. A single carrot, for example, contains 17 mg, and some studies have shown that a single carrot a day is sufficient to lower your risk of illness. It is recommended to eat at least two beta-carotene–rich foods daily.

VITAMIN E

The immune systems of most people decline with aging, but vitamin E appears to offer substantial protection against that decline. Like vitamin C and beta-carotene, vitamin E stops free radical formation. It also stimulates the production of natural killer cells that seek out and destroy viruses, bacteria, and cancer cells.

After taking supplements of vitamin E, immune cells multiply more rapidly in the face of a disease-causing agent, says Mohsen Meydani, Ph.D., associate professor of nutrition at the Antioxidant Research Laboratory, at Tufts University.

Vitamin E and Heart Disease

Atherosclerosis, or the formation of plaque, is the leading cause of heart disease and stroke. Vitamin E has been shown to be a powerful factor against heart and artery diseases by lowering blood cholesterol and protecting against the formation of plaque.

Sources

Vitamin E can be found in whole grains, especially wheat and bulgur; sunflower seeds; seafood, such as shrimp; and vegetable oils, especially olive and sesame oils.

Recommended Amounts

Although food can supply good sources of vitamin E, many scientists argue for supplementation because research is showing just how powerful its effects are above 60 mg a day.

Most people can get 30 mg a day of vitamin E by eating grains, seeds, and vegetable oils, which is more than adequate, since the RDA for vitamin E is 10 mg. Some scientists argue that supplementation is necessary for certain groups, especially the elderly or for those who do not eat a healthy diet. They recommend low doses of 60 to 200 mg per day.

VITAMIN B$_6$

Vitamin B$_6$, an antioxidant found in fish, brown rice, oats, whole wheat, walnuts, soybeans and soybean products (miso and tamari, for example), is essential for maintaining and restoring adequate immune function. B$_6$ is vitally important when the immune system is depressed or fighting any type of infection.

GLUTATHIONE

Glutathione prevents oxidation of cells and tissues and promotes the proliferation of chemical messengers within the immune system, especially interleukin. Glutathione, which is the most widely available antioxidant, is also the most abundant of the antioxidants in the bloodstream. Usually, the only deficiencies in Western countries occur in the elderly.

Sources

Glutathione is present in virtually all foods, but the best sources include fresh vegetables, fruits, beans, and animal food products. Processing can reduce glutathione quantities in food.

Recommended Amounts

There is no RDA or any known therapeutic quantity.

SELENIUM

Selenium, a mineral found in whole grains, seafood, and seeds, works in combination with vitamin E as an antioxidant, says Dr. Chandra. Selenium also protects against cancer and stimulates a stronger immune response to antigens.

Antioxidants work best when they work together, which is why many researchers say that there is no substitute for a healthy diet. Research that focuses exclusively on a single nutrient doesn't reveal how the body responds to the synergistic effects of multiple antioxidants, nor does it take into account how we normally obtain nutrition—that is, from food.

SYNERGISTIC EFFECTS OF ANTIOXIDANTS

Research has shown that when three of these antioxidants—vitamin C, beta-carotene, and vitamin E—are added to the diets of people, immune function improves significantly. One study showed that the number of T cells increased, that CD4s (the immune cell that declines dramatically in AIDS patients) increased, and the ratio between CD4 and immune-suppressor cells (CD8, which shuts off immune function) improved overall. Also, researchers have found that the effectiveness of lymphocytes in the presence of a disease-causing agent improved significantly when blood levels of these antioxidants was increased, according to an article in *Age and Aging* in 1991.

Minerals

Research is showing that minerals protect the membrane of immune cells, make the immune system more responsive to antagonisms, and assist in the production of immune cells. It is generally recommended that mineral intake not exceed the RDA. Most healthful diets contain enough minerals for health maintenance.

ZINC

Zinc protects against all forms of infection, especially in children. Deficiencies of zinc depress immune function and cause the thymus gland to atrophy. Since the thymus serves as a kind of training school for immune cells, any impairment of thymus function causes a general impairment of the immune system.

A study published in the *American Journal of Obstetrics and Gynecology* in November 1986 showed that deficiencies of zinc are associated with recurrent vaginal yeast infections in women. Children with depressed zinc levels suffer higher-than-average rates of infection. Zinc deficiency is also associated with prostate disease in men and higher rates or arthritis in both sexes.

Optimal zinc levels increase the number of circulating immune cells. Zinc also causes antibodies to mount a stronger attack against a disease-causing agent.

Sources

Pumpkin seeds; whole grains, such as brown rice, whole wheat, bulgur, whole wheat bread and flour; cashews; most beans, and black-eyed peas are good sources of zinc.

Recommended Amounts

Optimal levels of zinc range from 15 to 30 mg, easily obtained through a healthful diet. Zinc is a good example of how an important nutrient can become toxic at the wrong dose. Immune function is depressed at intake levels of 100 mg of zinc per day, a dosage often taken by people who take supplements.

CALCIUM

Essential for bones, teeth, and muscle, calcium also plays a role in maintaining a healthy immune response, according to Tufts researchers. Good sources include broccoli, collard greens, kale, sardines, and low-fat dairy products.

Recommended Amounts

The optimum daily amount for the average person is 1000 mg of calcium. For women of postmenopausal age, 1200 to 1500 mg is generally recommended.

IRON

"Iron is involved in more than 200 enzymes and is essential for mounting an immune response," said Dr. Chandra. Good sources include all animal foods, leafy greens, and sea vegetables, especially nori. Unless prescribed by a medical doctor, iron should not be supplemented. High iron levels are associated with an increased risk of cancer and liver disease.

A Low-Fat Diet

Fat depresses immune function by infiltrating the cell membrane of macrophages and other immune cells and prevents them from recognizing self from not-self. This allows viruses, bacteria, and even cancer cells to proliferate.

Fat is also a free radical producer and consequently a major contributor to aging and most major diseases, including heart disease, cancer, diabetes, and obesity. Fat decreases resistance to bacteria, viral infections, and tumors. It also depresses phagocyte cell activity. Phagocytes, like macrophages, consume many bacteria, viruses, and cancer cells.

Virtually every health authority, from the American Heart Association to the National Cancer Institute, has recommended that fat intake should be below 30 percent of total calories, and that 20 percent is probably closer to the ideal.

SPECIAL FOODS AND CANCER

Broccoli, cabbage, kale, brussels sprouts, collard greens, and mustard greens contain a group of compounds called indoles that may prevent tumor-causing estrogen from targeting the breast. In animal studies, indoles have been shown to switch on enzymes that protect against exposure to carcinogens.

These vegetables are also rich sources of another cancer fighter, sulforanphane. Sulforanphane has been called a "major and very potent" trigger for detoxifying tissues and blood and for promoting production of cancer-preventive enzymes, according to research published in the *Proceedings of the National Academy of Sciences*.

Another group of cancer-fighting nutrients, phytochemicals, are found in particularly abundant supply in beans, and especially in soybeans and soybean products, such as tofu, tempeh, natto, tamari, miso, and soy sauce. These foods contain a newly discovered compound called *genistein,* which prevents blood vessels from attaching to tumors and providing essential oxygen and nutrients for tumors to survive, according to an April 1993 article in *Proceedings of the National Academy of Sciences.* Soybeans also contain a substance called protease inhibitor, which interferes with cancer cell proliferation at both the early and later stages of development.

Other foods rich in phytochemicals and other cancer fighters are citrus fruits, carrots, parsnips, celery, and parsley. "To harness anticarcinogenic activity, a combination of these vegetables would probably work best," said Dr.

Herbert Pierson, a leading cancer researcher and formerly of the National Cancer Institute.

Finally, citrus fruits, which contain plenty of vitamin C, also offer a substance called D-limonene, which has been shown to interfere with cancer proliferation.

IMMUNE BOOSTER #2: CULINARY HERBS

A wide array of medicinal herbs are proving to have powerful immune-boosting and cancer-fighting properties, but new research is now showing that many culinary herbs may be just as powerful at promoting health. The most prominent of these is garlic.

According to Dr. Michael Wargovich, a leading authority on cancer at the M. D. Anderson Cancer Center in Houston, Texas, garlic promotes health in a wide variety of ways, but how it affects the immune system is still unknown. What is known is that garlic strongly affects liver function, causing it to metabolize and neutralize carcinogens that would otherwise produce cancer cells and tumors.

One of the liver's many jobs is to neutralize all poisons and foreign substances entering the body. Under ideal conditions, the liver recognizes cancer cells and treats them as toxins, converting them to soluble compounds that are easily eliminated from the body. In certain cases, however, the liver's actions on carcinogens actually promotes their toxicity. In effect, the liver can make carcinogens better at producing cancer.

The tars and nicotine of cigarettes, for example, are low-level poisons under ordinary circumstances. However, once they are metabolized by the liver, they become more reactive and, therefore, more effective at triggering cancer cells in the lungs and other organs. Garlic stimulates the liver to more effectively identify these poisons and turn them into harmless, water-soluble compounds.

Garlic also encourages a variety of detoxifying enzymes to be produced by the body, some of which directly attack cancer cells and tumors. Studies have found that the rates of stomach and colorectal cancers are lower among those who eat a lot of garlic. Scientists speculate that garlic may block the tumor-promoting effects of a certain group of fatty acids, called prostaglandins, which are hormonelike substances in the body. Prostaglandins may encourage tumor growth when they go unregulated.

The sulfur compounds found in garlic—allicin being the most widely known—are responsible for promoting the body's detoxifying activities. Allicin is most effective when eaten raw, but researchers at the National Cancer Institute say that garlic also has health-promoting effects when eaten cooked. Consequently, scientists are recommending that garlic be used both raw and cooked. Many of these sulfur chemicals are also found in onions, though apparently in smaller quantities.

"It seems that the stronger the food—and in the case of garlic, that means the smell—the stronger the health-enhancing effects are," said Dr. Wargovich.

Other important immune boosters and cancer fighters are shiitake mushrooms and their relatives, reishi mushrooms. Studies at the U.S. National Cancer Institute and the Japanese National Cancer Institute have established the shiitake mushroom as an immune booster, a cancer fighter, and a powerful cholesterol-lowering plant. Shiitake has antiviral and antibacterial properties; it also causes the immune system to mount a stronger attack against an invading antigen or a tumor. Both animal and human studies have shown that shiitake substantially lowers blood cholesterol; some research suggests that the cholesterol-lowering effect of shiitake extract—the concentrated form of the herb—may be as much as 25 percent when used over a couple of weeks. (See the herbs section in Part III of this book for more on herbs.)

Other culinary herbs that are now being touted as cancer fighters and immune boosters include:

Cumin: Israeli scientists have found that people who regularly add cumin to their food have lower rates of urinary tract cancers, including those of the bladder and prostate. Scientists in India confirmed these findings and discovered that cumin greatly increased the body's production of a detoxifying agent, GST, which is known to have strong cancer-inhibiting properties.

Turmeric: According to Dr. Wargovich and others, turmeric inhibits cancer at several sites in the body by disrupting certain chemical processes that would otherwise lead to cancer and support its growth.

Green tea: Japanese green tea contains antioxidants, flavonoids, and indoles, all of which stimulate the body's production of enzymes that block tumor formation.

Licorice: The sweet-tasting chemicals found in the licorice root have been found to inhibit skin cancer in animal studies.

Cinnamon: At the U.S. Department of Agriculture, botanist and herb researcher Jim Duke, Ph.D., has found that cinnamon increases the number of certain immune cells, called leukocytes. Research at the HNRC at Tufts has found that cinnamon triples insulin's ability to metabolize glucose, or blood sugar. By increasing the efficiency of insulin, cinnamon protects against diabetes and lowers hunger and sugar cravings, thus making it easier to control weight.

Mint: Dr. Duke reports that mint increases the number of phagocyte cells, which are capable of destroying pathogens, bacteria, and cancer cells.

Chamomile: The common herb tea speeds up a process called phagocytosis, or the proliferation of phagocyte cells.

IMMUNE BOOSTER #3: EXERCISE

Moderate exercise stimulates the production of a variety of immune cells and enhances the overall function of the immune system, according to a report published in the journal *Sports Science Review* on July 16, 1992.

Dr. Chandra reports that exercise balances hormones and improves the strength of lymphocytes, important immune cells that, like macrophages, attack viruses, bacteria, and cancer cells. Recent research from Loma Linda University reported that moderate exercise, which consisted of brisk walking, forty-five minutes per session, five times per week, increased natural killer cell activity.

Other studies have shown that moderate exercise also improves the ability of macrophage cells to neutralize bacteria and viruses. Moderate exercise is associated with lower incidences of the common cancers, such as those of the colon, prostate, and breast. Exercise experts report that as little as thirty minutes of walking per day, three to five times per week, is enough to boost cardiovascular fitness and immunity.

In fact, the walking doesn't even have to be all that brisk to have a positive effect. A study published in the *Journal of the American Medical Association,* on December 18, 1991, showed that strolling at a leisurely pace of about three miles per hour significantly increased high-density lipoproteins (the kind of cholesterol that protects against heart disease) in fifty-nine women, who walked between twelve and twenty minutes per session, three to four times per week.

Conversely, living by the old "no pain, no gain" cliché has been shown to depress the immune system. According to Dr. Chandra, research has consistently shown that excessive exercise, such as that experienced by marathoners, can depress immunity. Numerous studies have shown that moderate exercise is also associated with increased longevity.

IMMUNE BOOSTER #4: STRESS REDUCTION TECHNIQUES

Stress affects immunity in a number of ways, but primarily through the endocrine system by causing the secretion of immune-depressing hormones. Dealing with stress effectively is therefore essential in the maintenance of a healthy immune system. Among the best ways of doing that is through physical exercise, meditation, and relaxation techniques.

Researchers at the University of Miami Medical School have found that daily relaxation exercises—that is, the progressive releasing of tension in muscles throughout the body—caused CD4 cells to increase. The study was done on men with HIV, who normally experience a steady decrease in CD4 cells. When Gail Ironson, M.D., a psychiatrist at the University of Miami Medical School, and her colleagues followed up on the men a year later, they found that those men who continued to do some form of daily meditation or relaxation exercises were less likely to suffer from AIDS symptoms.

Other research has shown that meditation or relaxation exercises have increased immune cell activity in the face of an antigen. One study showed an increase in natural killer cells and greater proliferation of lymphocytes in medical school students who practiced a daily relaxation regimen.

In addition to these traditional exercises is a newly recognized relaxation tool for controlling stress and boosting immunity: writing in a journal about your feelings each day. One recent study showed that those who wrote about traumatic or painful events in their lives for four days, twenty minutes a day, increased T cells.

IMMUNE BOOSTER #5: SOCIAL SUPPORT

There is no denying that humans are social creatures, but we are only beginning to learn that social life is essential to our health, as well as our happiness. This is especially the case in times of a health crisis.

New research is showing that people with cancer who participate in support groups not only live longer but also experience an improvement in immune function. A study conducted at the University of California at Los Angeles on women with the early stages of skin cancer found that those who participated in a support group had much better scores on psychological tests and higher blood levels of natural killer cells than those who did not participate in such a group. Other research recently published in the British medical journal *The Lancet* supports these findings.

These studies hearken back to perhaps the most famous research demonstrating a link between social support and illness: the Alameda County study.

In 1979, researchers reported a study of 7,000 residents of Alameda County, California, who were followed over a nine-year period. The scientists found that those members of the community who were married or maintained strong ties to friends, social, religious, or community groups such as clubs, civic groups, or church membership, experienced lower rates of illness and greater longevity than those who were unmarried or socially isolated.

IMMUNE BOOSTER #6: INTIMACY

We call it "dying of a broken heart," and, indeed, the research consistently shows that the loss of a loved one is associated with depressed immune response and premature death. Studies have shown that bereavement specifically reduces the effectiveness of lymphocytes, a type of white blood cell essential to immune function. In some cases, the lymphocytes either fail to recognize an antigen or only mount a feeble attack. The net effect is that the person is incapable of warding off an illness that, for many, results in death.

Men, especially, are particularly vulnerable to illness when they live alone or lose a loved one. Dr. Maradee Davis and her colleagues at the University of California at San Francisco studied 7,651 adults and found that middle-aged men who were unmarried or divorced were twice as likely to die ten years sooner than men who were married or lived with their wives. That finding held true even after accounting for differences in economic status, smoking habits, drinking, obesity, and physical activity.

"Men who lived alone or with someone other than a spouse had significantly shorter survival times compared with those living with a spouse," Dr. Davis reported in her study, published in the *American Journal of Public Health* in March 1992. The pattern of early death was particularly strong among younger men. "The age-adjusted relative hazard of dying was highest in the youngest age group, 45 to 54 years, and decreased somewhat with increasing age."

Ironically, the same pattern did not exist among women. Dr. Davis speculates that the reason women fare better than men is because "women have better social support networks, are better at making friends, and seem to take better care of their health than men do."

These findings found remarkable resonance in a recent study conducted by Redford Williams, M.D., at the behavioral research department at Duke University Medical School. He found that those who suffer a heart attack and have no spouse or close personal friends are three times more likely to have a fatal heart attack within five years of the original event than those whose hearts are equally injured but are married or have intimate relationships.

The Duke University research is based on a nine-year follow-up study of 1,368 patients who were initially admitted to Duke for cardiac catheterization to diagnose heart disease.

For people with both minor and severe heart muscle damage due to a heart attack, the results were consistent. People generally face about a 40 percent chance of dying within five years. Dr. Williams found that those who were married or have a close intimate relationship reduced their risk of suffering a fatal heart attack to 20 percent, while those who lacked intimacy raised their chances of dying to 60 percent.

Other research has consistently supported these findings. Women with breast cancer who participate in a support group live longer than those who try to deal with the disease alone.

Scientists are discovering that not only are the recommendations of traditional healers effective, but so, too, are the guidelines for living offered by spiritual traditions. After reviewing the relationship of simple diet, meditation, and intimacy to longer life, Dr. Williams said, "It seems evident that the core teachings of most of our religions have been right all along."

THE KIDNEYS

Located in the middle of the back, well above the waistline, the kidneys are paired organs, each one about four to five inches long and weighing about six ounces. The kidneys filter the blood of waste. The basic functional unit of the kidneys is the nephron. In our youth, each of us has about 1 million nephrons in each kidney, but because of a wide assortment of insults—primarily diet- and stress-related—the number of nephrons decreases with age, until you have about 250,000 at the age of seventy. The kidneys are essential organs, although we can survive with only one kidney.

The kidneys perform the minute-to-minute miracle of removing all the constituents from the blood and then choosing which ones should be restored and which ones should be eliminated as part of the urine.

Among the most common disorders affecting the kidneys are stones, or calculi, made up primarily of oxalate, which comes from foods high in oxalic acid or calcium. Scientists do not know why kidney stones form but believe they come from a diet rich in oxalic acid (foods that contain oxalic acid include spinach, rhubarb, sesame seeds, and coffee), and low in water. They are especially prevalent in Third World countries that lack both protein and adequate water.

In Chinese medicine, stones are formed from deficient kidney qi, meaning the kidneys are functioning with less than optimal levels of energy. Kidney qi is reduced by diets rich in fat and sodium, along with lifestyles that include high stress and inadequate rest.

The Chinese also maintain that the kidneys nourish the inner ear and hearing mechanism with qi, or life force. When the kidneys are weak, they are unable to send adequate life forces to the inner workings of the ear, causing the accumulation of wax, cellular debris, and atherosclerosis, all of which impair hearing.

The kidneys are highly sensitive to excesses of fat and sodium. Fat causes cholesterol plaques to clog the tiny nephrons, or the basic filtering unit within the organs. This can destroy the kidneys. Sodium has a paradoxical relationship with the kidneys. Small to moderate amounts actually tonify and strengthen kidney function, according to Chinese medicine. But excesses cause too much contraction of the organs, thus preventing them from filtering waste from the body. This excessive contraction of the kidneys has the same effect as pinching a hose while water is running: pressure builds behind the pinch, resulting in high blood pressure.

Western science has shown that excess protein, particularly animal protein, damages the kidneys. Chinese medicine has long maintained the same per-

The Kidneys

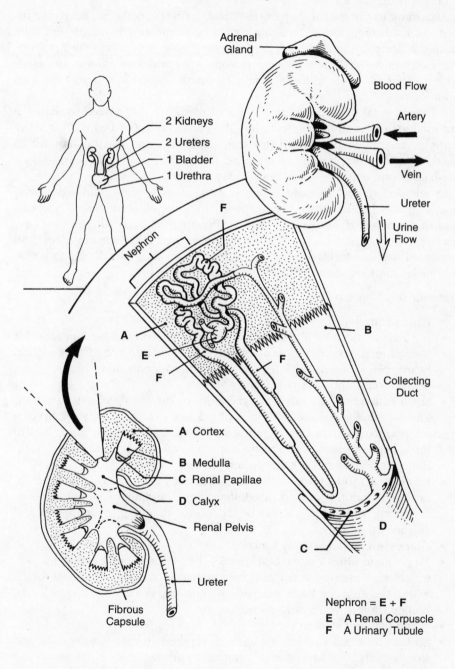

Adrenal
Gland

Blood Flow

Artery

Vein

Ureter

Urine
Flow

2 Kidneys
2 Ureters
1 Bladder
1 Urethra

Nephron

F

A

E

F

B

F

Collecting
Duct

A Cortex

B Medulla

C Renal Papillae

D Calyx

Renal Pelvis

D

C

Ureter

Fibrous
Capsule

Nephron = **E** + **F**

E   A Renal Corpuscle
F   A Urinary Tubule

spective, but maintains that small amounts of protein, especially the protein of beans, heals the kidneys.

According to Chinese and other traditional forms of medicine, beans are regarded as warming foods, meaning that they stimulate circulation and thus warm the body. They also contain moderate amounts of mono- and polyunsaturated fats, which lower cholesterol somewhat and thus assist in the elimination of fat from the kidneys. These fats make beans a rich and luscious food.

A fundamental principle in all traditional medicine is the need for balance and moderation in all things, including the consumption of beans. Too many beans or too much protein creates too much acid and can be harmful to health. Most Oriental healers recommend that small amounts of beans—from one-half to one cup—be eaten once a day.

In addition to the standard beans is tofu, a moderately refined soybean product that is rich in calcium and protein, and tempeh, a fermented soybean food that is rich in digestive enzymes. Finally, there is natto, a fermented soybean condiment used on rice and other grains and sometimes in soups. All fermented soybean foods assist in digestion by providing friendly bacteria that help make nutrients more available to the small intestine.

Diet and Foods to Eat

- Pure, clean water
- In Chinese medicine, beans are considered a powerful healing food for the kidneys. Among the most effective kidney strengtheners are adzuki beans, black beans, chickpeas, green and red lentils, navy beans, mung beans, limas, and split peas.
- Small amounts of sea salt tonify the kidneys, but too much salt can cause kidney damage. Use only a pinch of salt in cooking. Usually the tip of a teaspoon (less than one-eighth teaspoon) is necessary to cook two to three cups of grain. Avoid using salt at the table as a condiment.
- Barley is considered a kidney-strengthening herb.
- Fermented foods, such as tempeh, and small amounts of miso, tamari, or shoyu should be used in cooking. Small amounts (one tablespoon, two or three times per week) of sauerkraut also help to strengthen and cleanse the kidneys.
- Grapes strengthen kidney function.
- To promote urination, eat blackberries, blueberries, cranberries, and watermelon. Watermelon tea promotes urination and the release of toxins within the kidneys. It can be made by grinding dried watermelon seeds, boiling then in water, and then steeping.
- White fish and salmon
- Daikon root, a long, white radish, is reputed to melt fat deposits and stones and help to eliminate stagnation from tissues throughout the body. To make a traditional remedy to encourage urination and elimi-

nation, grate two to three tablespoons of fresh daikon into a cheesecloth sack. Squeeze the sack so that the daikon juice falls into a cup. Pour boiled water into the cup. Add one to two drops of shoyu or tamari. Drink twice a day. To dissolve blockages and stones in the kidneys, grate one to two tablespoons of daikon radish into a cup. Pour hot water into the cup. Add two drops of tamari or shoyu. Drink once or twice a day.

Foods to Reduce or Avoid

- Excessive amounts of salt
- Animal foods (especially eggs, pork, and cheese)
- Coffee (especially hard on kidneys)
- Alcohol
- Tobacco
- Cinnamon
- Cloves
- Ginger
- Hot spices
- Cold drinks
- Raw foods
- Use seaweed cautiously, in no more than one to two tablespoon-sized servings daily.

Herbs

- Burdock root is a hardy, medicinal food that has been revered by Chinese, European, and American healers for many centuries. Burdock is considered one of the strongest blood purifiers in the entire herb kingdom. It is used for a wide variety of disorders, but is generally recognized as one of the best herbs for breaking down and eliminating waste products from metabolism. In Chinese medicine, it is regarded as a strengthening herb for the entire urinary tract and sex organs. Pressure cook sliced burdock for fifteen minutes with sliced carrots and kombu seaweed in about one and one-half inches of water.
- Burdock tea detoxifies blood, stimulates and tonifies kidneys and bladder, and eliminates waste and stagnation within the kidneys. Boil one to two tablespoons of stems, twigs, and leaves in one cup of water, steep for ten minutes, and drink two or three times per day.
- Basil, used in cooking or boiled in water to make a tea, strengthens kidneys.
- Chamomile tea promotes dissolution of stones. It is commercially available in tea bags.
- A nettle root infusion is reputed to dissolve stones and eliminate blockages.

Supplements for the Kidneys

- Beta-carotene: 15–30 mg/day
- Vitamin B$_6$: 3 mg/day
- Vitamin C: 100 mg/day
- Vitamin E: 100–400 IU/day
- Magnesium: 100 mg/day

The Large Intestine

The large intestine is about six feet long, about two inches wide, and is the primary site of waste removal. The organ gathers unused and unwanted food material that has not been assimilated into the bloodstream in the small intestine. The mass is moved along its six-foot length by the large intestine's ability to expand and contract, which is called peristalsis. It also absorbs excess water back into the system, as well as a small amount of nutrients, then eliminates unabsorbed food material through the anus.

When constipation occurs, waste is reabsorbed via the lymph vessels that line the large intestine, and eventually the waste makes its way into the bloodstream, where it can cause problems elsewhere in the body. Constipation and inefficient bowel elimination has been linked to breast cancer and other serious illnesses.

The most important food constituent for promoting healthy large-intestine function is dietary fiber. An inadequate amount of fiber has been shown to be a contributing cause of constipation, diverticulosis, and colon cancer.

Diet and Foods to Eat

- Brown rice and sweet rice are regarded as herbs for the large intestine.
- Root vegetables, including carrots, daikon, ginger, turnips, parsnips, rutabagas, sweet potatoes, yams, and potatoes are all rich in fiber, and the colored vegetables also contain beta-carotene, a cancer-fighting antioxidant.
- Whole grain flours, rich in fiber, strengthen elimination and promote large intestine health.
- Leafy greens, especially watercress, cabbage, bok choy, and mustard greens
- Fruit, including cantaloupe, apples, persimmons, peaches, pears, strawberries, and citrus fruit
- Mushrooms
- Cruciferous vegetables, such as cauliflower, broccoli, watercress, kale, and collard greens are all rich in fiber, minerals, and a cancer-fighting substance called sulforanphane. (See the cancer-fighting foods in our section on the Immune System, in Part IV.)
- Food should be cooked (but not overcooked) as opposed to raw. Cooked food places less strain on the digestive tract.
- According to Chinese medicine, pungent flavor promotes peristalsis and large intestine function. (See the section on Chinese medicine.) Chinese medicine holds that each flavor serves as a mild stimulant to a specific organ or set of organs. Pungent-tasting foods stimulate large intestine function and strengthen the organ. Pungent foods include garlic, the

The Large Intestine

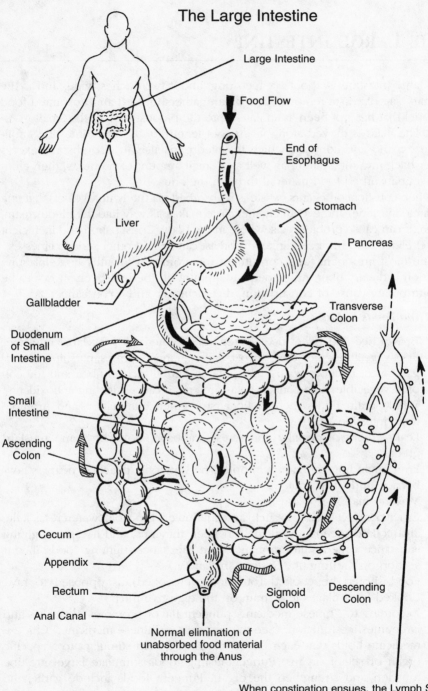

Large Intestine

Food Flow

End of Esophagus

Stomach

Liver

Pancreas

Gallbladder

Transverse Colon

Duodenum of Small Intestine

Small Intestine

Ascending Colon

Cecum

Appendix

Rectum

Anal Canal

Sigmoid Colon

Descending Colon

Normal elimination of unabsorbed food material through the Anus

When constipation ensues, the Lymph System reabsorbs waste into the bloodstream, causing problems in other body systems.

onion family, turnips, ginger, horseradish, cabbage, radishes, daikon, and white peppercorns.

- Cereal grasses including wheat, barley grass, spirulina, and chlorella

Herbs

- Yerba santa leaf
- Mullein leaf
- Nettles
- Chickweed
- Flaxseed
- Fennel
- Fenugreek
- Coltsfoot
- Elecampane root
- Bentonite clay cleanses waste and toxins from the large intestine and liver. (See the section on bentonite clay in Part III, Herbology, for instructions on use.)

Foods to Avoid

- Animal foods—meat and dairy—lack fiber. Undigested meat accumulates in the intestines, contributing to the formation of pockets, which gives rise to a number of illnesses, including diverticulosis and colon cancer.
- Refined flour products and processed foods lack fiber.
- Cigarettes contain carcinogenic tars and chemicals that combine with bile acids (produced by the liver) within the large intestine and promote the production of cancer cells and tumors. Cigarettes are also major free radical producers (see the nutrition section). Free radicals alter DNA within cells and promote mutations, uncontrolled growth, and cancer. Finally, cigarette smoke robs the body of oxygen, which science has shown promotes mutation of cells and production of cancer.
- Eggs contribute to constipation. Chinese medicine maintains that eggs are highly contracting, thus causing tension within the large intestine and mitigating its ability to expand and contract.
- Sugar expands and weakens the spleen, which in Chinese medicine provides life force or qi to the large intestine.
- Hot spices, such as chili peppers.

Exercise

- Walk daily. Walking assists the intestines in performing their peristaltic action.

THE LIVER

The liver cleanses the body of all the poisons that infiltrate it daily, including fat; cholesterol; alcohol; drugs (both pharmaceutical and recreational); artificial colors, flavors, and preservatives; airborne pollutants; and poisons in the water and food.

While the liver's ability to deal with these toxins is extraordinary, once the limits of its function are exceeded, these toxins accumulate in the organ and cause disease. However, the liver has the remarkable ability to regenerate itself. Up to two-thirds of the liver can be impaired, yet the organ can fully restore itself under the right conditions.

The substances and foods that pose the greatest threat to the liver are poisonous drugs, excessive use of recreational and pharmaceutical drugs, alcohol, foods high in fat, artificial ingredients, and cigarette smoking. Because the liver must deal with every toxin taken into the body, it is highly susceptible to the ravages of free radical formation, particularly the creation of scar tissue, a common reaction to free radicals or oxidation of tissues. (See the sections on nutrition and immune boosting.) Cigarette smoking, dietary fat, alcohol, radiation, all forms of pollution (air, water, and soil), pesticides, and other chemical toxins promote free radicals and create scarring within the liver. In addition, foods rich in fat block blood circulation within the liver. Fat is converted from fatty acids to low-density lipoproteins (LDLs) and high-density lipoproteins (HDLs) in the liver. Excessive fat makes this job all the more difficult.

On the other hand, diets rich in antioxidants and low in fat and chemical toxicity promote the regeneration of the liver. Vegetable foods that are rich in beta-carotene and vitamins C and E are particularly healing to the liver.

In addition, the Chinese system has maintained that anger is particularly damaging to the liver. Chinese healers maintain that anger injures the liver, and that as the liver weakens, the person experiences more anger, forming a vicious cycle. Anger, the Chinese maintain, prevents circulation of blood, lymph, and qi through the liver, this causing stagnation and forming the basis for disease. Conversely, a balanced temperament helps the liver restore harmony and maximum circulation.

Diet and Foods to Eat

- Whole wheat is considered a healing food for the liver in Chinese medicine. The Chinese maintain that wheat promotes circulation within the liver, optimizes liver qi, and promotes the elimination of toxins that have accumulated within the organ.
- Lima beans, green beans, and split peas

The Liver

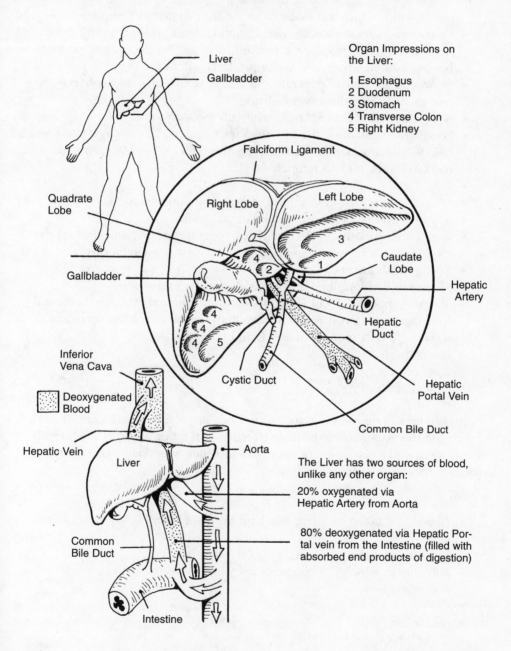

Liver
Gallbladder

Organ Impressions on the Liver:

1 Esophagus
2 Duodenum
3 Stomach
4 Transverse Colon
5 Right Kidney

Falciform Ligament

Right Lobe

Left Lobe

Quadrate Lobe

Caudate Lobe

Gallbladder

Hepatic Artery

Hepatic Duct

Cystic Duct

Inferior Vena Cava

Deoxygenated Blood

Hepatic Portal Vein

Common Bile Duct

Hepatic Vein

Aorta

Liver

Common Bile Duct

Intestine

The Liver has two sources of blood, unlike any other organ:

20% oxygenated via Hepatic Artery from Aorta

80% deoxygenated via Hepatic Portal vein from the Intestine (filled with absorbed end products of digestion)

- Leafy greens, especially broccoli, parsley, collard greens, and dark lettuce, such as romaine. Not only are these rich in nutrients and fiber, which help eliminate waste from the liver, but they also provide lots of antioxidants, which are essential to the liver's efforts to heal itself.
- Carrots and carrot juice are rich in antioxidants and, according to Chinese medicine, carrots are a healing food for the liver. They promote healing and elimination of waste products within the liver.
- Seaweeds are rich in minerals and A and B vitamins, and enhance immunity and strengthen liver function.
- Squash is rich in antioxidants, especially beta-carotene.
- Foods that strengthen the intestinal tract, especially the large intestine, help to take the burden off the liver. These foods include miso and fermented foods, such as tempeh.
- Tofu
- Wheat germ is rich in vitamin E, a powerful antioxidant.
- Spirulina and chlorella are rich in antioxidants.
- Garlic improves the liver's ability to recognize carcinogens and rid the blood of these harmful chemicals. (See the section on immune boosters.)
- Young, fresh greens
- Sprouts and chlorophyll-rich foods, especially mung beans.
- Mugwort mochi: (Mochi is pounded sweet rice; it is available in natural food stores. Mugwort is an effective herb for the liver.) Cut up mochi in squares; boil in soup, so it is soft and dumplinglike.
- Rice vinegar
- Light cooking
- Raw vegetables

According to Chinese medicine, sour foods are regarded as cleansing and purging to the liver. Among the most effective sour foods to eat for liver health are grapefruit, lemons alone or squeezed in water, sauerkraut, green apples, sour cherries, sour oranges, and limes.

Herbs

- Dandelion, taken as a tea, has long been regarded as a powerful liver cleanser.
- Burdock root tea
- Milk thistle, which can be combined with dandelion, helps liver cleanse and rebuild itself.
- Garlic
- Celandine
- Culler's root
- Goldenseal

Supplements

- Beta-carotene: 15–30 mg/day
- Vitamin E: 100–400 IU/day

Foods to Avoid

- Reduce or avoid red meat, eggs, whole-milk products, peanut and other nut butters, and nuts.
- Alcohol generally should be avoided, although beer is preferable because of its lower alcohol content and because the presence of barley promotes both kidney and liver function; limit drinks to two or less per day.
- Refined foods that are high in artificial ingredients
- Recreational and pharmaceutical drugs
- Coffee and caffeinated soft drinks
- Sugar

THE LUNGS

Lungs capture oxygen, which in turn provides energy, and then release carbon dioxide, which is the "exhaust" from cells. Oxygen is exchanged for carbon dioxide in tiny sacs called alveoli. In order for this exchange to take place efficiently, good circulation within the lungs is essential. All airborne toxins, cigarette smoke, and high-fat foods are especially harmful to the lungs.

Studies have shown that lung cancer rates are higher among cigarette smokers who eat a diet richer in fat than those who smoke and eat low-fat diets. In fact, before the Japanese started to eat more fat from animal foods, they had extremely low rates of lung cancer, even though Japan has the most cigarette smokers per capita in the world.

As with other organs, a great threat to the health and capacity of the lungs is free radical formation. To some extent, free radicals are inescapable, since they are a natural by-product of cellular and immune activity. Consequently, everyone loses some lung capacity with aging. However, to some extent, exposure to free radical producers can be controlled by limiting the source of free radicals such as cigarettes and other airborne pollutants, which are particularly prevalent in cities, foods rich in fat and cholesterol, and toxic chemicals in water (use a home filtration system to avoid possible contaminants). Especially important is eating foods rich in antioxidants, especially beta-carotene and vitamins C and E, all of which reduce the damage from a wide assortment of free radical producers, including cigarettes, airborne pollutants, and high-fat diets. Plant foods that are rich in antioxidants, especially leafy green vegetables, are especially healing to the lungs.

Foods to Eat

- Brown rice is considered an herb for the lungs, according to Chinese medicine. Other healing grains include barley, oats, and millet. The Chinese maintain that the qi, or life force, in rice goes directly to the lungs and promotes the increase in life force to these organs. In doing so, brown rice enhances lung function and assists the lungs in resisting the normal degeneration of aging. It also enhances the elimination of waste products from the lungs.
- Leafy green vegetables, especially mustard greens, kale, watercress, cabbage, and dark lettuce. The Chinese maintain that the qi in green leafy vegetables causes the lungs to open up and promotes circulation, just as the qi causes a leaf to open, allowing its own fluids to circulate freely through its vessels.

The Lungs

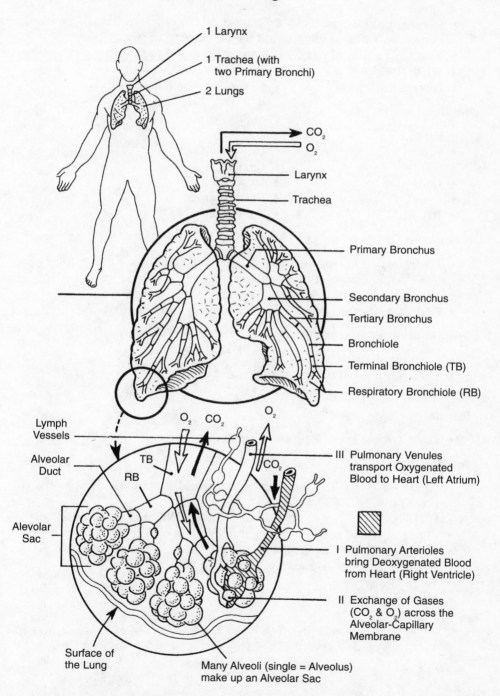

1 Larynx

1 Trachea (with two Primary Bronchi)

2 Lungs

CO₂
O₂

Larynx

Trachea

Primary Bronchus

Secondary Bronchus

Tertiary Bronchus

Bronchiole

Terminal Bronchiole (TB)

Respiratory Bronchiole (RB)

Lymph Vessels

Alveolar Duct

Alveolar Sac

Surface of the Lung

O₂ CO₂   O₂   CO₂

TB

RB

III Pulmonary Venules transport Oxygenated Blood to Heart (Left Atrium)

I Pulmonary Arterioles bring Deoxygenated Blood from Heart (Right Ventricle)

II Exchange of Gases (CO₂ & O₂) across the Alveolar-Capillary Membrane

Many Alveoli (single = Alveolus) make up an Alveolar Sac

- Lotus root has long been regarded by the Chinese as a stimulus to the lungs, especially promoting elimination of waste.
- Onions, turnips, cauliflower, Chinese cabbage, and celery all promote circulation within the lungs and the elimination of waste.
- Root vegetables, especially daikon, carrots, and parsnips
- White fish, such as cod, flounder, halibut, and scrod
- Ginger, freshly grated as a condiment on vegetables

Herbs

- Ginger
- Fennel
- Dill
- Coriander
- Basil
- Bay leaf

- Garlic
- Horseradish
- Cinnamon
- Licorice
- Black pepper
- Cardamom

Foods to Avoid

- Foods high in fat, including excess amounts of red meat and whole-milk products, are harmful to the lungs.
- Fried foods
- Excessive amounts of oil, especially oils high in saturated fats

Other Substances to Avoid

- Cigarette smoke
- Exhaust fumes from buses, trucks, and cars
- Fumes from toxic chemicals

Exercise

- Daily aerobic exercise, such as walking

Supplements

- Liquid chlorophyll, 1 tsp. per day (optional if spirulina or chlorella is taken)
- Spirulina, 1 tsp. per day (optional if chlorophyll or chlorella is taken)
- Chlorella, 1 tsp. per day (optional if spirulina or chlorophyll is taken)
- Calcium: 500–800 mg/day
- Beta-carotene: 15–30 mg/day
- Zinc: 15 mg/day
- B complex

THE LYMPH SYSTEM

The lymph system is related to both the circulatory and immune systems. Like the circulatory system, the lymph system is a vast network of vessels that run from head to foot, limb to limb. These vessels permeate every organ in your body and visit the neighborhoods of every cell. Unlike the circulatory system, however, the lymph has no heart. Lymph is moved through its vessels by various forms of pressure exerted through breathing, physical movement, exercise, muscular activity, and the intestines.

The lymphatic system is also an essential part of the immune system. If waste is not moved from tissues, the immune system must continually attack waste products and diseases that lodge in the tissues—everything from flu viruses and food poisons to carcinogens and cancer cells. If these harmful elements are not moved out of the body, they will eventually overrun the system. Gradually, the immune system is debilitated by the mounting poisons and aberrant cells, until such disease-causing agents manifest as a major illness.

WHAT IS LYMPH?

Originally, lymph is tissue fluid (also called interstitial fluid), the liquid essence of the body that occupies the spaces between cells and connective tissues. It is like our internal biological lake, in which cells appear like islands, here and there. Tissue fluid is essentially blood plasma. Consequently, it possesses most blood constituents, including oxygen, immune cells, antibodies, blood proteins, and nutrients—everything but the red blood cells. It also contains all of the poisons that arrive in our blood, tissues, and cells via our diets, water, and air. These pollutants, of course, are myriad: pesticides, herbicides, artificial coloring agents, carbon dioxide, carbon particles, heavy metals, cellular debris, dust, bacteria, viruses, and cancer cells. People who live in cities are literally stuffed with air pollutants each day, poisons that make their way into the lungs and bloodstream and eventually to cells and tissue fluids.

Enter the lymph. As we said, lymph was originally tissue fluid, which becomes lymph once it enters the lymphatic capillaries, lymph vessels, and nodes. The lymph system has three functions, essentially: It moves the life-giving constituents—oxygen, nutrition, immune cells, and antibodies—to cells and tissues; it transports the waste and poisons away from cells and tissues, as well as fats and cholesterol from the intestines; and finally, the lymph nodes constantly react to and neutralize toxins, pathogens, and cancer cells. Thus, the lymph is one of the body's pipelines of life (another being the blood), while doubling as the body's sewer system. It literally moves the waste out of the tissues, away from cells, and back into the bloodstream to be cleansed by

The Lymph System

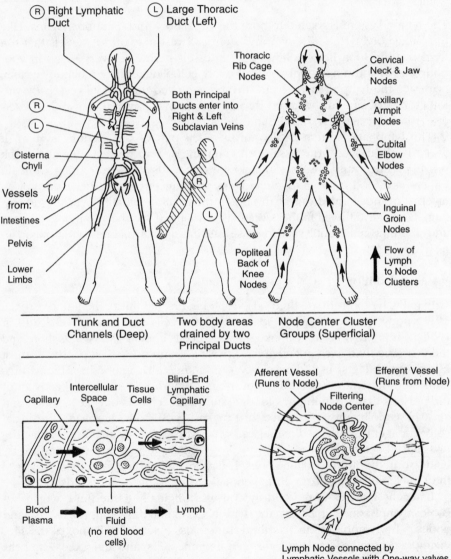

(R) Right Lymphatic Duct

(L) Large Thoracic Duct (Left)

Thoracic Rib Cage Nodes

Cervical Neck & Jaw Nodes

Both Principal Ducts enter into Right & Left Subclavian Veins

Axillary Armpit Nodes

Cubital Elbow Nodes

Cisterna Chyli

Vessels from:

Intestines

Pelvis

Lower Limbs

Inguinal Groin Nodes

Popliteal Back of Knee Nodes

Flow of Lymph to Node Clusters

Trunk and Duct Channels (Deep)

Two body areas drained by two Principal Ducts

Node Center Cluster Groups (Superficial)

Afferent Vessel (Runs to Node)

Efferent Vessel (Runs from Node)

Filtering Node Center

Capillary

Intercellular Space

Tissue Cells

Blind-End Lymphatic Capillary

Blood Plasma → Interstitial Fluid (no red blood cells) → Lymph

Filtration of Blood Fluid

Lymph Node connected by Lymphatic Vessels with One-way valves the liver and kidneys. Useful blood constituents are recycled and waste is eliminated. It's a two-pronged attack, a healer and a cleanser. Truly, this is a miraculous part of the body, a system that virtually all of us ignore until it becomes a problem.

A SYSTEM OF VESSELS AND NODES

Lymph vessels range throughout the body. At intervals along these vessels are lymph nodes, which are larger bodies of lymphatic tissue that contain lymphocytes (white blood cells), antibodies, and other immune constituents. Bacteria, viruses, cancer cells, and biological waste enter these lymph nodes and are destroyed by an army of immune cells and antibodies awaiting them in the nodes. Clusters of large lymph nodes are located in the sides of the neck and under the jaw; the armpits; front of the rib cage; and along the groin. Smaller nodes are located at the back of the head, elbows, shoulders, and backs of the knees. Millions of even smaller ones are positioned throughout the body.

It is the larger lymph nodes in the neck and under the jaw that we are all so familiar with. When these nodes are backed up and infected, we often refer to them as "swollen glands."

Naturally, the ideal situation is to keep the lymph moving so that the waste enters the bloodstream and is eliminated from the body. But here's the trick nature has played on all of us: There are only two small doors from which lymph can exit the lymph system and enter the bloodstream. And they are tiny doors, indeed.

"All lymph vessels lead eventually to the right lymphatic and thoracic ducts, which empty into the right and left subclavian veins, respectively, where the lymph reenters the blood stream," wrote Edwin B. Steen and Ashley Montagu in their preeminent two-volume work *Anatomy and Physiology.*

Each of those doors—the right lymphatic and thoracic ducts—is the width of a pencil. These are the only two places where all the accumulated lymph can be released from the lymphatic vessels and into the bloodstream, where it's cleansed and eliminated from the body. Because they are located in the neck, behind the clavical bones, gravity is working against us.

In addition to the host of poisons we must deal with daily is the fact that most of us experience periodic or chronic stress. Stress causes muscle tension, which prevents lymph from moving freely along its vessels. Hence, the lymph becomes stagnant. And we have such problems with our immune systems today not only because the lymph is stagnant, but because today's toxins are unlike anything human biology has encountered before. PCPs, heavy metals, radioactive particles, and a host of artificial chemicals are just a few of the consequences of our modern technology. In the face of these poisons, the immune system must maintain much higher levels of activity and efficiency than those of previous generations.

When the lymph is blocked, these poisons accumulate in lymph vessels and nodes. As the toxins multiply—we consume more and more of them daily—they eventually overrun the system. Ultimately, they manifest as some form of sickness, ranging from a mild illness—a cold, virus, or flu—to chronic disease—allergies, eczema, headaches, mononucleosis, lung and endocrine disorders—to the life-threatening, such as cancer.

Remarkably, the immune system is capable of neutralizing and eliminating the toxins we have consumed. The human body possesses powers of self-healing that no one has fully understood, or appreciated. The first step in marshaling these healing forces is to get the lymph—and the waste it carries—moving again. This will allow us to eliminate much of the toxicity that currently stagnates within our system and must be dealt with by our immune function. Once this is accomplished, we can focus our healing powers more efficiently on whatever health issue we face, and thus begin to restore health.

Therefore, we have to be especially conscious of pumping lymph by the only methods that we are capable of, which are:

- Daily exercise
- Deep breathing
- Muscle relaxation
- Bowel movement
- A healthful diet, rich in fiber
- Massage and acupressure

Below are recommendations for keeping the lymph system flowing.

Foods to Eat

- Whole grains, especially brown rice, whole wheat, barley, millet, corn, oats, rye, and buckwheat; all rich in fiber, complex carbohydrates, vitamins, and minerals
- A wide assortment of vegetables, including leafy greens, round vegetables, and roots; all rich in fiber, complex carbohydrates, vitamins, and minerals
- Fruit; rich in fiber and many vitamins and minerals
- Low-fat animal products to enhance circulation of lymph

Note: These foods will promote healthy bowel function, which pumps lymph and prevents it from stagnating in organs and tissues.

Foods to Avoid

- Refined foods, made with processed flour products, which promote constipation
- Foods high in fat, which are difficult to digest and eliminate

- Excessive meat and animal foods, which are difficult to digest and promote constipation
- Sugar, which promotes constipation and swelling of lymph nodes

Chemical Substances to Avoid

- Over-reliance upon laxatives. They weaken colon function and promote constipation. Instead, rely upon a high-fiber diet to support healthy elimination.

Note: See our chapter on natural solutions to constipation.

Exercise

- Daily walking, if weather permits
- Bicycle riding
- Any sport activity that is aerobic

Physiotherapy

- Therapeutic massage; any of the deep tissue, muscular massage techniques; see those described in Part III under Massage.
- Acupressure

Reproductive Health: Female

Virtually all female reproductive problems and hormone-dependent cancers, such as those of the breast and uterus, are related to the excess production of estrogen by a woman's body.

Research has shown that high levels of circulating estrogens are associated with:

- Early menarch (first menstrual period): Girls on a high-fat diet routinely get their first periods at age twelve, while those on a low-fat diet get their first periods, on average, at the age of sixteen. Early menarche is associated with an increased risk of breast cancer.
- PMS, or premenstrual syndrome (painful and irregular periods, associated with irritability, emotional disturbances, and headaches): PMS occurs when estrogen levels peak; the higher the estrogen levels, the more severe the symptoms.
- Heavy, irregular, or painful menstrual periods: High estrogen levels overstimulate ovaries and sex organs, causing heavy, irregular, or painful periods.
- Fibroids of the uterus: High levels of estrogen cause the creation of noncancerous growths within the uterus. The growths vary in size, but can become bigger than a grapefruit. Not surprisingly, fibroids often disappear after menopause, when estrogen levels decline.
- Fibrocystic breast disease: Women typically experience breast sensitivity and tenderness during their menstrual periods, when estrogen levels are highest. Excess stimulation of estrogen by the breast tissue causes the tissues to become swollen and sensitive. Such stimulation results in scar tissue, causing milk ducts to become blocked and cysts to form. Fibrocystic breast disease is associated with a higher risk of breast cancer.
- Breast, endometrial (uterine), and ovarian cancers: High estrogens are associated with an increased risk of all three cancers.
- Late menopause: Menopause is delayed when estrogen levels remain high in a woman's body.

THE MAJOR CAUSE OF HORMONAL IMBALANCE: DIETARY FAT

The most common reason estrogen levels become excessive is because there is too much fat in the diet. Dietary fats are stored in fat cells. Those cells produce estrogen. The more fat you eat, the more estrogen your body produces.

A healthy body circulates estrogen only once. The liver places a chemical substance on the estrogen that prevents it from being reabsorbed by the small intestine, which means that it is eliminated from the body through the large

Female Reproduction

Female Pelvic Region with Sex Organs

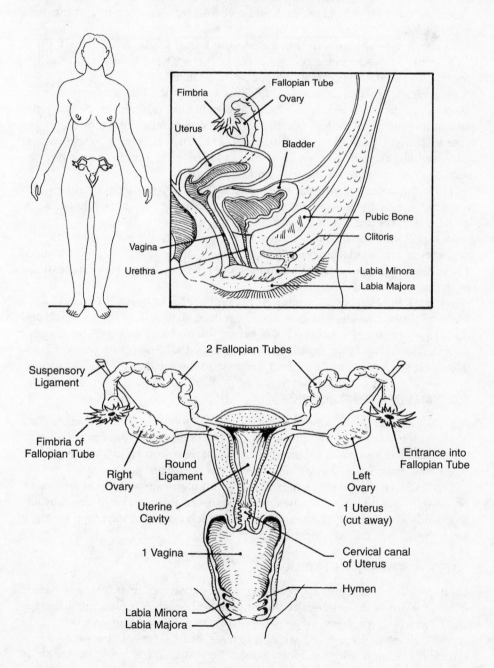

intestine. Unfortunately, a diet rich in fat, animal protein, and refined foods promotes the production of intestinal bacteria (clostridia species) that have the ability to remove that reabsorption-blocking enzyme from the estrogen, which
means the body is able to take up and recirculate a given quantity of estrogen
many times.

Estrogen acts like growth hormone in the breast tissue, causing milk ducts
and lymph tissues to close off and form pockets. These tissues can then become waste dumps for cancer-producing substances.

In addition, dietary fat causes the liver to produce bile acids, which are
used by the body to emulsify, digest, and eliminate fats. Anaerobic bacteria,
also in the intestines of those on diets high in meat and animal foods, are also
able to convert bile acids into estrogen-like hormones. These estrogens also
circulate within the body, causing the stimulation of hormone-sensitive tissues, such as the ovaries, breasts, and the uterus.

Thus, the more fat you eat, the more estrogens your body produces, the
more frequently those same estrogens are circulated, and more bile acids are
converted into estrogen-like hormones.

Research has consistently shown that women on a low-fat diet have far
lower estrogen levels in their bloodstreams than women on high-fat diets.
They also have lower rates of hormone-dependent diseases, including cancers
of the ovaries, uterus, and breast.

As Dr. John McDougall reports in his book, *The McDougall Program for a
Healthy Heart,* women can dramatically reduce their risk of hormone-related
disorders—including cancers of the breast, uterus, and ovaries—by keeping
their estrogen levels low. Research has shown that a 17 percent reduction in estrogen causes a fourfold to fivefold decrease in the incidence of breast cancer.

FIBER ELIMINATES ESTROGENS

A high-fiber diet is the key to reducing estrogens in the body. Dietary fiber
binds with estrogens in the intestinal tract and eliminates them from the body.
Numerous studies have reported that vegetarian women eliminate two to
three times more estrogen in their feces than nonvegetarians.

Studies have shown that when women with high estrogen levels are placed
on a high-fiber, low-fat diet, their blood levels of estrogen drop dramatically.
One study showed that women who follow such advice reduce their estrogen
levels by 50 percent in twenty-two days.

NATURAL SOURCES OF ESTROGEN

Many women who are approaching menopause or already have passed
through it are being encouraged to undertake hormone replacement therapy
(HRT) as a way of preventing osteoporosis, maintaining higher levels of the
"good" cholesterol (or HDL, which prevents heart disease), and warding off
symptoms of menopause. Unfortunately, there is a considerable downside to

hormone replacement therapy. Numerous studies have found that HRT increases a woman's risk of breast cancer by about 50 percent. If the hormone therapy does not include progesterone, it will increase a woman's risk of uterine cancer twentyfold. To reduce the risk of a woman contracting uterine cancer, doctors prescribe progesterone, another female hormone, which mitigates the harmful effects of the estrogens.

In addition to the risk of disease, many women report a wide array of uncomfortable side effects from the drugs, including breast tenderness, monthly bleeding, cramping, bloating, PMS, irritability, headaches, and depression. New research is showing, however, that the risk of disease and many of the side effects actually stem from the type of hormones being prescribed.

A common hormonal prescription for HRT is *Premarin,* which contains an estrogen extracted from the urine of pregnant mares, along with *Provara,* which is a synthetic progesterone.

There are three types of estrogen produced by a woman's body: estradiol, estrone, and estriol. Of those three, estriol is produced in the greatest quantities; about 80 percent of a healthy woman's estrogen is composed of estriol. Not only have scientists found that estriol is the mildest estrogen of the three types, but it is the only one that is noncancerous. Indeed, new research has found that estriol may prevent cancer. The two forms of estrogen that predominate in HRT prescriptions, however, are estradiol and estrone, both of which have been shown to promote cancer. One of the ways estriol prevents cancer, scientists now believe, is that it blocks estradiol and estrone from entering the cells through the estrogen-receptor sites on the cell wall. This prevents these harmful estrogens from getting inside the cell and causing cancer-producing mutations within the DNA.

Critics of the pharmaceutical industry, which continues to produce estradiol and estrone prescriptions, have noted that the drug companies do not mass-produce estriol because they cannot place a patent on the hormone. Estradiol and estrone can be patented because it is derived from horses and altered sufficiently to be called synthetic. Synthetic drugs can be patented.

A growing number of doctors have now begun to specifically prescribe estrogens that are composed of 80 percent estriol, 10 percent estradiol, and 10 percent estrone, or what are called *tri-estrogens.*

In addition to tri-estrogens, specialized pharmacies are also producing natural progesterone from plants, or phytoestrogens, specifically from yams. This natural progesterone is identical to the hormone produced by a woman's body. New research has shown that it causes an increase in bone density, prevents menopausal symptoms, and has none of the side effects that artificial estrogen has.

You can learn more about the advantages of plant-based hormone therapy in *Natural Progesterone,* by John Lee, M.D., and *Women's Bodies, Women's Wisdom,* by Christiane Northrop, M.D.

Among the pharmacies for tri-estrogens and natural progesterone most widely recommended by doctors are:

Women's International Pharmacy
5708 Monona Drive
Madison, WI 53716-3152
(800) 279-5708

Biotanica
Sherwood, Oregon
(800) 572-4712

International Academy of Compounding Pharmacists
P.O. Box 1365
Sugarland, TX 77487
(800) 927-4227

Diet and Foods to Eat

- Plant foods, such as whole grains, vegetables, beans, yams, and soybean products—including tempeh and tofu—contain phytoestrogens, which are taken up by cells and block harmful estrogens from being absorbed. All bean products, including tofu and tempeh, are especially high in phytoestrogens.
- Barley
- Beans
- Leafy green vegetables, such as collard greens, kale, mustard greens, broccoli, cabbage, and others are especially rich in minerals, which strengthen kidneys.
- Sterility is a deficiency of kidney yang, or the warm, outgoing, fiery energy that flows from the kidneys. To strengthen the outgoing energy and warmth (yang) of a woman's kidneys, use the following herbs in cooking: cloves, fenugreek seeds, fennel seeds, anise seeds, black peppercorns, ginger (dried is better), cinnamon bark, walnuts, black beans, onion family (garlic, onions, chives, scallions, and leeks), quinoa, chicken, trout, and salmon.

See also the sections on infertility and menopause in Part II and the section on strengthening the kidneys in Part IV.

Foods to Avoid

- Cooling foods, especially raw fruits, raw foods, excessive salt, and excessive amounts of seaweed (only one tablespoon, four or five times per week)
- Animal foods, especially meat, poultry, eggs, fats, and oils
- Spices and stimulants

- Alcohol
- Cheese, milk, and dairy products block circulation in the tiny capillaries that provide blood and oxygen to organs.
- Sugar, refined flour products, honey, chocolate, and all soft drinks containing sugar
- Avoid excess salt. Never use salt at the table.

REPRODUCTIVE HEALTH: MALE

Male sexual function depends on optimal circulation within the sex organs. The two greatest impediments to circulation are dietary fat and stress. Fat blocks blood flow within the tiny capillaries that bring blood and oxygen to the testes and penis, resulting in a range of disorders, including prostate disease, cancer, sexual dysfunction, and impotence.

Stress causes muscles within the pelvis to contract. As these muscles remain contracted over time, they squeeze blood vessels, thus blocking the optimal flow of blood and immune cells, oxygen, and nutrition to cells and tissues. These muscles also contract around lymph vessels. Lymph removes waste from the cells, tissues, and organs. When lymph is blocked, waste accumulates within tissues and forms the basis for disease. The blockage of blood and lymph may increase the likelihood of infection, especially within the prostate gland, one of the most common reasons for prostate swelling.

Both dietary fat and stress also alter the hormonal environment. Fat affects testosterone in men, just as it does estrogen in women. The more meat and fat in the diet, the higher the testosterone levels, and particularly a by-product of testosterone metabolism called dihydrotestosterone. High levels of dihydrotestosterone play a role in the onset of disorders of the prostate, according to numerous studies, including an in-depth report entitled, "Prostate Cancer: A Current Perspective," published in 1991 in the *American Journal of Epidemiology.*

Epidemiological studies have shown consistently that men with diets high in animal proteins and fat have higher rates of prostate cancers than those whose diets include higher amounts of vegetables and lower amounts of fat and animal proteins. Japanese men, who historically have had low rates of prostate disease, have seen the incidence of prostate cancer climb steadily since World War II as their consumption of meat has increased.

Other dietary factors that may also promote disorders of the prostate include cigarette smoking, excessive alcohol consumption, and lack of dietary beta-carotene.

Traditional therapies, especially those of naturopathy, maintain that minerals, particularly zinc, are essential to healthy sexual function, and vitamin E is essential to the health and vitality of the prostate gland and sexual vitality.

In Chinese medicine, the health of male sex organs depends on the strength of the kidneys and liver. The kidneys provide life force, or qi, to the sex organs. They are said to be responsible for the development of the sex organs while either the male or female child is a fetus, as well as maintaining the health and vitality of the sex organs during maturity. The liver plays an important role, as well. The liver meridian, which is the channel of qi that supports the organ, runs from the middle of the thorax, in the area of the liver, loops upward, and then down the front of the body, curving inward at the groin and running directly through the testes. Since meridians appear as mirror images of each other on each side of the body, the liver meridian runs in the same pattern on both the left and right side of the body, thus running through each of the two testes. The liver meridian also provides qi to the prostate gland in men. This means that the health of the liver, and the amount of qi running through the liver meridian, is directly responsible for the health of the male sex organs.

The Chinese maintain that each organ is supported by certain emotional conditions, as well as damaged by imbalanced emotions. The kidneys are harmed by excessive fear or stress, while the liver is injured by excessive anger. Both of these emotions can also be injurious to the sex organs, particularly prolonged stress, which weakens kidneys and eventually drains the life force from the sex organs.

As for specific conditions affecting male sexuality, Chinese medicine asserts that premature ejaculation is caused by a deficiency of the holding and contracting force within the kidneys, also called *kidney yin*. Sterility is seen as a deficiency of warming, outgoing, or fiery energy that flows from the kidneys, also called *kidney yang* in Chinese medicine. Foods that strengthen kidney yin and yang are listed below.

In addition to diet are lifestyle factors, particularly exercise. Research has shown that men who engage in vigorous aerobic exercise at least three times per week have lower rates of prostate cancer than those who live more sedentary lives. Exercise increases circulation throughout the male sex organs. It also reduces testosterone and its by-product, dihydrotestosterone, which has been shown to cause prostate disease and prostate cancer.

See also the sections on prostate, impotence, and infertility in Part II, as well as the section on the kidneys in Part IV.)

Diet and Foods to Eat

- Barley is considered an herb for the kidneys and sex organs in Chinese medicine.
- Beans are considered a healing herb for the kidneys.
- Leafy green vegetables, such as collard greens, kale, mustard greens, broccoli, cabbage, and others are especially rich in minerals, which strengthen kidneys.
- Sea vegetables such as nori (sushi nori requires no preparation; simply open the package and wrap brown rice or other grains or noodles within and eat), wakame (especially good in soup), kombu (in stews), and arame (as a vegetable) are very strengthening to kidneys.
- Root vegetables, including carrots, daikon (eat only twice per week; more can increase elimination and weaken kidneys), parsnips, rutabagas, and turnips
- Burdock root: Pressure cook in one inch of water with carrots cut up in coins. Burdock root can be a powerful herb for cleansing and strengthening the kidneys and sex organs.

- Pumpkin seeds are rich in vitamin E and zinc, which strengthen male sex organs.
- Black sesame seeds strengthen kidneys.
- Foods that strengthen kidney yin include beans, especially black beans; black sesame seeds; fish; sea vegetables (one to two tablespoons per day); small amounts of sea salt (use only in cooking; never use at the table as a condiment); and barley.

Herbs

- Saw palmetto is especially good for swelling of the prostate.
- Nettle
- Echinacea, when prostate infection occurs

Foods to Avoid

- Cooling foods, especially raw fruits, raw foods, excessive salt, and excessive amounts of seaweed (only one tablespoon, four or five times per week)
- Animal foods, especially meat, poultry, eggs, fats, and oils
- Spices and stimulants
- Alcohol
- Cheese, milk, and dairy products block circulation in the tiny capillaries that provide blood and oxygen to organs.
- Sugar, refined flour products, honey, chocolate, and all soft drinks containing sugar

Exercise

- Aerobic exercise daily maximizes circulation throughout the body, including within sex organs: walk, jog, run, bicycle, and participate in other aerobic sports.
- Yoga especially stretches muscles in the pelvis and relieves stress.
- Stretching exercises, especially the back, pelvis, and backs of legs

Supplements

- Minerals, especially zinc: 15 mg/day

Probiotics

- Chlorella is especially good for prostate problems.

Mind/Body

- Relaxation techniques to relieve stress
- Meditation, prayer

THE SKIN

The skin is the body's largest organ, responsible for an array of essential bodily functions, including breathing oxygen, eliminating carbon dioxide and other forms of waste, acting as a shield against toxins from outside, and helping to maintain body temperature. The skin is continually repairing and renewing itself. It responds almost instantly to sudden changes in emotions, and it is the body's main organ of sexual attraction.

The surface layer of the skin, which is composed of cells, sweat pores, and sebaceous glands, is covered with a thin sheath of dead cells, which are continually being pushed up to the surface from below. If the dead cells are not removed, they can reduce and even block the skin's effort to breathe and eliminate waste.

At the surface lies a slightly acidic coating of oil, called the *acid mantle,* which can protect the skin against some bacteria. Below the surface is a complex of sweat and oil glands, hair follicles, blood vessels, nerves, and muscle tissue. These are held together by a tough connective tissue called *collagen,* which runs in strands or fibers. The relative health of your collagen determines the contour of your skin, how wrinkled and lined it is. Healthy collagen is often called *soluble collagen,* because it can absorb and hold moisture.

Below the collagen is a layer of fat and muscle, which also provides some contour and acts as a cushion and as insulation.

The two major skin problems most people face are wrinkling, due to age, and blemishes, or acne.

Aging of the skin occurs when collagen becomes hard and crosslinked with neighboring collagen fibers. This prevents it from holding water and plumping up. Instead, it collapses on itself, binds with other collagen fibers, and forms a kind of fishnet below the surface of the skin, which is manifested as wrinkles. The cause of this crosslinking is a process called oxidation or *free radical formation.* (See the section on the immune system.) What actually happens is that the atoms of human tissue begin to decay, or lose electrons. Once an electron is lost, the atom attempts to regain its electrical balance by stealing one or more electrons from neighboring atoms. This stealing creates a chain reaction in which atoms are changing their structures and forming bonds that would not otherwise occur. The net effect is a chaos of crosslinking collagen fibers, revealed on the skin's surface as wrinkles.

Actually, free radical formation is now regarded as the basis for most, if not all, forms of aging. According to scientists at the University of Southern Alabama Medical School and the University of California at Davis, free radicals are linked to as many as sixty illnesses, including cancer, heart disease,

Alzheimer's disease, Parkinson's disease, cataracts, arthritis, and immune disorders.

Acne occurs when oil, called sebum, blocks the pores and hair follicles at the skin's surface, thus preventing the skin from eliminating oil and waste. This causes waste to accumulate in the pores, resulting in pockets of infection that manifest as red sores, boils, and pimples. Acne does not occur when the pores remain unblocked.

Adolescents experience more acne than adults because of a rapid increase in the production of the male hormone androgen, which is present in both sexes but more abundant in males. Androgen causes the body to produce more sebum, which results in a greater number of blocked pores and blemishes.

BASIC SKIN CARE

Skin care specialists maintain that before using any specific product for aging or acne, everyone should follow a basic skin care regimen.

Properly Clean the Skin

Skin experts recommend avoiding soap because of its high pH (potential hydrogen, which determines the relative acidity or alkalinity of any substance), which dries skin and diminishes its life expectancy. The pH spectrum runs from 0 to 14; anything above 7 is considered alkaline; anything below 7 is acid. The skin's surface is mildly acidic, having a pH of around 5. Most soaps are well over 7, and some as high as 10. Soaps with a high pH will not only dry the skin out but eliminate its acid mantle.

Skin cleansers that contain vegetable oils, such as coconut oil, and water, combine with sebum and allow it to be dissolved and rinsed away. At the same time, water dissolves dirt.

Effective skin cleansers, also known as sufactants, can contain a number of different vegetable oils, including coconut, sesame, or palm oils. These are safe and effective cleansers and have a relatively low pH. Stearic acid, a fatty acid derived from vegetable oils, is used in some natural skin care products to provide a pearly firmness.

Seaweeds are increasingly used as skin cleansers, as well. Their high mineral content stimulates circulation, helps eliminate toxins imbedded in the skin, and leaves the skin feeling smooth. Seaweeds can, to some extent, remineralize the skin, thus strengthening its immune and healing functions.

Research into the use of seaweeds in skin care products has just begun (they are also used in shampoos), but chemists are excited about their many possible applications.

Facial Scrubs

Use a facial scrub that contains a mild abrasive. These abrasives vary in coarseness, ranging from a very mild base of oatmeal or ground-up almonds to coarser materials, such as silica (a finely ground sand) or the shells of almonds, apricots, or walnuts.

"There have been a number of studies examining the relative smoothness and blemishing of men's and women's skin," said Mike Bathledge, a chemist at Earth Science, a natural cosmetic company in Minneapolis. "What they have found is that men have fewer blemishes and smoother skin than women. Now, that's ironic because women are spending all this money on these skin care products, so you'd think their skin would be healthier. But what's been found is that men are exfoliating their faces every day by shaving. Men are taking off that top layer of dead cells every day with their razors, allowing their skin to breathe and eliminate waste much easier. So I recommend that women use a mild abrasive scrub on their faces, once every other day or so, which will do the same thing."

Experts in the natural cosmetics industry point out that European women have been using exfoliants for decades. Many natural cosmetics companies offer a light peel that contains papaya extract (papain) that lifts off dead cells. This peel, unlike an exfoliant, should only be used once a week.

After the skin is thoroughly clean, a skin toner or rinse that has an astringent effect closes pores, tightens the skin, and helps to keep it from being exposed to many of the toxins floating in the air. There are a wide variety of toners, but most skin care specialists recommend avoiding those that contain alcohol, which dries the skin and harms the soluble collagen below.

Witch hazel turns up in a lot of natural skin care products, especially toners. Witch hazel has a strong astringent effect, but can dry out the skin somewhat if it is used in high quantities. Most natural cosmetics companies use only small amounts of witch hazel and combine it with moisturizing nutrients and herbs, such as vitamin E, geranium, or honey, that balance its drying effects.

Other common herbs in toners are lemon, ivy, sage, nettle, and burdock.

Moisturizers

Moisturizers, also known as humectants, attract moisture to the skin's surface and hold it there; moisturizers make the skin softer and prevent it from drying and chapping, thus slowing the aging process.

There are a wide variety of moisturizers, ranging from the simple—vegetable glycerin and rose water—to the expensive, such as hyaluronic acid, which costs about $6,000 a kilo. You don't need a lot of hyaluronic acid, but even a little is going to cost a lot.

In between those two are the less expensive though still effective jojoba oil, vitamin E oils, sorbitol (derived from plants), honey, aloe vera, and iris. Aloe vera is one of those plants that seems to have been designed by nature to treat human skin conditions. Since ancient times, it has been used effectively to treat everything from dry skin, burns, and insect bites to skin irritations, acne, cuts, and abrasions.

Iris is another plant that has remarkable moisture-controlling properties. Despite the fact that the iris grows best in hot, dry climates, the plant itself is surprisingly moist, even watery. The secret seems to lie in the rhizome's ability to store water and release it in quantities that balance the prevailing atmospheric conditions.

Some moisturizers may cause problems, however. Mineral oil, used in many mass-market skin care products, is a petrochemical that can dry the skin, block pores, and prevent it from breathing and eliminating waste.

One of the most common moisturizers in natural cosmetics, NaPCA (or sodium PCA), may cause an allergic reaction in a minority of people. NaPCA, which is highly touted by many natural cosmetics companies, is derived from an amino acid (pyroglutamic acid). It is produced in human tissue but synthesized in the laboratory. It is highly effective at attracting moisture to the surface of the skin. Some critics maintain, however, that NaPCA has caused some people to suffer allergic reactions. Many people have used NaPCA with satisfaction, and it continues to be one of the industry's most popular products.

ANTIAGING

The aging of skin tissue can be slowed and even improved by halting free radical formation, which means preventing the breakdown and decay of tissues. Studies have shown, however, that certain nutrients can stop free radicals from forming. Foods rich in beta-carotene (the vegetable source of vitamin A) and vitamins E and C donate electrons to imbalanced atoms, thus restoring health and harmony to tissues throughout the body. Natural cosmetic companies place an abundance of these nutrients, called antioxidants, in many of their skin care products, including cleansers, toners, and moisturizers.

The science is well established that these nutrients do, indeed, stop free radical formation, whether they are taken in the diet or applied directly to the skin.

Skin specialists report that the depths such products penetrate varies widely, depending on the size of the molecule, the temperature of the skin, and other factors. Diets rich in antioxidants provide these substances to the bloodstream, thus getting to tissues throughout the body, including the deeper reaches of the skin. Scientists are quick to point out that if people really want to take good care of their skin and slow the aging process, they will reduce fat, artificial ingredients, and chemical pollutants, all of which stimulate free radical formation.

NATURAL TREATMENTS FOR ACNE

Among the most effective herbs for treating blemishes and acne are the following:

- Yarrow heals and acts as a blood styptic, a substance that reduces blood flow and inflammation to the area.
- Calendula heals, soothes, is antiseptic, and anti-inflammatory.
- Camomile soothes the skin and makes it smooth.
- Sage heals, is antiseptic, anti-inflammatory, and kills bacteria.
- The antioxidants, beta-carotene and vitamins E and C, heal, support the immune response, and prevent further infection.
- Tea tree oil is derived from the leaves of the *Melaleuca alternifolia* tree, a species found only on the north coast of New South Wales, Australia. Tea tree oil is a broad-spectrum fungicide and antiseptic that has been effective against a wide variety of skin problems and infections. Among the recommended uses are to treat acne; bee stings and insect bites; burns; vaginal infections, including candidiasis; gum disease; toothache; athlete's foot; infections under the fingernails; lice and scabies; and sunburn. Some recommend that tea tree oil be put in steam and inhaled to treat throat infections and sinus problems.
- Clay: There are a variety of clays—green, red, black, and yellow—but all of them draw oil, bacteria, and dirt from the pores of skin. Clay pulls at the skin and increases circulation, which causes deeper cleaning and rapid healing.

THE SMALL INTESTINE

The small intestine digests and absorbs nutrients from food. Enzymes are released in the small intestine to help break down foods and make nutrients more available to the tiny fingerlike projections, called villi, which absorb the nutrients in the food.

The small intestine is about twenty-two feet long, and approximately 1.5 inches in diameter. It runs from the stomach to the large intestine, coiling throughout the lower abdomen. The organ is divided into three sections: The duodenum is a short, curved tube, about ten inches long, that is attached to the stomach and receives both the bile and pancreatic ducts; it extends to the jejunum, which is about nine feet long and coils upward to the left; the jejunum attaches to the ileum, which is about 12 feet long, and coils downward to the right.

The ileum joins the large intestine at a bulblike structure called the cecum. Within the cecum is the ileocecal valve, which is a barrier created by a pair of lips within the intestinal canal that prevent food from flowing back into the small intestine once it reaches the colon. The innermost lining of the small intestine is permeated with villi.

The small intestine contains trillions of bacteria, though the initial stages of the organ—the duodenum and parts of the jejunum—are essentially sterile due to the acid secretions from the stomach. Still, some bacteria do get past the stomach and, once inside the intestines and beyond the acid environment, begin to multiply.

The kinds of bacteria within the intestines vary among individuals according to the types of diets consumed and the amounts of antibiotics and other medications taken (many of which destroy healthful bacteria). Much friendly bacteria exists in the intestines that assist in the breakdown of food and digestion, making nutrients more accessible to the bloodstream.

Among the more common species of bacteria that reside in both the small and large intestine are *Escherichia coli,* usually called *E. coli; Candida albicans,* or yeast; and *lactobacteria,* of which *lactobacillus* is a widely known strain. Harmful bacteria, such as *E. coli* and *Candida albicans,* secrete toxins that if produced in sufficient quantities can cause disease.

Lactobacteria, on the other hand, are helpful to the body; they produce some vitamins, such as vitamin K, and digestive enzymes, which assist in the breakdown of foods. Studies have shown that diets rich in animal foods, especially red meats, increase the population of harmful bacteria—and their disease-producing secretions—in the large and small intestine.

Intestinal transit-time (the time elapsed between consumption of food and elimination) depends a lot on the overall health of the intestines and the kinds

The Small Intestine

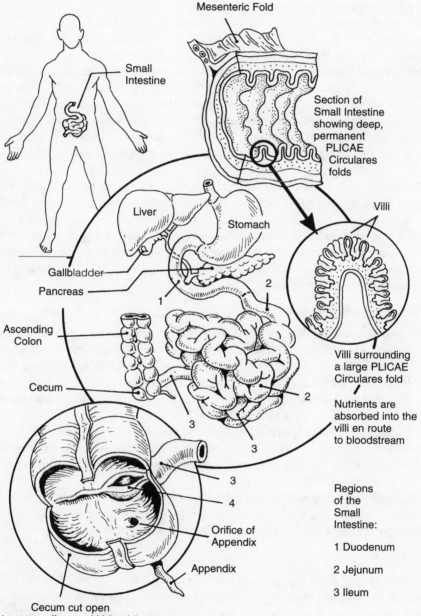

Small
Intestine

Mesenteric Fold

Section of
Small Intestine
showing deep,
permanent
PLICAE
Circulares
folds

Liver

Stomach

Villi

Gallbladder

Pancreas

1

2

Ascending
Colon

Cecum

2

3

3

3

Villi surrounding
a large PLICAE
Circulares fold

Nutrients are
absorbed into the
villi en route
to bloodstream

3

4

Orifice of
Appendix

Appendix

Regions
of the
Small
Intestine:

1 Duodenum

2 Jejunum

3 Ileum

Cecum cut open
to expose Ileocecal Valve (4)

of foods consumed. Fiber-rich foods move quickly through the organ, but heavier, fat-rich foods take far more time. On the average, food spends about four to six hours in the stomach; another five to six hours in the small intestine; and another fifteen to twenty-four hours in the large intestine, before it is finally eliminated from the body.

The small intestine is rarely affected by tumors, and cancer of the small intestine is uncommon, at least as a point of origin. (Malignancies that originate elsewhere in the body can spread to the organ, however.)

The small intestine is viewed in Chinese medicine as a yang (or expanded) organ and part of the fire element in the theory of the five elements. It is associated with summer, the season during which it receives its optimal amount of qi. If appropriate measures are taken, the small intestine and heart can be more easily healed in the summer months; conversely, if these organs are abused, symptoms tend to appear and can be severe during the summer season.

The small intestine receives its optimal amounts of life force during the hours of 1 P.M. to 3 P.M. (See the Chinese clock in the section on Chinese Medicine in Part III.)

The emotion associated with a balanced fire element is joy. Imbalances in the small intestine, especially a deficiency of qi, show up as a lack of joy and even depression. People with excessive small intestine qi are often overly emotional and even hysterical.

General Recommendations

- Chew every mouthful of food at least thirty-five times each. Chewing breaks down food and makes it easier on the stomach and small intestine to digest. Saliva assists in the digestion of carbohydrates. Saliva also makes the food more alkaline, which creates less gas. (Gas is experienced in the stomach and intestine, of course, but it is caused by spleen imbalances, according to the Chinese.)
- Walk daily, weather permitting. Walking increases oxygen intake and circulation, which improves small intestine function. Aerobic exercise is wonderful for the fire element; it strengthens and helps to cleanse organs of waste.
- Laugh. According to Chinese medicine, laughing, joy, and having fun all heal both the heart and small intestine by concentrating qi, or life force, in the middle of the body, especially in the heart and small intestine.

Foods to Eat

- Corn on the cob; whole corn; and glutinous millet
- Squash (acorn, buttercup, butternut, hubbard, and summer squash)
- Asparagus, broccoli, brussels sprouts, chicory, collard greens, carrots, dandelion, endive, okra, and scallions

- Seeds: sunflower and sesame seeds, both in small amounts and very well chewed
- Apricots, raspberries, strawberries, and raisins
- Red lentil beans
- Miso or tamari broths, with small amounts of wakame seaweed (about 1 tablespoon-size shard of seaweed per cup of soup), and vegetables. Miso and tamari create alkaline broths that soothe and tonify the small intestine, stomach, and spleen. They contain digestive bacteria and enzymes that assist digestion. For indigestion, chronic stomach and small intestine problems, a light miso soup (¼ teaspoon of miso per cup of soup) in the morning will help to alleviate stomach and digestive problems.
- Shrimp, in moderate amounts (Shrimp is moderately high in cholesterol, which in small amounts can stimulate the fire element, but when eaten too frequently can dull and weaken the heart and small intestine.)
- Fibrous foods: To cleanse and strengthen the small intestine, be sure that the diet is composed chiefly of whole grains, fresh vegetables, and fruits. These foods are rich in fiber and assist in cleansing the small intestine of fat deposits and undigested waste.

Foods to Avoid

- Red meat and all fatty animal foods. Fat requires greater quantities of bile acids (see Large Intestine), which create and exacerbate ulcers and any inflammation.
- Avoid spices, especially hot spices, which irritate the intestinal lining and cause greater acid reactions in the stomach. Hot spices are fire foods, but clearly too much fire to create a balanced condition in the small intestine and heart.
- Avoid highly acidic foods, such as peppers, eggplants, and tomatoes, until symptoms abate.

Supplements

- Beta-carotene, or the vegetable source of vitamin A: 10–20 mg per day
- Thiamine: 1.5 mg per day
- Riboflavin: 1.8 mg per day
- Vitamin B_6: 2–10 mg per day
- Vitamin B_{12}: 2–10 mg per day
- Niacin: 20 mg per day
- Vitamin C: 100 mg per day
- Vitamin E: 60–400 mg per day

Herbs

- Chamomile tea (soothes and heals): one cup per day
- Dandelion tea (cleanses blood of toxins): one cup, three times per week

- Gingerroot tea (stimulates digestion and circulation): one cup, two times per week
- Goldenseal (tea or infusion; heals and cleanses blood): one cup per day three times per week for a three-week period. If you would like to continue using, wait one week and resume the three-week regimen.
- Slippery elm (tea or infusion; heals and cleanses blood): one cup three times per week for three weeks. If you would like to continue using, wait one week and resume the three-week regimen.

Note: The medicinal teas—dandelion, goldenseal, and slippery elm—can be taken on the same day.

The Spleen

From the perspective of Western medicine, the spleen is responsible for introducing immune cells into the blood, for cleansing the blood of cellular debris, for recovering hemoglobin, and for storing blood.

From the Chinese perspective, the spleen is the primary organ of digestion; it transforms nutrients into qi, or life force; it governs the orderly flow of blood throughout the body; it nourishes the four limbs and flesh with qi; it discerns the five tastes—bitter, sweet, pungent, salty, and sour; and it is responsible for our capacity to perceive creative ideas and have understanding for others.

The spleen distributes qi to the small and large intestine. The quality of that energy—whether it is smooth and fluid or unstable and chaotic—will determine how well or how poorly we digest food and eliminate waste. This, all digestive issues are seen in Chinese medicine as related to the health of the spleen.

All forms of gas—belching, flatulence, rumbling stomach—are spleen related. So, too, are heartburn, acid indigestion, and nausea. These symptoms indicate a spleen imbalance, usually an excess of energy that the spleen cannot distribute in an orderly fashion. When the spleen passes excessive or chaotic energy on to the large intestine, the result will likely be diarrhea or spastic colon.

When the spleen is chronically weak or deficient, it may not be able to absorb and distribute the qi that emanates from many foods, especially spices, sugar, and wine, foods that the Chinese maintain injure the spleen. Usually this kind of spleen deficiency causes intermittent or chronic constipation. In this case, the spleen is simply unable to pass sufficient qi on to the large intestine. When the intestine receives inadequate life force, it is unable to do its job.

The spleen is strengthened by alkaline foods and especially by chewing food thoroughly. Chewing mixes the food thoroughly with saliva, which alkalizes it and makes it more harmonious to the spleen. Chew thirty-five to fifty times a mouthful to strengthen the spleen.

The following foods and lifestyle recommendations can help to strengthen the spleen and overcome the kinds of health issues related to spleen imbalances.

Foods to Eat

- Millet and sweet corn are regarded as herbs for the spleen. Other healing grains include barley, oats, rice (both brown and basmati), and wheat.
- Squash, like millet and sweet corn, is a healing food for the spleen. All

The Spleen

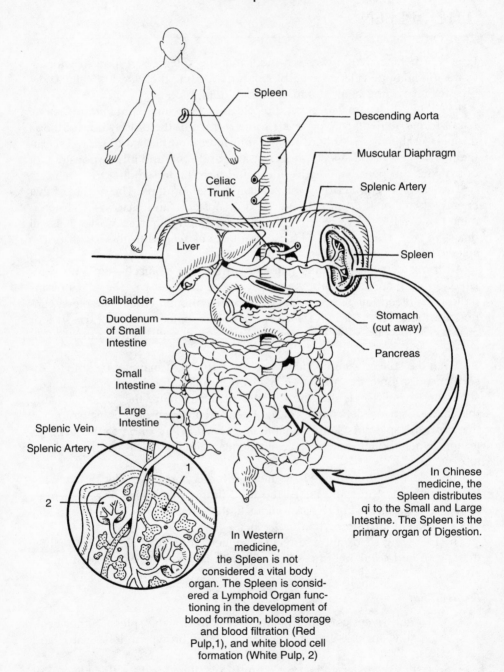

Spleen

Descending Aorta

Muscular Diaphragm

Splenic Artery

Celiac Trunk

Spleen

Liver

Gallbladder

Duodenum of Small Intestine

Stomach (cut away)

Small Intestine

Pancreas

Large Intestine

Splenic Vein

Splenic Artery

1

2

In Western medicine, the Spleen is not considered a vital body organ. The Spleen is considered a Lymphoid Organ functioning in the development of blood formation, blood storage and blood filtration (Red Pulp,1), and white blood cell formation (White Pulp, 2)

In Chinese medicine, the Spleen distributes qi to the Small and Large Intestine. The Spleen is the primary organ of Digestion.

forms of squash can have a therapeutic effect: acorn, butternut, buttercup, hubbard, hokkaido, pumpkin, and spaghetti squash.

- Leafy greens, especially collard greens
- Other healing vegetables: asparagus, broccoli, brussels sprouts, cabbage, collard greens, cucumbers, cauliflower, celery, green beans, lettuce, okra, peas, parsley, and green peppers
- Roots, such as parsnips, sweet potatoes, yams, and rutabagas
- Chickpeas
- Shiitake and button mushrooms
- Sweet fruits, such as apples, sweet oranges, raisins, grapes, melons, cherries, avocados, figs, pears, sweet oranges, plums, prunes, and raisons
- White fish and shrimp
- Miso soup: Have a small bowl with wakame seaweed daily. Both miso and seaweed contain salt. To avoid excess salt consumption, use one-quarter teaspoon of miso per cup of soup; use one tablespoon-sized shard of wakame per cup of soup.

Make a special drink to strengthen spleen. Chop into small pieces one squash, two carrots, two parsnips, and one onion. Boil until the entire mash becomes liquid. Keep adding water to ensure that the vegetables are fully dissolved or leave only a residue of fiber at the bottom of the pot. Drink two or three times daily for hypoglycemia, sugar cravings, and spleen imbalances.

For indigestion, gas, and upset stomach, eat one umeboshi plum, a Japanese pickled plum that is available in most health food or natural food stores. The plum alkalizes the stomach and calms the spleen, thus balancing the energy that the spleen sends to the large intestine.

Further Dietary Recommendations

- Avoid extremely hot or cold beverages. Especially avoid excessively cold beverages that shock the system.
- Avoid eating while emotionally upset or under stress. Stress dramatically affects digestion and can lead to stomach upset, constipation, or diarrhea.
- Do not eat standing up. Always sit while eating.
- Avoid drinking during meals. Liquids dilute the stomach juices, preventing complete digestion.
- Avoid overeating. Excess food burdens organs and makes all forms of indigestion, constipation, and diarrhea more likely.
- When suffering from indigestion or stomach upset, reduce highly acidic foods, including tomatoes, eggplant, citrus fruit, and spices.

THE STOMACH

The stomach is a muscular sac, shaped like a boxing glove, with the fat end at the top attached to the esophagus, and the narrow end, at the bottom, attached to the duodenum, or the first stage of the small intestine. An adult's stomach holds about three pints of food. Its purpose is to store food; secrete digestive juices; stir the food into a creamy mass called *chyme;* begin the breakdown of protein for assimilation by the small intestine (the only nutrient even partially digested by the stomach); and secrete the churned mass into the small intestine for absorption. The stomach itself is composed of circular and longitudinal muscles, which enable it to mix and dissolve the food and then push it into the duodenum.

Assisting the stomach in its job of breaking down food particles and churning the mass into chyme is an array of digestive juices, among which are pepsin, used to break down and help assimilate protein; intrinsic factor, used to assist in the absorption of vitamin B_{12}; and hydrochloric acid, which kills bacteria within the food. The stomach begins secreting these digestive juices the minute you see or smell food, or begin eating.

Though protein is partially digested by the stomach, the other two macronutrients—carbohydrates and fats—are digested primarily in the mouth and/or small intestine. Carbohydrates, found primarily in grains, vegetables, and fruits, are broken down by the enzyme amylase in the mouth; they are further broken down in the small intestine and then absorbed. Fat is digested exclusively in the small intestine.

Fat, refined carbohydrates, coffee, tea, tobacco, sugar, alcohol, spices, fried foods, and many drugs—including aspirin—all increase production of stomach acids, which in turn increase the likelihood of indigestion and other stomach disorders, including ulcers. Excessively salted, pickled, and smoked foods have all been shown to increase the risk of stomach cancer. Finally, milk products can also cause stomach problems for people who are lactose intolerant. Lactose, the sugar found in milk, requires the enzyme lactase, which the body uses to digest milk products. A great many ethnic groups throughout the world lose that enzyme after they are weaned from mother's milk, which makes further consumption of milk products problematical. About forty percent of Eastern Europeans, seventy percent of African Americans, and most Asians are lactose intolerant.

Stomach ulcers are caused when the stomach's protective mucous lining is worn away. This exposes the sensitive tissue below the mucous membrane to the powerful stomach acids, which can eat away at the tissues, cause a sore that eventually can bleed and become life-threatening. Stomach ulcers have three primary causes: cigarette smoking; infection from bacteria that eat away at the stomach lining; and overuse of nonsteroidal anti-inflammatory drugs (NSAIDs), such as aspirin and ibuprofen.

The Stomach

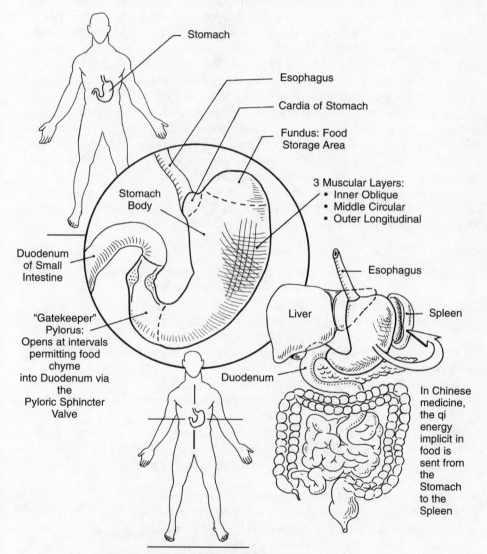

Stomach

Esophagus

Cardia of Stomach

Fundus: Food
Storage Area

Stomach
Body

3 Muscular Layers:
• Inner Oblique
• Middle Circular
• Outer Longitudinal

Duodenum
of Small
Intestine

Esophagus

Liver

Spleen

"Gatekeeper"
Pylorus:
Opens at intervals
permitting food
chyme
into Duodenum via
the
Pyloric Sphincter
Valve

Duodenum

In Chinese
medicine,
the qi
energy
implicit in
food is
sent from
the
Stomach
to the
Spleen

In Chinese medicine, the stomach
is seen as the center of man's being,
the physical and psychological balance
point. Also the resonator of life experience
and emotional equilibrium

In Chinese medicine, the stomach is seen as the repository of food matter, while the energy implicit within the food—its life force, or qi—is sent from the stomach to the spleen. The spleen is seen as the governor of digestion, say the Chinese, because it disperses qi throughout the digestive tract and thus provides the life force needed to assimilate nutrition and eliminate waste. The Chinese also maintain that the stomach function can be seen metaphorically as representing our ability to take in a wide array of life experiences. Someone with a strong stomach can enjoy a wide variety of foods, which means that, metaphorically, the person can also enjoy many types of experiences. A person with a weak stomach, however, must limit what he eats, and usually is picky about the conditions in which he finds himself.

The Chinese also state that our emotional equilibrium is dependent upon having a strong stomach. Located in the center of the body, the stomach is seen in Oriental medicine as part of one's center of being, the physical and psychological balance point. The Chinese say that when the stomach is weak or troubled, the entire body and mind are destabilized.

The following foods to eat and avoid, as well as the lifestyle recommendations listed below, are designed to help strengthen the stomach and prevent stomach disorders.

Patterns of Eating

- Eat four to six small meals through the day, rather than three larger meals. This will place less stress upon the stomach.
- Do not overeat.
- Chew each mouthful thirty-five to fifty times each. The more you chew, the less stress you put upon your stomach.
- Minimize fat. Foods rich in fat increase stomach acid and the likelihood of stomach disorders.
- Eat protein and starchy foods in separate meals.
- Proteins, fats, and starches combine best with green and nonstarchy vegetables.
- Eat alkalizing foods, such as those that contain small amounts of salt, first, as opposed to those containing fat, protein, or sugar.
- Eat fruit and sweetened foods alone, immediately after a meal or, worse, before a meal.
- Eat melons alone because they digest very quickly.
- Avoid drinking fruit juice for at least two hours after eating a meal containing starch and four hours after a meal containing protein.
- Avoid excessively cold drinks.

Foods to Eat

- Whole grains, cooked with a pinch of sea salt to alkalize them
- Millet and sweet rice, which are considered in Chinese medicine to be medicinal and especially healing for the stomach, spleen, and pancreas

- Barley, which treats indigestion from starchy food stagnation or poorly tolerated mother's milk in infants
- Collard greens
- Squash, which is especially healing for the stomach, spleen, and pancreas, according to Chinese medicine
- Apples, which inhibits growth of ferments and disease-producing bacteria in the intestines
- Ginger. Eat ginger freshly grated in tea, or in capsule form, or chew a small piece. Studies have shown that ginger settles the stomach and overcomes nausea.
- Grapefruit peel, which moves and regulates spleen-pancreas digestive energy and is good for getting rid of gas
- Lemon and lime, especially for those who eat a high-fat, high-protein diet; alleviates flatulence and indigestion
- Umeboshi plums, sometimes called "Japanese Alka-Seltzer." Take 1 plum or half-teaspoon of umeboshi paste. Will cure most dyspepsia in 10 minutes.
- Carrots, which treat indigestion, excess stomach acid, and heartburn

Foods to Reduce or Avoid

- Coffee, tea, and other caffeinated beverages
- Meat (rich in fat)
- Dairy (rich in fat); also, lactose creates stomach disorders for lactose-intolerant people
- Eggs (rich in fat)
- Poor-quality oils (all oils are liquid fat)
- Sugar
- Spicy foods
- Fried foods
- Alcohol
- Mints, which have been shown to create regurgitation of stomach juices and heartburn
- Highly acidic foods, such as tomatoes, eggplant, and peppers

Chemicals to Avoid

- Limit over-the-counter medications, including aspirin. The anti-clotting effects of aspirin can promote bleeding of the stomach, inflammation (or gastritis), and bleeding ulcers.
- Ibuprofen and other nonsteroidal anti-inflammatory medicines, which also contribute to stomach distress, especially for those with existing stomach problems

Mind/Body

- Meditation
- Positive imaging routines
- Progressive relaxation exercises

(These and other methods of promoting internal harmony and balance can be found in the section on Faith in Part III.)

Resources for Natural Foods, Herbs, Supplements, and Natural Healing Products

MAIL-ORDER SOURCES OF NATURAL AND ORGANIC FOODS:

Mothers & Others for a Livable Planet
40 W. 20th St.
New York, NY 10011
888-ECO-INFO

Mountain Ark Trading Co.
799 Old Leichester Hwy.
Asheville, NC 28806
800-643-8909

Wellspring Natural Food Company
Mail Order Catalog
P.O. Box 2473
Amherst, MA 01004
800-578-5301

MAIL-ORDER AND TOLL-FREE SOURCES FOR FRESH PACKAGED HERBS AND SUPPLEMENTS

Castle Gray
800-987-3747
Vitamins, supplements, herbs
Over 1,000 cruelty-free products for
body care

Gaia Herbs
12 Lancaster County Rd.
Harvard, MA 01451
800-831-7780

The Herb Pharm
P.O. Box 116
Williams, OR 97544
800-348-4372

Hi-Life Vitamins
800-622-8877
Vitamins and supplements

Health Depot
800-786-4611
Vitamins, herbs, and supplements

Herbs, Etc.
1345 Cerrillos Rd.
Santa Fe, NM 87505
888-694-3727

L & H Vitamins
37-10 Crescent St.
Long Island City, NY 11101
800-221-1152

San Francisco Herb Company
250 14th St.
San Francisco, CA 94103
800-227-4530

Solgar Vitamin and Herb Co.
500 Willow Tree Rd.
Leonia, NJ 07605
Supplements, herbs, and natural products

Vitamin Discount Connection
645 Kolter Dr., #2
Indiana, PA 15701
800-848-2110

The Vitamin Shoppe
4700 Westside Ave.
North Bergen, NJ 07047
800-497-1122
Vitamins and supplements

Vitmin Trader
6501 4th St. NW
Albuquerque, NM 87107
800-334-9300

Wellness Health Pharmacy
800-227-2627
Nutritional supplements, vitamins, and health information

MAIL-ORDER AND TOLL-FREE SOURCES FOR NATURAL ESTROGENS, PROGESTERONES, AND BOTANICALS

Biotanica
Sherwood, Oregon
800-572-4712

Healthy Directions, Inc.
800-722-8008
A source of Pro-Gest cream

Women's International Pharmacy
5708 Monona Drive
Madison, WI 53716-3152
800-279-5708
Source of natural estrogens, estriol, tri-estrogen, natural progesterone, and other hormone preparations

International Academy of
Compounding Pharmacists
P.O. Box 1365
Sugarland, TX 77487
800-927-4227
Provides names of pharmacists in your area who prepare natural and customized hormone formulae

INDEX